Musculoskeletal Disorders: Diagnosis, Prevention and Treatment

Musculoskeletal Disorders: Diagnosis, Prevention and Treatment

Editor: Bran Conley

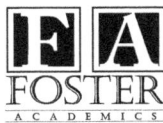

FA FOSTER
ACADEMICS

www.fosteracademics.com

www.fosteracademics.com

F A
FOSTER
A C A D E M I C S

Cataloging-in-Publication Data

Musculoskeletal disorders : diagnosis, prevention and treatment / edited by Bran Conley.
    p. cm.
Includes bibliographical references and index.
ISBN 978-1-63242-767-0
1. Musculoskeletal system--Diseases. 2. Musculoskeletal system--Diseases--Diagnosis.
3. Musculoskeletal system--Diseases--Prevention. 4. Musculoskeletal system--Diseases--Treatment.
I. Conley, Bran.
RC925.7 .M87 2019
616.7--dc23

© Foster Academics, 2019

Foster Academics,
118-35 Queens Blvd., Suite 400,
Forest Hills, NY 11375, USA

ISBN 978-1-63242-767-0 (Hardback)

Contents

Preface

The system of the human body, which provides humans with the ability to move using their muscular and skeletal systems, is known as human musculoskeletal system. It provides movement, support, form, and stability to the body. Pain, injuries and disorders related to this system are called musculoskeletal disorders. Enthesopathy, Achard syndrome, joint effusion, lumbar disc disease, Sever's disease, Zenker's paralysis and winged scapula are some of the common examples of musculoskeletal disorders. The assessment of musculoskeletal disorders follows a physical examination and a review of symptoms and pain, medical history, intensity of pain, as well as an examination of recreational and occupational hazards. Various diagnostic tests such as X-ray and MRI also help specialists in establishing a diagnosis. The treatment of musculoskeletal pain is often addressed through a prescription of anesthetic and anti-inflammatory drugs, targeted exercises, physical therapy and occupational therapy, chiropractic care, acupressure and acupuncture, etc. This book explores all the important aspects of musculoskeletal disorders in the present day scenario. It strives to provide a fair idea about this subject and to help develop a better understanding of the diagnosis, prevention and treatment of various musculoskeletal disorders. With state-of-the-art inputs by acclaimed medical experts, this book targets students and professionals.

Significant researches are present in this book. Intensive efforts have been employed by authors to make this book an outstanding discourse. This book contains the enlightening chapters which have been written on the basis of significant researches done by the experts.

Finally, I would also like to thank all the members involved in this book for being a team and meeting all the deadlines for the submission of their respective works. I would also like to thank my friends and family for being supportive in my efforts.

Editor

Emotional distress was associated with persistent shoulder pain after physiotherapy: a prospective cohort study

Kaja Smedbråten*⬤, Britt Elin Øiestad and Yngve Røe

Abstract

Background: There is a paucity of research on the association between psychological factors and persistent shoulder pain. The aim of this study was to investigate whether emotional distress was associated with pain intensity and self-reported disability after physiotherapy treatment in patients with shoulder pain.

Methods: Data from 145 patients treated at physiotherapy outpatient clinics aged ≥18 years with self-reported pain in the shoulder or arm, and movement activity problems related to the upper-extremity, were included. Outcome measures were pain intensity measured by Numeric Pain Rating Scale and disability measured by Patient Specific Functional Scale. Demographic and clinical characteristics, including emotional distress measured by Hopkins Symptom Checklist – 25, were obtained at study onset. Association between characteristics at study onset and pain and disability after physiotherapy treatment were analysed using multiple linear regression and a backward manual elimination method. The final models were adjusted for age and sex.

Results: Higher emotional distress at study onset (B 1.06, 95% CI 0.44 to 1.68) was associated with higher pain intensity after the physiotherapy treatment ($P = 0.001$). Emotional distress was not associated with self-reported disability after the physiotherapy treatment.

Conclusion: This study found that emotional distress at study onset was associated with shoulder pain intensity after physiotherapy treatment, but not with disability. The findings indicate that emotional distress should be included in the initial physiotherapy examination of shoulder pain.

Keywords: Shoulder pain, Emotional distress, Physiotherapy

Background

Shoulder pain is a common disorder in the general population, with a point prevalence ranging from 6.9 to 26%, and a lifetime prevalence from 6.7 to 66.7% [1]. In many patients, the shoulder pain is long lasting, and 41% of the patients report persistent symptoms one year after they initially sought help for their problem [2]. Exercise therapy is a common treatment modality for shoulder pain, and there is evidence to support that physiotherapist-prescribed exercise decreases pain and improves function at short-term follow-up [3, 4]. However, the evidence of its long-term effectiveness has been questioned [5].

A systematic review of prognostic factors in patients with acute and subacute non-traumatic shoulder pain found strong evidence that high scores on the Shoulder Pain and Disability Index (SPADI), more shoulder pain, and a longer duration of complaints were associated with persistent shoulder pain [6]. Moderate evidence was found for male gender, age > 55 years, poor general health, a gradual onset of complaints, longer duration of sick leave, the perception of high job demand, low perceived social support, and the number of visits to a general practitioner [6]. The authors of the review suggested that the lack of identified psychosocial prognostic factors could be due to little use of questionnaires containing these functions in shoulder pain populations [6].

A recent cohort study, which included a range of biopsychosocial factors, found that psychological factors were

* Correspondence: kajasmedbrat@gmail.com
Department of Physiotherapy, Faculty of Health Sciences, OsloMet – Oslo Metropolitan University, Pb 4, St.Olavs plass, 0130 Oslo, Norway

consistently associated with the outcome of physiotherapy for patients with shoulder pain [7]. The psychological factors that were associated with a better outcome at six weeks and six months were higher pain self-efficacy and patient expectations of 'complete recovery' in comparison to 'slight improvement' as a result of physiotherapy treatment [7]. The association between emotional factors and the outcome of physiotherapy in patients with shoulder pain has been scarcely investigated in epidemiological research. The aim of this study was to investigate whether emotional distress was associated with pain intensity and self-reported disability after physiotherapy treatment in patients with shoulder pain.

Methods

This study was a prospective cohort study of consecutive patients treated at two student clinics located at the Department of Physiotherapy at OsloMet – Oslo Metropolitan University in Norway between September 2013 and September 2016. Patients receiving physiotherapy at the two clinics answered questionnaires for the FysioPol database. The FysioPol database contains pre- and post-treatment information about the patients treated at the student clinics, and was established in order to measure the quality of treatment and facilitate research at the department [8]. The database includes information on socio-demographic status and characteristics of the patients' complaints such as pain duration, pain intensity, disability, medication and emotional distress. The data is collected through electronic questionnaires.

The patients were treated by physiotherapy students in their second or third study year, under supervision of a teacher. The treatment period was intended to be up to nine weeks. The treatment consisted of individualised exercise therapy. In addition, some of the patients reported that they had received information, advice and manual techniques such as massage and stretching.

Patients aged 18 years or older with self-reported pain in the shoulder or arm were included. We excluded patients who did not report any movement activity problems related to the upper-extremity in the Patient Specific Functional Scale (PSFS) [9]. Patients who were unable to read and understand Norwegian were excluded.

The study protocol was considered by the Regional Committee for Medical and Health Research Ethics in Norway (REC), which concluded that the study did not require ethical approval. The study was approved by the Norwegian Centre for Research Data (NSD). All patients had signed a written, informed consent form.

Outcome measures

The primary outcome in this study was the Numeric Pain Rating Scale (NPRS) [10]. The NPRS is an 11 point scale where 0 indicates no pain, and 10 indicates the worst imagined pain. In this study, the scale was used as a measure of pain intensity during the last week. The PSFS was used as a secondary outcome [9]. In this questionnaire, the patients wrote down up to three activities they found impossible or had difficulty doing because of their problem. The difficulty associated with each activity was rated on a scale from 0 (impossible to perform the activity) to 10 (no difficulty, or at the same level as before the pain occurred). The average rating of the activities was used in the analyses as a measure of self-reported disability [11, 12]. Only scores from activities that had been rated both before and after treatment were included in the calculation of the average score.

Potential prognostic factors

The set of variables considered as potential prognostic factors was obtained by the FysioPol-questionnaire package at study onset, including clinical characteristics identified with prognostic value in previous research, and demographic factors. The Hopkins Symptom Checklist-25 (HSCL-25) [13] was used as a measure of emotional distress. The questionnaire aims to assess symtomps of anxiety, depression and somatization. HSCL-25 is a shorter version of the Symptom Checklist 90 (SCL-90) and consists of 25 items that are rated from 1 (not at all) to 4 (very much). The total score was obtained by averaging the scores, and ranged between 1 and 4. A maximum of five missing items were accepted. A higher total score indicates a higher level of emotional distress. The Norwegian version of the HSCL-25 has been used in several studies of musculoskeletal pain [14–17]. Evidence of psychometric properties of HSCL-25 in the population of patients with shoulder pain is to our knowledge lacking. Other clinical characteristics considered as potential prognostic factors included pre-treatment pain intensity measured by NPRS; pre-treatment disability measured by PSFS; duration of pain divided into 0–3 months, 4–12 months and more than 12 months; use of pain relieving drugs divided into less than every week and every week or more; concomitant neck pain; and number of pain sites divided into two pain sites or less and three pain sites or more. The demographic factors included age, sex, body mass index (BMI), level of education, work status, relationship status and smoking status. Level of education was divided into lower level (≤ 13 years) and college / university (> 13 years). Work status was divided into working and not working. Students were included in the working group, which consisted of both full time and part time working patients, while retirees were included in the not working group, which also included unemployed patients and patients on full time sick leave and disability pension.

Statistical analyses

Descriptive data are presented as number of patients and percentages, means and standard deviations or medians and interquartile range. Paired t-tests were used to identify changes from pre- to post- treatment measures of pain intensity and self-reported disability. Characteristics of the individuals who were lost to follow-up were compared to pre-treatment characteristics of the study sample. The groups were compared on pain intensity, disability, emotional distress and age using independent t-tests, and sex using a Chi-square test.

Simple linear regression analyses were performed to examine the relationship between each of the potential prognostic factors and the outcome (the NPRS and the PSFS). The variables with a statistically significant relationship with the outcome at the 20% level ($P < 0.20$) [18] were considered for the final multiple regression models. A backward manual elimination method was used to remove those variables with the highest P-value, one by one. The elimination was repeated until the remaining variables in the models were all statistically significant at the 5% level ($P < 0.05$). To prevent elimination of a variable at one step in the analysis process being crucial, the variables removed on backward elimination were all re-entered in the models one by one, and remained in the models if they were statistically significant at the 5% level. The multiple regression models were adjusted for age and sex.

Assumptions for the regression models were assessed. Correlation analyses were performed for all the independent variables and the correlation had to be less than 0.7 between the variables to be entered in the models [18]. An extreme value in the variable of BMI (> 39) was interpreted as an univariate outlier, due to a standardized score in excess of 3.29, disconnected from the other standardized scores [18]. Since a BMI-value of > 39 may involve other health problems than the ones investigated in this study, and the case therefore may not be a part of the population we intended to investigate, the case was excluded.

SPSS version 24 was used for all of the statistical analyses.

Results

Altogether, 251 patients reported shoulder- or arm pain during the inclusion period and were eligible for participation (Fig. 1). Of these, 209 patients met the inclusion criteria, but 30.6% did not answer the post- treatment questionnaires. Thus, 145 patients were included in the study. The patients lost to follow-up did not differ in age, sex, pain intensity, disability or level of emotional distress at study onset compared to the study sample ($P > 0.05$) (see Additional file 1 Table S1). The demographic and clinical characteristics of the patients at study onset are shown in Table 1. The study group had an average level of emotional distress of 1.6 (SD 0.5). The average pre-treatment pain intensity was 4.9 (SD 2.3), and the average self-reported disability was 4.5 (SD 2.0).

The median length of the treatment period was 5 weeks (IQR 3 to 6) (n=112). The patients had a statistically significant improvement in pain intensity from pre- to post-treatment ($P < 0.001$) of 2.0 (SD 1.9) points. The patients had also a statistically significant improvement in self-reported disability (P < 0.001) of 1.7 (SD 2.7) points. The average post-treatment pain intensity was 2.9 (SD 2.1) (n=140) and the post-treatment self-reported disability was 6.2 (SD 2.6) (n=133).

The results from the simple linear regression analyses between potential prognostic factors and pain intensity after treatment are presented in Table 2. A number of

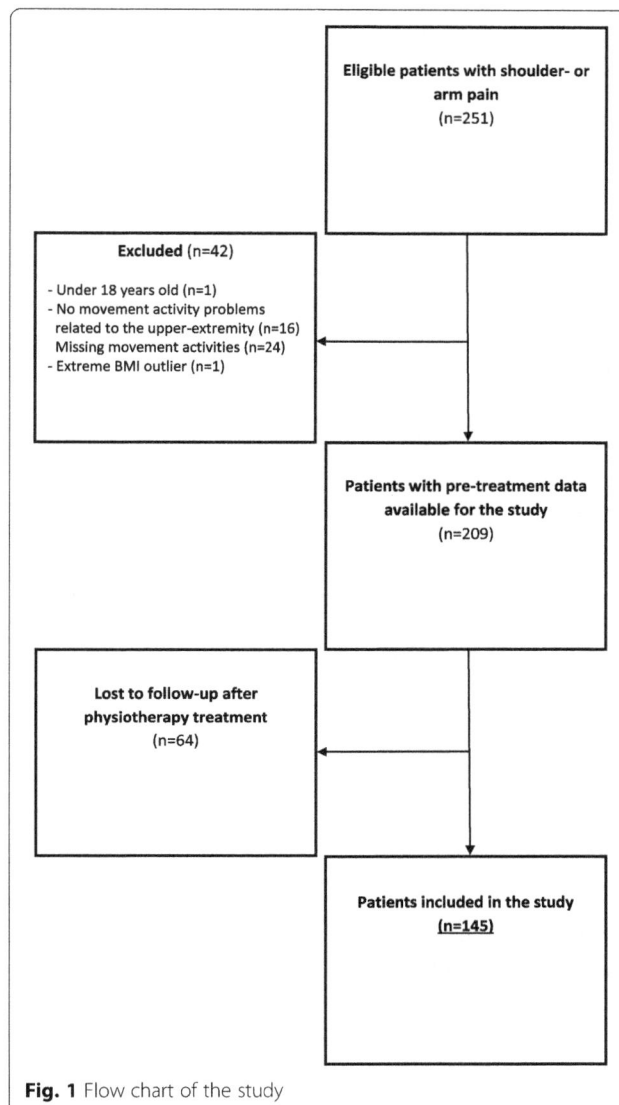

Fig. 1 Flow chart of the study

Within the flow chart:

- Eligible patients with shoulder- or arm pain (n=251)
- Excluded (n=42)
  - Under 18 years old (n=1)
  - No movement activity problems related to the upper-extremity (n=16) Missing movement activities (n=24)
  - Extreme BMI outlier (n=1)
- Patients with pre-treatment data available for the study (n=209)
- Lost to follow-up after physiotherapy treatment (n=64)
- Patients included in the study (n=145)

Table 1 Characteristics of the study sample at study onset ($n = 145$)

Variables	Frequency (%)	Mean (SD)
Age		44.0 (15.4)
Sex, female (missing: 2)	104 (71.7)	
BMI (missing: 25)		24.7 (3.7)
Education		
≤ 13 years	45 (31.0)	
College /university	98 (67.6)	
(Missing: 2)		
Work status		
Working or being in education	119 (82.1)	
Not working	26 (17.9)	
Relationship status		
In a relationship	75 (51.7)	
Not in a relationship	68 (46.9)	
(Missing: 2)		
Smoking (missing: 2)	12 (8.3)	
Emotional distress (HSCL-25)[a] (1–4)		1.6 (0.5)
Pain intensity (NPRS)[b] (0–10) (Missing: 18)		4.9 (2.3)
Disability (PSFS)[c] (0–10)		4.5 (2.0)
Duration of pain		
0–3 months	28 (19.3)	
4–12 months	39 (26.9)	
> 12 months	78 (53.8)	
Use of pain relieving drugs		
Every week or more	31 (21.4)	
Less than every week	113 (77.9)	
(Missing: 1)		
Concomitant neck pain	60 (41.4)	
Number of pain sites		
> 2 sites of pain	24 (16.6)	
≤ 2 sites of pain	121 (83.4)	

[a] HSCL-25 = Hopkins Symptom Checklist – 25, the average of 25 questions rated between 1: not at all, 4: very much
[b] NPRS = Numeric Pain Rating Scale, 0: no pain, 10: worst imagined pain
[c] PSFS = Patient Specific Functional Scale, the average of up to three activities rated between 0: impossible to perform the activity, 10: no difficulty, or at the same level as before the pain occurred

factors showed a statistically significant association at the 20% level with pain intensity after treatment. These were: emotional distress, pre-treatment pain intensity, pre-treatment disability, duration of pain for more than 12 months in comparison to 0 to 3 months, use of pain relieving drugs, concomitant neck pain, number of painful sites, sex, BMI and work status. In the final multiple model, higher emotional distress, higher pre-treatment pain intensity and duration of pain for 4 to 12 months

in comparison to 0 to 3 months were associated with higher pain intensity after treatment (Table 2).

The results of the simple linear regression analyses between potential prognostic factors and disability after treatment (PSFS) are presented in Table 3. A number of factors showed a statistically significant association at the 20% level with disability after treatment. These were: emotional distress, pre-treatment pain intensity, pre-treatment disability, duration of pain for more than 12 months in comparison to 0 to 3 months, use of pain relieving drugs, concomitant neck pain, number of painful sites, age, education, work status and smoking status. In the final multiple model, higher pre-treatment disability, duration of pain for more than 12 months in comparison to 0 to 3 months, concomitant neck pain and a lower level of education (≤ 13 years) were associated with higher self-reported disability after treatment (Table 3).

Discussion

This study showed that higher emotional distress at study onset, in combination with higher pre-treatment pain intensity and duration of pain for 4 to 12 months in comparison to 0 to 3 months, was associated with a poor outcome in terms of pain intensity after physiotherapy in patients with shoulder pain. Emotional distress was not associated with self-reported disability.

Pain outcome

In a recent systematic review of prognostic factors for shoulder pain, strong evidence was found that high scores on the SPADI questionnaire, more shoulder pain, and a longer duration of complaints, were associated with persistent shoulder pain [6]. In contrast to the results of the present study, the systematic review did not find any evidence that psychological factors were associated with shoulder pain. However, the authors of the systematic review claimed that psychosocial factors might have been underestimated due to limited use of questionnaires containing these functions in shoulder pain populations [6].

Emotional distress was investigated in two previous studies on shoulder pain, which found no association with outcome [16, 17]. One of the studies comprised patients with diagnosed subacromial pain in secondary care [16], the other study included patients with diagnosed rotator tendinosis in primary care [17]. The inconsistencies between these studies and the present findings might be explained by differences in the study populations; the present study was a cohort study comprising patients with self-reported shoulder or arm pain.

Furthermore, the present findings are not consistent with those in a previous study on patients presenting new episodes of shoulder- or low back pain to their general practitioner [19]. Interestingly, the cohort study

Table 2 Linear regression of pain intensity after treatment (NPRS) and potential prognostic factors

	Simple regression		Final multiple regression model [b] N=122	
	B (95% CI)	P-value	B (95% CI)	P-value
Emotional distress (HSCL-25)	2.05 (1.49 to 2.60)	P < 0.001	1.06 (0.44 to 1.68)	P = 0.001
Pre-treatment pain intensity (NPRS)	0.58 (0.45 to 0.71)	P < 0.001	0.46 (0.32 to 0.61)	P < 0.001
Pre-treatment disability (PSFS)	−0.22 (− 0.39 to − 0.05)	P = 0.012		
Duration of pain				
0–3 months [a]				
4–12 months	0.34 (−0.72 to 1.39)	P = 0.528	0.93 (0.07 to 1.78)	P = 0.033
> 12 months	0.75 (− 0.18 to 1.69)	P = 0.112	0.75 (− 0.01 to 1.50)	P = 0.053 [c]
Use of pain relieving drugs (0,1)	1.62 (0.78 to 2.46)	P < 0.001		
Concomitant neck pain (0,1)	1.34 (0.65 to 2.03)	P < 0.001		
Number of painful sites (0,1)	1.09 (0.16 to 2.02)	P = 0.022		
Age	−0.01 (− 0.03 to 0.02)	P = 0.508		
Sex (0,1)	0.88 (0.12 to 1.64)	P = 0.024		
BMI	0.09 (−0.02 to 0.20)	P = 0.100		
Education (0,1)	−0.45 (− 1.22 to 0.32)	P = 0.250		
Work status (0,1)	−0.99 (− 1.90 to − 0.09)	P = 0.032		
Relationship status (0,1)	0.00 (− 0.70 to 0.70)	P = 0.997		
Smoking (0,1)	0.77 (−0.50 to 2.05)	P = 0.233		

Duration of treatment was not associated with pain intensity after treatment (P = 0.951)
[a] Reference category
[b] Adjusted for age and sex
[c] Before the model was adjusted for age and sex, duration of pain > 12 months was associated with pain intensity after treatment (P < 0.05)
NPRS = Numeric Pain Rating Scale. HSCL-25 = Hopkins Symptom Checklist – 25. PSFS = Patient Specific Functional Scale
Use of pain relieving drugs (0: < once a week, 1: ≥ once a week). Concomitant neck pain (0: no, 1: yes). Number of painful sites (0: ≤ 2 painful sites, 1: > 2 painful sites). Sex (0: male, 1: female). Education (0: ≤ 13 years, 1: College / University). Work status (0: not working, 1: working full time, part time or being in education). Relationship status (0: not in a relationship, 1: in a relationship). Smoking (0: no, 1: yes)

found that for the shoulder pain patients, no psychological factors were associated with persistent symptoms or disability after three months, with the exception of catastrophizing, which in patients with a long duration of pain at study onset (≥ 3 months) was associated with persistent symptoms [19]. However, it is worth noting that the patients in this study had no distress at baseline, measured by a subscale of the Four-Dimensional Symptom Questionnaire [20], while the patients in our study had an average level of 1.6 (SD 0.5) on the HSCL-25. This might explain the difference in findings. Another possible reason for different results might be that factors associated with persistent pain after an exercise therapy intervention differ from factors associated with pain after other types of treatment.

Nevertheless, a recent cohort study from the UK reported that other psychological factors than distress, such as patient expectations of recovery and pain self-efficacy, were associated with the level of pain and disability after physiotherapy in patients with shoulder pain [7]. Although the study did not identify any association between anxiety and depression and

outcome, the authors suggested that this could be due to a low number of included patients with extreme anxiety and depression [7]. Based on the findings of the study, the authors concluded that when assessing people with musculoskeletal shoulder pain and considering referral to physiotherapy services, psychosocial and medical information should be considered [7].

Disability outcome
Our data showed no association between emotional distress at study onset and self-reported disability after treatment. The factors associated with higher post-treatment disability were higher pre-treatment disability, duration of pain for more than 12 months in comparison to 0 to 3 months, concomitant neck pain and a lower level of education. The results indicate that patients with a history of chronic shoulder pain and disability may have a poor outcome in terms of disability regardless of emotional distress.

Our findings that emotional distress was associated with pain, but not with disability, are difficult to explain. One explanation might be that mental functions are more directly associated with the

Table 3 Linear regression of disability after treatment (PSFS) and potential prognostic factors

	Simple regression		Final multiple regression model [b] N = 130	
	B (95% CI)	P-value	B (95% CI)	P-value
Emotional distress (HSCL-25)	− 1.62 (− 2.43 to − 0.81)	P < 0.001		
Pre-treatment pain intensity (NPRS)	−0.16 (− 0.36 to 0.04)	P = 0.123		
Pre-treatment disability (PSFS)	0.45 (0.24 to 0.66)	P < 0.001	0.32 (0.10 to 0.53)	P = 0.004
Duration of pain				
0–3 months [a]				
4–12 months	−0.12 (−1.43 to 1.19)	P = 0.859	−0.60 (− 1.81 to 0.61)	P = 0.327
> 12 months	−1.23 (− 2.39 to − 0.06)	P = 0.039	−1.17 (− 2.24 to − 0.11)	P = 0.031
Use of pain relieving drugs (0,1)	−1.68 (− 2.72 to − 0.65)	P = 0.002		
Concomitant neck pain (0,1)	− 1.47 (−2.36 to − 0.59)	P = 0.001	−1.14 (− 2.01 to − 0.28)	P = 0.010
Number of painful sites (0,1)	−0.97 (− 2.15 to 0.21)	P = 0.106		
Age	−0.02 (− 0.05 to 0.01)	P = 0.191		
Sex (0,1)	−0.54 (− 1.53 to 0.45)	P = 0.283		
BMI	−0.08 (− 0.21 to 0.05)	P = 0.235		
Education (0,1)	1.20 (0.25 to 2.15)	P = 0.014	0.94 (0.03 to 1.84)	P = 0.042
Work status (0,1)	2.04 (0.90 to 3.18)	P = 0.001	1.13 (−0.15 to 2.41)	P = 0.083 [c]
Relationship status (0,1)	0.04 (−0.87 to 0.95)	P = 0.928		
Smoking (0,1)	−1.64 (−3.19 to −0.08)	P = 0.039		

Duration of treatment was not associated with disability after treatment (P = 0.407)
[a] Reference category
[b] Adjusted for age and sex
[c] Before the model was adjusted for age and sex, work status was associated with disability after treatment (P < 0.05)
PSFS = Patient Specific Functional Scale. HSCL-25 = Hopkins Symptom Checklist – 25. NPRS = Numeric Pain Rating Scale
Use of pain relieving drugs (0: < once a week, 1: ≥ once a week). Concomitant neck pain (0: no, 1: yes). Number of painful sites (0: ≤ 2 painful sites, 1: > 2 painful sites). Sex (0: male, 1: female). Education (0: ≤ 13 years, 1: College / University). Work status (0: not working, 1: working full time, part time or being in education). Relationship status (0: not in a relationship, 1: in a relationship). Smoking (0: no, 1: yes)

experience of pain, than with disability. However, a cross-sectional study on people with chronic shoulder pain found that psychological distress was correlated with disability, but not with pain [21], which indicate that the relationship between distress, disability and pain may be complex.

Limitations
This study has some limitations that should be considered. Firstly, since the inclusion of patients was based on self-reported shoulder- or arm pain, we were not able to discriminate between localised shoulder pain and pain related to the shoulder, arm and hand. Secondly, a number of patients who met the inclusion criteria were excluded from the analyses due to loss to follow-up or missing values in some of the variables. However, the patients lost to follow-up did not differ from the study sample on characteristics such as sex, age, pain intensity, disability or emotional distress at study onset. A third concern involves the duration of treatment. There was a variety in duration of treatment, with a median of 5 weeks of physiotherapy (IQR 3 to 6). A period of

12 weeks of physiotherapy is often suggested for patients with shoulder pain [22]. Future research could establish whether the results after a longer follow-up differ from the results in this study.

Implications for practice and research
The results of this study showed that emotional distress at study onset was associated with the intensity of shoulder pain after physiotherapy. Psychological factors in general are little emphasised in the examination of shoulder pain, and it is rather the structural and biomechanical aspects of the condition that are usually considered in clinical decision-making. The findings of this study support, however, that emotional distress should be considered in the initial physiotherapy examination of shoulder pain.

Emotional distress may be a cause or a consequence of shoulder pain, and whether the treatment should be directed towards reducing distress is not possible to tell based on the present findings. Nevertheless, findings of a meta-analysis on neck and back pain indicate that psychological distress mediates the relationship between pain and disability [23]. Future research is needed to investigate the relationship between emotional distress, pain and disability. The research should identify whether targeting emotional distress in shoulder pain rehabilitation is likely to improve the outcome for shoulder patients with a high degree of emotional distress, to identify whether and how to best individualise the treatment for these patients.

Conclusion

This study found that higher emotional distress, in combination with higher pain intensity and duration of pain for 4 to 12 months in comparison to 0 to 3 months, was associated with a poor outcome in terms of shoulder pain intensity after physiotherapy, but not with disability. The present findings indicate that emotional distress should be included in the initial physiotherapy examination of shoulder pain.

Abbreviations
HSCL-25: Hopkins Symptom Checklist – 25; NPRS: Numeric Pain Rating Scale; PSFS: Patient Specific Functional Scale; SPADI: Shoulder Pain and Disability Index

Acknowledgements
The authors would like to thank the members of the FysioPol project group who supported us and gave us permission to make use of the data in the FysioPol database. We would also like to thank the physiotherapists who collected the data and made it possible for us to perform this study.

Authors' contributions
KS, YR and BEØ contributed in the planning process and designing of the study. KS performed the statistical analyses. All authors drafted, read and approved the manuscript.

Competing interests
The authors declare that they have no competing interests.

References
1. Luime JJ, Koes BW, Hendriksen IJ, Burdorf A, Verhagen AP, Miedema HS, et al. Prevalence and incidence of shoulder pain in the general population; a systematic review. Scand J Rheumatol. 2004;33(2):73–81. https://doi.org/10.1080/03009740310004667.
2. van der Windt DA, Koes BW, Boeke AJ, Devillé W, De Jong BA, Bouter LM. Shoulder disorders in general practice: prognostic indicators of outcome. Br J Gen Pract. 1996;46(410):519–23.
3. Hanratty CE, McVeigh JG, Kerr DP, Basford JR, Finch MB, Pendleton A, et al. The effectiveness of physiotherapy exercises in subacromial impingement syndrome: a systematic review and meta-analysis. Semin Arthritis Rheum. 2012;42(3):297–316. https://doi.org/10.1016/j.semarthrit.2012.03.015.
4. Littlewood C, Ashton J, Chance-Larsen K, May S, Sturrock B. Exercise for rotator cuff tendinopathy: a systematic review. Physiotherapy. 2012;98(2):101–9. https://doi.org/10.1016/j.physio.2011.08.002.
5. Page MJ, Green S, McBain B, Surace SJ, Deitch J, Lyttle N, et al. Manual therapy and exercise for rotator cuff disease. The Cochrane Database Syst Rev 2016;6:Cd012224. https://doi.org/10.1002/14651858.CD012224.
6. Struyf F, Geraets J, Noten S, Meeus M, Nijs JA. Multivariable prediction model for the chronification of non-traumatic shoulder pain: a systematic review. Pain physician. 2016;19(2):1–10.
7. Chester R, Jerosch-Herold C, Lewis J, Shepstone L. Psychological factors are associated with the outcome of physiotherapy for people with shoulder pain: a multicentre longitudinal cohort study. British J Sports Med. 2018;52(4):269–75. https://doi.org/10.1136/bjsports-2016-096084.
8. Tveter AT, Major DH, Grotle M. FysioPol; a new electronic database for development of quality and knowledge in physiotherapy. Fysioterapeuten. 2015;9:8.
9. Stratford P, Gill C, Westaway M, Binkley J. Assessing disability and change on individual patients: a report of a patient specific measure. Physiother Can. 1995;47(4):258–63. https://doi.org/10.3138/ptc.47.4.258.
10. Downie WW, Leatham PA, Rhind VM, Wright V, Branco JA, Anderson JA. Studies with pain rating scales. Ann Rheum Dis. 1978;37(4):378–81. https://doi.org/10.1136/ard.37.4.378.
11. Hefford C, Abbott JH, Arnold R, Baxter GD. The Patient-Specific Functional Scale: validity, reliability, and responsiveness in patients with upper extremity musculoskeletal problems. The Journal of Orthopaedic and Sports Physical Therapy. 2012;42(2):56–65. https://doi.org/10.2519/jospt.2012.3953.
12. Koehorst ML, van Trijffel E, Lindeboom R. Evaluative measurement properties of the Patient-Specific Functional Scale for primary shoulder complaints in physical therapy practice. The Journal of Orthopaedic and Sports Physical Therapy. 2014;44(8):595–603. https://doi.org/10.2519/jospt.2014.5133.
13. Derogatis LR, Lipman RS, Rickels K, Uhlenhuth EH, Covi L. The Hopkins Symptom Checklist (HSCL): a self-report symptom inventory. Behav Sci. 1974;19(1):1–15. https://doi.org/10.1002/bs.3830190102.
14. Grotle M, Vollestad NK, Veierod MB, Brox JI. Fear-avoidance beliefs and distress in relation to disability in acute and chronic low back pain. Pain. 2004;112(3):343–52. https://doi.org/10.1016/j.pain.2004.09.020.
15. Johansen JB, Roe C, Bakke ES, Mengshoel AM, Storheim K, Andelic N. The determinants of function and disability in neck patients referred to a specialized outpatient clinic. Clin J Pain. 2013;29(12):1029–35. https://doi.org/10.1097/AJP.0b013e31828027a2.
16. Engebretsen K, Grotle M, Bautz-Holter E, Ekeberg OM, Brox JI. Predictors of shoulder pain and disability index (SPADI) and work status after 1 year in patients with subacromial shoulder pain. BMC Musculoskelet Disord. 2010;11:218. https://doi.org/10.1186/1471-2474-11-218.
17. Brox JI, Brevik JI. Prognostic factors in patients with rotator tendinosis (stage II impingement syndrome) of the shoulder. Scand J Prim Health Care. 1996;14(2):100–5. https://doi.org/10.3109/02813439608997078.
18. Tabachnick BG, Fidell LS. Using multivariate statistics. 6th ed. Boston: Pearson; 2013.
19. van der Windt DA, Kuijpers T, Jellema P, van der Heijden GJ, Bouter LM. Do psychological factors predict outcome in both low-back pain and shoulder pain? Ann Rheum Dis. 2007;66(3):313–9. https://doi.org/10.1136/ard.2006.053553.
20. Terluin B, Rhenen WV, Schaufeli WB, De Haan M. The Four-Dimensional Symptom Questionnaire (4DSQ): measuring distress and other mental health problems in a working population. Work & Stress. 2004;18(3):187–207. https://doi.org/10.1080/0267837042000297535.
21. Badcock LJ, Lewis M, Hay EM, McCarney R, Croft PR. Chronic shoulder pain in the community: a syndrome of disability or distress? Ann Rheum Dis. 2002;61(2):128–31. https://doi.org/10.1136/ard.61.2.128.
22. Klintberg IH, Cools AMJ, Holmgren TM, Holzhausen A-CG, Johansson K, Maenhout AG, et al. Consensus for physiotherapy for shoulder pain. Int Orthop. 2015;39(4):715–20. https://doi.org/10.1007/s00264-014-2639-9.
23. Lee H, Hubscher M, Moseley GL, Kamper SJ, Traeger AC, Mansell G, et al. How does pain lead to disability? A systematic review and meta-analysis of mediation studies in people with back and neck pain. Pain. 2015;156(6):988–97.

2

Missed fractures of the greater tuberosity

Umile Giuseppe Longo[1,2]*⑩, Steven Corbett[2] and Philip Michael Ahrens[2]

Abstract

Background: Fractures of the greater tuberosity may result from a variety of mechanisms. Missed injury remains a persistent problem, both from a clinical and medico-legal point-of-view. Few studies on this topic are available in the literature. We present the clinical and radiological findings of a consecutive series of 17 patients who were diagnosed and managed with undisplaced greater tuberosity fractures.

Methods: A retrospective study of a consecutive series of 17 patients who sustained an occult greater tuberosity fracture were performed. Patients sustained a traumatic occult greater tuberosity fracture, underwent shoulder radiographs after trauma in 5 days and they were diagnosed as negative by a consultant radiologist. All patients received a standard assessment using MRI (Magnetic Resonance Imaging) scans Each patient was evaluated for arm dominance, trauma history, duration and type of symptoms and post-treatment Oxford Shoulder Score.

Results: At the final follow up the mean OSS (Oxford Shoulder Score) was 38.3 (range 17–46; SD 9.11). Three patients required a glenohumeral joint injection for post-traumatic pain and stiffness and three patients required subacromial decompression for post-traumatic impingement.

Conclusions: Though undisplaced greater tuberosity fracture can be managed non-operatively with good results, patients with persistent post-traumatic shoulder pain, tenderness and limitation of shoulder function warrant investigation with MRI to identify occult fractures. Prompt identification of these fractures can facilitate patient treatment and counselling, avoiding a source of patient dissatisfaction and litigation.

Keywords: Shoulder, Fractures, Greater tuberosity, Management, Occult

Background

Fractures of the greater tuberosity may result from a variety of mechanisms. The most common are avulsion injuries such associated with anterior shoulder dislocation, or direct trauma, as might occur in a fall on the shoulder or with hyperabduction and impaction of the greater tuberosity against the surrounding bone structures [1, 2]. These fractures can be misdiagnosed, as radiographs of the shoulder are often insufficient to confirm the diagnosis [2], especially in the case of undisplaced fractures and if the radiographic series does not include an anteroposterior (AP) view with the arm in external rotation [2, 3]. Patients may complain of persistent rotator cuff symptoms and may be referred for further examination. Missed injury remains a persistent problem, both from a clinical and medico-legal point-of-view. Few studies on this topic are available in the literature.

We present the clinical and radiological findings of a consecutive series of 17 patients who were diagnosed and managed with undisplaced greater tuberosity fractures.

Methods

Few months ago we decided to publish a retrospective study of a consecutive series of patients who sustained an occult greater tuberosity fracture and were managed at our institution between 2006 and 2008. All patients gave written consent to participate in the study. The study was submitted and approved by the ethics committee of "Campus Bio Medico" of Rome.

Eligibility criteria

Patients were included in the study if (1) they sustained an occult greater tuberosity fracture, (2) they had a traumatic shoulder injury, (3) they underwent shoulder radiographs after trauma in 5 days and they were

* Correspondence: g.longo@unicampus.it
[1]Department of Orthopaedic and Trauma Surgery, Campus Bio-Medico University, Via Alvaro del Portillo, 200, 00128 Rome, Italy
[2]Shoulder Unit, Hospital of St John and St Elizabeth, 60 Grove End Road, London, UK

diagnosed as negative by a consultant radiologist, (4) the treating physician initially managed all the patients as a soft tissue injury, (5) all the diagnoses were made on the basis of an MRI performed within 6 weeks of the initial trauma, and (6) no previous history of shoulder symptoms.

An occult greater tuberosity was defined as the MRI findings of oedema in the greater tuberosity at T2-weighted images associated with a fracture line and/or cortical breach [4]. A crescent or oblique line of decreased signal intensity can be found at T1- or T2-weighted images of patients with greater tuberosity fracture [4].

The indication for MRI was shoulder pain associated with the clinical finding of tenderness on palpation of the greater tuberosity in the presence of negative radiographs.

Patients were excluded from the study if they had (1) associated rotator cuff tear, (2) previous surgery on the affected shoulder, (3) a displaced fracture of the greater tuberosity, (4) Hill-Sachs lesions or evidence of shoulder dislocation, (5) a glenoid rim fracture, (6) no history of trauma.

Patient demographics

Seventeen patients met the inclusion criteria. 6 patients were managed primarily by the authors, and 11 patients were secondary referred to them. All the patients were initially managed non-operatively. Of the 17 included patients, 16 agreed to participate in the study. 1 patient made a formal complaint against the initial treating physician and he declined to participate in the study. 3 patients agreed to participate in the study, but they moved abroad and were not contactable for final follow-up. Finally 13 patients were analyzed. The dominant arm was involved in 12 patients. Mechanism of index injury and associated shoulder MRI findings are reported in Table 1 for each patient.

Evaluation

Clinical evaluations were performed at a mean of 15 months (range, 3–44 months) from the diagnosis. Arm dominance, clinical history and post-treatment Oxford Shoulder Score were evaluated for each patient.

Imaging

Standard radiographs were performed for all patients in anteroposterior projections and a scapular lateral view or an axillary view.

MRI scans consisted of oblique coronal, oblique sagittal, and axial T2-weighted spin-echo MRIs (repetition time, 3200 milliseconds; echo time, 85 milliseconds).

Functional assessment

The Oxford shoulder score (OSS) was used to evaluate shoulder function. OSS is a patient-based questionnaire used to assess shoulder pain and function. The final score had a range from 12 (least difficulties) to 60 (most difficulties) [5, 6].

Non-operative management

A sling without pillow in slight internal rotation was used for 4 weeks. The sling was removed during bathing and exercises. Patients performed active elbow flexion and extension and pendular exercises as tolerated from the day of diagnosis [7].

At 4 weeks, the sling was discontinued and active assisted shoulder flexion, extension, abduction, external rotation and internal rotation were commenced. Isometric strengthening was not begun until 6 weeks post-injury, at which point we began rehabilitation of the rotator cuff, deltoid, and scapular stabilizers according to a validated protocol (http://www.moonshoulder.com/impactstudy.html).

Results

Of the 17 included patients, 16 agreed to participate in the study. 1 patient made a formal complaint against the initial treating physician and he declined to participate in the study. 3 patients were not contactable for final follow-up.

8 of the 17 patients had a sports related injury.

Our average follow up was 16.5 months, with all patients having 6 months or more follow up, except one patient who was fully recovered at 3 months with an OSS of 46. The internal consistency of OSS score was measured by the Cronbach's alpha, with 0.89 at the pre-operative assessment and 0.92 at 6-month follow-up. A coefficient of test-retest reliability of 6.8 was obtained using the Bland and Altman method. A significant correlation was obtained with Constant score, SF36 and Health Assessment Questionnaire Disability Index. The sensitivity to change of the study questionnaire was examined by comparing scores before and 6 months after operation, and it showed that the OSS is sensitive to clinical changes [5, 6]. The OSS in our patients showed good long term clinical results.

An issue which we highlight is that 3 of our patients were not able to attend for the final follow up, and we had to rely on the latest available clinical outpatient follow up result.

After trauma, all patients had pain in elevation and external rotation of the humerus. At diagnosis, all patients had minimal or no displacement of the fracture fragment. All fractures were undisplaced; therefore non-operative management was performed. Of the 16 included patients, OSS data were available for 13 of

Table 1 MRI findings for each patient

Patients	Affected/Dominant limb	Duration of follow-up (months)	Interval from initial injury to diagnosis	Referral	Associated injury at MRI	Type of primary injury	Treatment	Complications	Worker claim compensation	OSS
1	R/R	9 months	12 days	Secondary	None	Fall from scaffold	nonoperative, plus 1 glenohumeral joint injection	Stiffness at 6 weeks post-treatment, resolved at the final follow up	No	41
2	L/R	8 months	3 days	Primary	None	Rugby	nonoperative	No	No	46
3	R/R	8 months	67 days	Secondary	Partial thickness supraspinatus tear	Patagonian twister	nonoperative plus 1 glenohumeral joint injection 3 months after injury	Stiffness at 3 months post-treatment, resolved at the final follow up	No	31
4	L/R	8 months	60 Days	Secondary	None	Rugby army	nonoperative plus 1 glenohumeral joint injection 3 months after injury	Stiffness 3 months post-treatment, resolved at the final follow up	No	45
5	R/R	12 months	42 days	Secondary	None	Fall	nonoperative	No	No	31
6	R/R	15 months	28 days	Secondary	None	Direct fall on the right shoulder while cycling	nonoperative	No	No	46
7	R/R	11 months	8 days	Primary	Subscapularis tear	Fall down steps	nonoperative	No	No	Abroad
8	L/R	8 months	8 days	Primary	None	Fall	nonoperative	No	No	Declined
9	R/R	10 months	3 weeks	Primary	None	Fall on ice	nonoperative	No	No	Abroad
10	R/R	44 months	3 months	Secondary	None	Fall playing soccer	nonoperative	Post-traumatic impingement managed with subacromial decompression	No	Abroad
11	R/R	10 months	8 weeks	Secondary	None	Motocycle road traffic accident	nonoperative	No	No	30
12	R/R	46 months	2 months	Secondary	None	Fall while skiing	nonoperative	Post-traumatic impingement managed with subacromial decompression	No	48
13	L/L	6 months	3 months	Secondary	None	Fall while skiing	nonoperative	No	No	17
14	R/R	17 months	3 weeks	Primary	None	Bicycle road traffic accident	nonoperative	No	No	38
15	L/R	18 months	5 weeks	Secondary	None	Bicycle road traffic accident	nonoperative	No	No	44
16	L/R	3 months	1 day	Primary	None	Fall down stairs	nonoperative	No	No	46
17	R/R	20 months	4 months	Secondary	None	Fall from ladder	nonoperative	Post-traumatic impingement managed with subacromial decompression	No	35

them. At the final follow up the mean OSS was 38.3 (range 17–46; SD 9.11).

Data on demographics, interval from initial injury to diagnosis, associated injury at MRI, type of primary injury, treatment and complications are reported in Table 1. Figures 1 and 2 depicts the typical radiographic and MRI findings in these patients.

Following initial treatment all fractures united with no secondary displacement. Three patients required gleno-humeral joint injections for post traumatic stiffness between 6 and 12 weeks post injury and three patients required arthroscopy and subacromial decompression for post-traumatic impingement between 9 and 20 months post injury.

Discussion

The main finding of this study is that in the majority of patients with a traumatic undisplaced fracture of the greater tuberosity, non-operative management was effective, allowing a safe and prompt return to activities.

Isolated fractures of the greater tuberosity account for approximately 20% of all proximal humeral fractures and are associated with a glenohumeral dislocation in approximately 10—30% of cases [2]. Kim et al. [8] reported that isolated greater tuberosity fractures occurs frequently in male patients with a mean age of 42.8 years. Moreover patients with isolated greater tuberosity

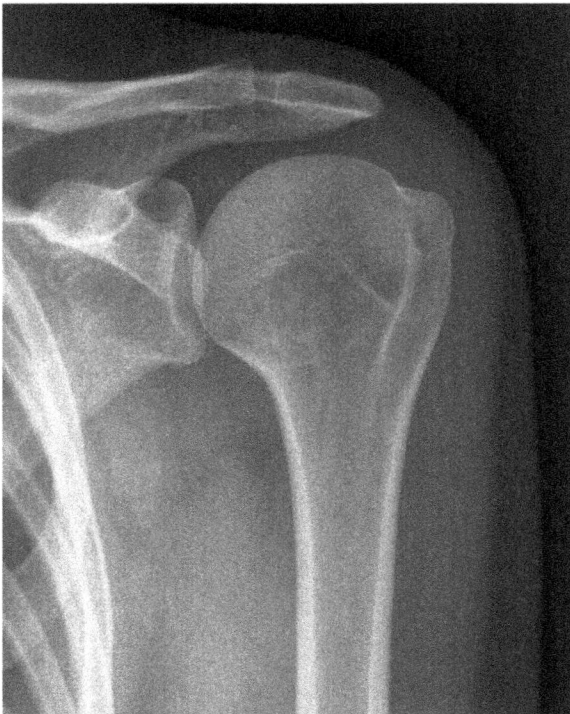

Fig. 2 MRI showing a visible fracture line of undisplaced greater tuberosity due to bony reabsorption at the fracture line

fractures had fewer medical comorbidities than those with surgical neck fractures [8]. Tuberosity avulsion or fracture may occur after a fall onto an outstretched upper extremity due to an eccentric load applied by the attached rotator cuff on the tuberosity, often in the setting of a traumatic glenohumeral dislocation. The majority of greater tuberosity fractures are undisplaced, however the impingement of the tuberosity against the acromion or the impact against the anteroinferior glen-oid during glenohumeral dislocation/subluxation could cause the inferior displacement of the tuberosity [8].

Non-displaced or minimally displaced (< 5 mm) fractures of the greater tuberosity are usually treated non opera-tively. Indications for surgery is a displacement > than 5 mm and take into account factor such as fracture characteristics and patient characteristics (age, comor-bidities, extremity dominance, pre-injury shoulder and individual level of function, local bone quality). Surgery may be performed with an open techniques with a standard deltopectoral approach or through a deltoid splitting approach or with an arthroscopically assisted technique.

According to our experience is rare that, if the arm is placed at the patient's side in a sling without pillow in slight internal rotation, an undisplaced fracture become displaced.

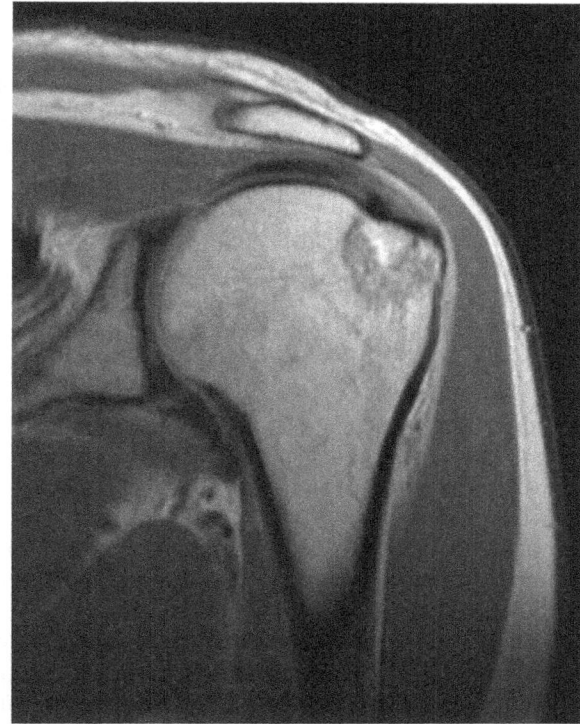

Fig. 1 Shoulder radiographs of a patient with undisplaced greater tuberosity fracture

Also, we used validated questionnaire-based outcome measures.

Patients with painful abduction and external rotation after shoulder trauma with no abnormality on plain radiographs should be always considered as potentially to have sustained an undisplaced greater tuberosity fracture. A consistent clinical finding that may differentiate from a rotator cuff injury is tenderness laterally over the greater tuberosity. Poor quality of radiographs, lack of the external rotation view or lack of clinical experience could be causes of missed diagnosis. MR examination subsequently performed due to persisting symptoms, revealed the fracture in all patients. Therefore, MRI should be always performed in patients with persistent pain, bony tenderness and decreased range of motion despite negative plain radiographs. This can avoid missed diagnosis and a potential source of patient dissatisfaction satisfaction and litigation.

Prevalence of rotator cuff tear associated with occult fractures of the greater tuberosity was lower than reported in literature (2 of 17 patients in our series), even though our series is too small to draw definitive conclusions. The involvement of the rotator cuff in previous reports was found in 11 of 24 patients, and 7 of 25 patients. Further studies are needed to better understand the relationship of symptoms caused by trauma and the presence of partial tendon tears, with or without fracture [4, 9–12].

The majority of patients were asymptomatic at the final follow up. Therefore healing of undisplaced greater tuberosity fracture is reliably achieved with non-operative treatment and surgical intervention should be only considered in case of persisting pain and shoulder function.

Strengths of the present study are that 2 fully trained shoulder surgeons performed all the diagnosis and treatment, and that the follow up evaluations were performed by an independent assessor.

Conclusions

In conclusion, undisplaced greater tuberosity fractures may be managed non-operatively with good results in the majority of cases. Nevertheless, shoulder MRI is warranted to confirm the diagnosis in patients with persistent post-traumatic shoulder pain and limitation of shoulder function with negative radiographs. Prompt identification of these fractures can facilitate patient management and information, particularly in counselling patients regarding the risk of stiffness and post-traumatic impingement. This will avoid a source of patient dissatisfaction and litigation.

Abbreviations
AP: Anteroposterior; MRI: Magnetic Resonance Imaging; OSS: Oxford Shoulder Score; SD: Standard deviation

Authors' contributions
UGL made substantive intellectual contributions to the published study and wrote the paper, SC and PMA analyzed the data, PMA contributed to statistical analysis. All authors read and approved the final manuscript.

Competing interest
UGL is a member of the Editorial Board of BMC Musculoskeletal Disorders. The remaining authors declare that they have no conflict of interest.

References
1. Hu C, Zhou K, Pan F, Zhai Q, Wen W, He X. Application of pre-contoured anatomic locking plate for treatment of humerus split type greater tuberosity fractures: A prospective review of 68 cases with an average follow-up of 2.5 years. Injury. 2018;49(6):1108–12.
2. Gruson KI, Ruchelsman DE, Tejwani NC. Isolated tuberosity fractures of the proximal humeral: current concepts. Injury. 2008;39(3):284–98.
3. Reinus WR, Hatem SF. Fractures of the greater tuberosity presenting as rotator cuff abnormality: magnetic resonance demonstration. J Trauma. 1998;44(4):670–5.
4. Gumina S, Carbone S, Postacchini F. Occult fractures of the greater tuberosity of the humerus. Int Orthop. 2009;33(1):171–4.
5. Longo UG, Saris D, Poolman RW, Berton A, Denaro V. Instruments to assess patients with rotator cuff pathology: a systematic review of measurement properties. Knee Surg Sports Traumatol Arthrosc. 2011;20(10):1961–70.
6. Longo UG, Vasta S, Maffulli N, Denaro V. Scoring systems for the functional assessment of patients with rotator cuff pathology. Sports Med Arthrosc. 2011;19(3):310–20.
7. Longo UG, Franceschi F, Berton A, Maffulli N, Droena V. Conservative treatment and rotator cuff tear progression. Med Sport Sci. 2012;57:90–9.
8. Kim E, Shin HK, Kim CH. Characteristics of an isolated greater tuberosity fracture of the humerus. Journal of orthopaedic science: official journal of the Japanese Orthopaedic Association. 2005;10(5):441–4.
9. Longo UG, Franceschi F, Spiezia F, Marinozzi A, Maffulli N, Denaro V. The low-profile roman bridge technique for knotless double-row repair of the rotator cuff. Arch Orthop Trauma Surg. 2011;131(3):357–61.
10. Longo UG, Salvatore G, Rizzello G, Berton A, Ciuffreda M, Candela V, Denaro V. The burden of rotator cuff surgery in Italy: a nationwide registry study. Arch Orthop Trauma Surg. 2017;137(2):217–24.
11. Del Buono A, Oliva F, Longo UG, Rodeo SA, Orchard J, Denaro V, Maffulli N. Metalloproteases and rotator cuff disease. J Shoulder Elb Surg. 2012;21(2):200–8.
12. Longo UG, Berton A, Khan WS, Maffulli N, Denaro V. Histopathology of rotator cuff tears. Sports Med Arthrosc Rev. 2011;19(3):227–36.

3

Minimally invasive direct lateral interbody fusion in the treatment of the thoracic and lumbar spinal tuberculosisMini-DLIF for the thoracic and lumbar spinal tuberculosis

Fengping Gan, Jianzhong Jiang, Zhaolin Xie, Shengbin Huang, Ying Li, Guoping Chen and Haitao Tan[*]

Abstract

Background: To investigate the clinical efficacy of minimally invasive direct lateral approach debridement, interbody bone grafting, and interbody fusion in the treatment of the thoracic and lumbar spinal tuberculosis.

Methods: From January 2013 to January 2016, 35 cases with thoracic and lumbar spinal tuberculosis received direct lateral approach debridement, interbody bone grafting, and interbody fusion. Of the 35 cases, 16 patients were male and 19 were female and the median age was 55.2 (range 25–83). The affected segments were single interspace, and the involved vertebral bodies included: 15 cases of thoracic vertebrae (1 cases of $T_{5/6}$, 2 cases of $T_{6/7}$, 4 cases of $T_{7/8}$, 3 cases of $T_{8/9}$, 5 cases of $T_{9/10}$) and 20 cases of lumbar spine (2 cases of $L_{1/2}$, 6 cases of $L_{2/3}$, 6 cases of $L_{3/4}$, 6 cases of $L_{4/5}$). After MIDLIF operation, all the patients received medication of four anti-tubercular drugs for 12 to18 months.

Results: The patients were followed up for 7 to 40 months with an average of 18.5 months. The visual analogue scale (VAS) at the last follow-up was 2.8 ± 0.5, which was significantly different from the preoperative VAS (8.2 ± 0.7). After MIDLIF, there was 5 cases occurred with transient numbness in one side of the thigh or inguinal region, and 10 cases suffered from flexion hip weakness. All the bone grafts were fused within 6~ 18 months (average of 11. 5 months) after the operation.

Conclusion: Minimally invasive lateral approach interbody fusion technology have the advantage of less injury and quick recovery after surgery, which is the effective and safe treatment for thoracic and lumbar spinal tuberculosis.

Keywords: Thoracic and lumbar spinal tuberculosis, Direct lateral interbody fusion (DLIF), Minimally invasive surgery

Background

In recent years, with the change of living environment, the epidemic situation of tuberculosis (TB) is still grim. China ranks second next to India among 22 high-burden countries despite decades' effort on TB control [1]. The complications of Spinal tuberculosis including instability of the spine, spinal deformity and spinal cord compression, and even paralysis. Surgical therapy is recommended and required after the above complications occur [2]. However, traditional surgical treatment has the features of large trauma and slow postoperative recovery. Therefore, the development and application of various techniques in spinal surgery have provided new treatments for minimally invasive surgery for spinal tuberculosis. In our hospital from January 2013 to January 2016, there was 35 cases who treated with minimally invasive direct lateral approach tuberculosis debridement, bone grafting and internal fixation, and got a nice effect.

Methods

General information

A total of 35 cases (16 men and 19 women), whose age ranged from 25 to 83 years old (mean 55.2 years old), were investigated in this study. Clinical manifestations in the 35 patients included back pain, anorexia, fatigue,

* Correspondence: tanhaitao99@hotmail.com
Department of Orthopaedics, Guigang City People's Hospital, No. 99-1 Zhongshan Rd, Guigang 537100, People's Republic of China

low-grade fever and sweats. There were 10 cases with spinal cord injury, and according to the Frankel grading [3], 4 cases of C class, and 6 cases of D class. The course of disease ranged from 3 months to 5.2 years, with an average of 13 months. The conventional digital X - line (DR), computed tomography (CT) and magnetic resonance imaging (MRI) examinations were performed before the operation, and then combination of the results of erythrocyte sedimentation rate (ESR) to produce a diagnosis as spinal tuberculosis. All the cases were confirmed by pathology. The affected segments were single interspace between adjacent vertebrae, and the involved vertebral bodies included, 15 cases of thoracic vertebrae (1 cases of $T_{5/6}$, 2 cases of $T_{6/7}$, 4 cases of $T_{7/8}$, 3 cases of $T_{8/9}$, 5 cases of $T_{9/10}$) and 20 cases of lumbar spine (2 cases of $L_{1/2}$, 6 cases of $L_{2/3}$, 6 cases of $L_{3/4}$, 6 cases of $L_{4/5}$). Preoperative ESR was 46~110 mm/h, with an average of 71 mm/h. The preoperative mean progression of the Cobb angle was 25.2° (5°~48°) [4].

The inclusion criteria: ① patients with thoracic vertebrae tuberculosis from T5 to T11, and thoracolumbar tuberculosis from L1 to L5. ② patients who had necrotic bone, paravertebral abscess with segmental instability. ③ The lesions which were located in the anterior or middle regions of the spine.

Exclusion criteria: ①The lesions which were located in interspace between the L5 and S1 or above T5 thoracic, and thoracolumbar from T11 to L1. ② The lesions involvement of the posterior column (spinal accessory been affected), and projecting into spinal canal need posterior decompression. ③ open pulmonary tuberculosis. ④ multi-segmental or discontinuous spinal tuberculosis.

Therapeutic method
Preoperative preparation
All the patients were treated with preoperative anti tuberculosis agents for more than 2 weeks before operation, including isoniazide (300 mg/d), rifampicin (450 mg/d), ethambutol (750 mg/d), streptomycin (750 mg/d) or pyrazinamide (15~30 mg/kg/day). During treatment, all the patients should receive periodic review of ESR, liver and kidney function, and the patient with the improvement of general condition (including mental, appetite etc.) would undergo surgery and were given glutamine to strengthen parenteral nutrition. The patients with the poor situation were given blood transfusions, Human Albumin etc. to support treatment.

Main instrument of experiment
Direct lateral interbody fusion (DLIF; Medtronic Sofamor Danek, Inc. Memphis, TN, USA) and Extreme lateral interbody fusion (XLIF; NuVasive, Inc., San Diego, California) side path minimally invasive fusion system

are both used in side channel minimally invasive channel. Intraoperative neurological monitoring of patients was performed using the NIM-Eclipse (Medtronic, Medtronic Inc., Jacksonville, FL).

Operation method
After tracheal intubation general anesthesia, patients keeping 90 degree lateral position. The side that had bone destruction serious and more pus was chosen as surgical approach. DR marking surface location of vertebral disease, the lumbar bridge was aligned to the lesion segment of the vertebral body. Center on the waist bridge, the head and end of the operation table were both decreased about 40 degrees, and then properly fixed position. Preoperative C arm fluoroscopy determine and mark segmental lesions, and taking directly external incision of the abeam peritoneum in lumbar, about 5 cm, skin incision subcutaneous. In the C arm X-ray fluoroscopy guided, the blunt dissection of abdominal muscle layer (obliquus externus abdominis and obliquus internus abdominis) through the incision, the guide needle from the retroperitoneal space passed through the psoas muscle into the symptomatic vertebrae. The thoracic spine using the anterior lateral approach of the thoracic cavity, and taking a lateral oblique incision (about 6-8 cm) in midaxillary line which located on the upper interspace of the lesions interspace. Skin and subcutaneous incision, intercostal muscles and parietal pleura incision. Into the chest, separating the pleura. After lung protection with wet gauze, pushing forward the small S hook to show the lesion of intervertebral space. The guide wire was placed into vertebra clearance, and the C arm X-ray machine side perspective was used to determine the position of the positioning needle to ensure it was located in the middle position. Along the guide pin are inserted into the expansion sleeve and tubular separating hook, connecting to free arm and fixed. Proper opening of the lesion to reveal the intervertebral space, removal of paravertebral abscess and caseous material. Spatula, rongeur and chisel were used to remove lesions of intervertebral disc and necrosis of bone until health bone appearance. Rely on the spinous process of top pressure and intervertebral spreader correction of kyphosis, measuring bone groove length, implantation the same length autologous iliac bone grafting (18 cases), or select the appropriate length and diameter of titanium mesh (17 cases), in which 12 cases with the autogenous iliac bone implanted in titanium mesh bone graft and 5 cases with allogeneic freeze-dried bone cut into strips pieces implanted in titanium mesh bone graft, compaction and imbedding bone groove.

Internal fixation: 20 cases who showed no obvious osteoporosis and the stability of the spine is relatively small were treated with lateral anterior vertebral plate fixation, and 10 cases who showed serious damage of vertebral and intervertebral with posterior pedicle screw fixation,5 cases who did not showed serious damage but with obvious osteoporosis with lateral nail bar fixation. After irrigating the incision, streptomycin (1 g) and isoniazid (0.5 g) were placed in the gap. Thoracic vertebra and lumbar incision placement of closed thoracic drainage tube and drainage tube, respectively, and closed the incision. Intraoperative EMG monitoring was performed in all the 30 cases to avoid spinal cord and lumbosacral plexus injury.

Postoperative treatment

Postoperative routine treatment with antibiotics for 48 h, and thoracic cavity closed drainage tube was removed at 24~ 48 h after operation. During the postoperative 3–4 days, the patients were standing, walking and walking under the protection of a brace, and wearing a brace for 3 months. Continued anti-tuberculosis treatment for 12~ 18 months, regular review of liver, kidney function and ESR. The X-ray and CT examinations were performed at postoperative 1, 3, 6, 12 months and the last follow-up to evaluate bone fusion. The detailed surgical results of the 35 patients were presented in Table 1.

Declarations

This study obtained the written permission from all the participant.

Results

The operation time ranged from 79 to 129 min, with an average of 94 min, and the perioperative blood loss was 200~ 600 ml, with an average of 320 ml. All cases were followed up for an average of 18.5 months (range from 7 to 40 months). After operation, the symptoms of back pain improved obviously, and the VAS score (2.3 ± 1.4) at the last follow-up was significantly lower than the preoperative score (8.2 ± 1.1). All wounds healed by first intention without any incision related complications, and no pulmonary infection, respiratory failure and other complications occurred. There was 5 cases occurred with transient numbness in one side of the thigh or inguinal region. Of the 5 cases, there was 4 cases, whose symptoms disappeared after 1~ 12 months of Neurotrophic therapy, and there was 1 cases, whose the symptoms of numbness were relieved after 12 months treatment, but did not disappear completely. There was 10 cases that suffered from flexion hip weakness and were recovered at 1~ 3 months without treatment. All patients had a good internal fixation at the last follow-up without complications such as loosening and breakage. The bone grafts were fused for 6~ 18 months, with an average of 11.5 months.

As shown in Fig. 1, a 63 years old the female patient with thoracic spinal tuberculosis at $T_{7/8}$ received digital X - line (DR), computed tomography (CT) and magnetic resonance imaging (MRI) examinations before the operation. Preoperative CT scan image showed bone defect at $T_{7/8}$ with disc space narrowing and preoperative MRI image showed $T_{7/8}$ vertebral tuberculosis with paraspinal abscess. The patient underwent minimally invasive direct lateral approach debridement, interbody bone grafting, and interbody fusion surgery (the autogenous iliac bone implanted in titanium mesh bone graft.), and Fig. 2 showed the working channel established in the operation and postoperative X-ray after withdrawal the working channel. The operation time was 86 min, and the perioperative blood loss was 550 ml (intraoperative blood loss 300 ml and postoperative blood loss 250 ml). After operation, the symptoms of back pain improved obviously, and the 1 week postoperative score (4.5) and 1 month postoperative score (1.8) were both significantly lower than the preoperative VAS score (8.9). Postoperatively 18 months and 24 months, the patient received DR and CT again, respectively, and the results indicated the good bone fusion and good position of internal fixation (Fig. 3).

Discussion

Spinal tuberculosis (TB) is the most common form of extra-pulmonary tuberculosis, accounting for approximately 1 to 3% of all tuberculosis cases [5], and has a great impact on the quality of life, which can lead to paralysis. Spinal tuberculosis is local infection in systemic tuberculosis, the effective drug treatment is to kill *Mycobacterium tuberculosis*. Mild spinal TB respond well to the standard antituberculosis therapy, and early mild spinal tuberculosis with nutrition support and reasonable anti tuberculosis drugs and other conservative treatment can be cured [6].

The surgical treatment of spinal tuberculosis requires complete debridement, interbody fusion and internal fixation, and it can shorten the course of disease and reduce the fatality rate. But the traditional anterior spine fusion for the treatment of spine TB have large trauma, which will affect the treatment and rehabilitation of spinal tuberculosis [7–9]. Interventional therapy is a minimally invasive treatment method between conservative treatment and surgical treatment. Guided by CT and B-ultrasound, percutaneous micro-invasive treatment of local abscess and catheter drainage has the advantages of convenient operation, safe and effective, and less trauma, and is an effective and safe operation treatment for spinal tuberculosis abscess, especially be suitable for the general condition of patients [10]. But the postoperative problems were serious, such as the long indwelling drainage tube brings inconvenience to the life, the

Table 1 The surgical results of 35 patients

No.	Gender	Age range	Segment lesion	Operation method	Follow-up time(month)	Pre-operation VAS score	Post-operation VAS score
1	male	26–30	L1/2	lateral anterior vertebral plate fixation	7	7	0
2	female	26–30	T7/8	posterior pedicle fixation	12	9	1
3	female	41–45	L2/3	lateral anterior vertebral plate fixation	18	8	1
4	female	61–65	T8/9	lateral anterior vertebral plate fixation	18	8	2
5	male	51–55	L4/5	lateral anterior vertebral plate fixation	24	9	1
6	male	46–50	T9/10	lateral nail bar fixation	21	8	0
7	female	76–80	T5/6	posterior pedicle fixation	15	8	2
8	female	66–70	L3/4	lateral anterior vertebral plate fixation	18	9	1
9	male	61–65	L4/5	lateral anterior vertebral plate fixation	22	7	0
10	male	56–60	T7/8	posterior pedicle fixation	20	6	2
11	female	46–50	L4/5	posterior pedicle fixation	36	8	1
12	male	31–35	T9/10	lateral anterior vertebral plate fixation	32	9	2
13	female	41–45	L1/2	lateral nail bar fixation	30	7	1
14	male	36–40	T7/8	lateral anterior vertebral plate fixation	24	7	1
15	male	76–80	L3/4	lateral nail bar fixation	22	8	3
16	female	81–85	T8/9	lateral anterior vertebral plate fixation	28	6	2
17	female	71–75	L3/4	lateral anterior vertebral plate fixation	24	7	0
18	female	61–65	T6/7	lateral anterior vertebral plate fixation	12	8	1
19	male	51–55	L4/5	lateral anterior vertebral plate fixation	18	7	0
20	female	56–60	T9/10	lateral nail bar fixation	18	9	1
21	male	46–50	L2/3	posterior pedicle fixation	24	7	1
22	male	31–35	L4/5	lateral anterior vertebral plate fixation	28	7	0
23	female	76–80	T6/7	lateral anterior vertebral plate fixation	36	8	2
24	female	71–75	L2/3	lateral anterior vertebral plate fixation	36	6	1
25	male	66–70	L3/4	posterior pedicle fixation	24	8	0
26	male	36–40	T8/9	lateral nail bar fixation	12	7	1
27	female	46–50	L4/5	lateral anterior vertebral plate fixation	28	8	1
28	female	56–60	L2/3	lateral anterior vertebral plate fixation	18	7	2
29	female	76–80	T7/8	posterior pedicle fixation	18	7	2
30	male	61–65	L3/4	posterior pedicle fixation	20	7	1
31	female	66–70	T9/10	lateral anterior vertebral plate fixation	24	6	1
32	female	66–70	L2/3	lateral anterior vertebral plate	24	9	3

Table 1 The surgical results of 35 patients *(Continued)*

No.	Gender	Age range	Segment lesion	Operation method	Follow-up time(month)	Pre-operation VAS score	Post-operation VAS score
				fixation			
33	male	56–60	L3/4	posterior pedicle fixation	12	9	2
34	female	51–55	L2/3	posterior pedicle fixation	30	8	1
35	male	51–55	T9/10	lateral anterior vertebral plate fixation	12	7	2

*visual analogue scale: VAS

repeated blockage and the falling off of drainage tube, the retrograde infection and the long treatment cycle. In addition, the indications for interventional therapy are narrow and only applicable to the more abscess and which located in middle column of anterior spinal column. It is not suitable for the patients with instability, kyphosis, spinal cord compression, and the abscess locating in the spinal canal. Since the first thoracoscopic anterior spinal surgery performed by Mack in the early 1990s, thoracoscopic assisted anterior spinal surgery has developed rapidly. It has been developed from simple anterior discectomy and debridement to anterior spinal instrumentation and reconstruction, and has applications in a wide range of fields. A large number of literatures have confirmed its minimal invasion, safety and efficacy [11–13]. However, due to the higher requirements of surgical techniques, the need for more departments, longer learning curve, expensive equipment and other factors, there are also limitations of clinical application.

Direct lateral approach interbody fusion (DLIF) is a new technology in recent years. It used a minimally invasive approach single channel side could complete interbody fusion of single/multi segmental lumbar, restore intervertebral height, expand the nerve root canal, which achieved indirect decompression, alleviate root irritation symptoms, at the same time correction of scoliosis, vertebral tilt, slip deformity, rearrange and stabilize the spine. It was reported that DLIF was mainly applied in spinal degenerative diseases [14, 15]. Our hospital used DLIF in spinal degenerative disease which obtained good effect, and then it was applied in spinal tuberculosis. We have summarized some advantages of the minimally invasive direct lateral approach debridement, interbody bone grafting, and interbody fusion as following:① direct lateral small incision was about 5 ~ 6 cm, and only blunt separation of muscle fiber gap can reach directly to the affected vertebrae, which greatly reduced the incidence of other complications caused by surgical trauma. Since the direct access to the vertebral space which does not require destruction of any bony structure, the stability of the spine was better protected, and there was no risk of injury to important structures such as the large vessels and spinal cord without anterior or posterior approach. ②It can in the limited range of incision exposure reached complete debridement and bone graft and anterior lateral plate or vertebral pedicle screw fixation.

Our experience included:① strictly grasp the indications, mainly for $T_4 \sim T_{11}$ segment tuberculosis and $L_2 \sim L_5$ segment tuberculosis, the lesions confined to the anterior and middle column and did not involve in the spinal canal and posterior column, and not need a posterior spinal canal decompression; ②accurate

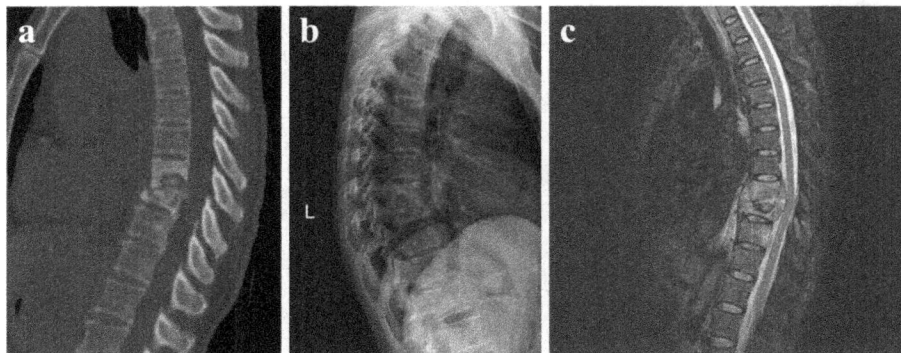

Fig. 1 A patient with thoracic spinal tuberculosis at T7/8 received digital radiography (DR), computed tomography (CT) and magnetic resonance imaging (MRI) examinations before the operation. **a** Preoperative CT scan image showed bone defect at T7/8 with disc space narrowing. **b** Preoperative DR image. **c** Preoperative MRI image showed T7/8 vertebral tuberculosis with paraspinal abscess

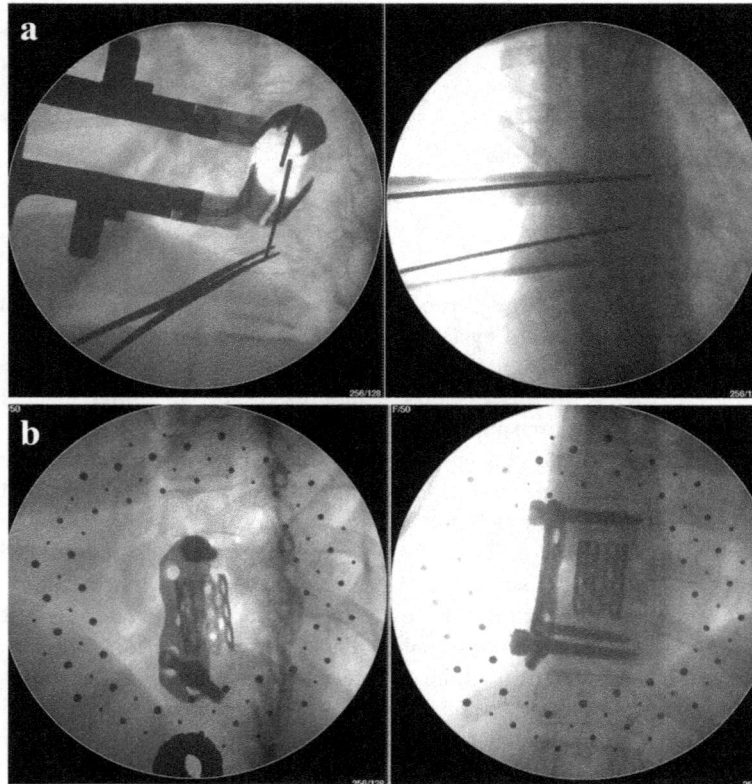

Fig. 2 X-ray fluoroscopy of working channel in the operation. **a** The working channel established in the operation. **b** Postoperative X-ray after withdrawal the working channel

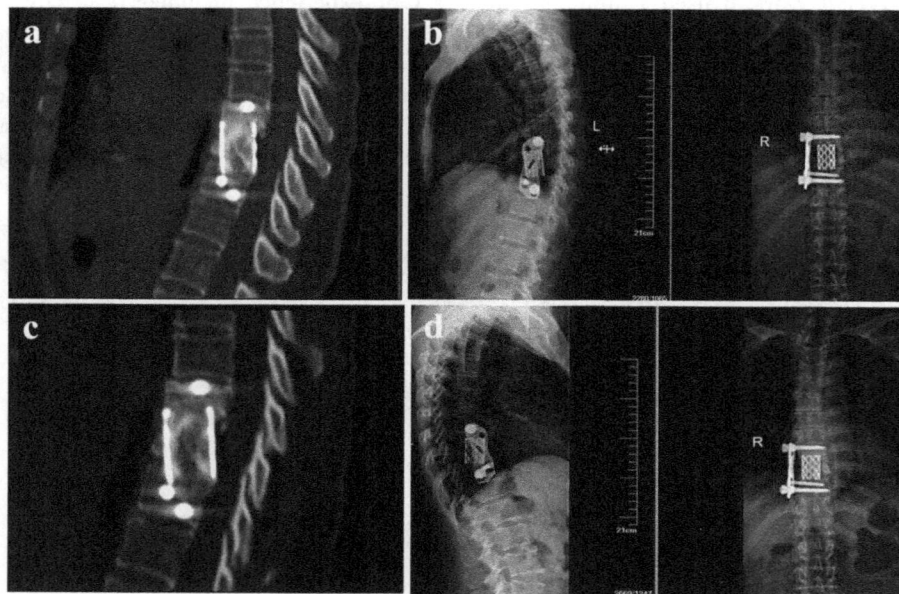

Fig. 3 Postoperative DR and CT images showed good position of internal fixation and good bone fusion, respectively. **a** CT images of postoperative 18 months. **b** DR images of postoperative 18 months. **c** CT images of postoperative 24 months. **d** DR images of postoperative 24 months

positioning of the preoperative and intraoperative opening baffle, it was arranged in the lateral 1/3 of the vertebral body to avoid injuring the lumbosacral plexus; ③ the most frequently reported complications of lumbar lateral extreme lateral interbody fusion (XLIF) was transient numbness in one side of the thigh or inguinal region and flexion hip weakness the with incidence rate of 1 ~ 60.1% [16]. In our study, there was 5 cases occurred with transient numbness in one side of the thigh or inguinal region, and the incidence rate was 14.3%. There was 10 cases suffered from flexion hip weakness, and the incidence was 28.6%. The main preventive measures are intraoperative electromyography (EMG) monitoring to avoid the injury of lumbosacral plexus during establishing passage. Most of the scholars emphasized that the application of EMG monitoring is very important to establish a safe approach [17]. EMG real-time monitoring can detect the distance between the expansion tube and nerve. The primary expansion tube inserted or opened every time was monitored by EMG, when the distance was 1 cm and nerve would send an alarm signal, the more closer and the more dense alarm. The signals by EMG guided the doctor to take measures to avoid the nerve, which greatly reduced the risk of lumbar plexus injury. Uribe et al. [18] reported that the application of electromyography can reduce nerve injury rate (less than 1%). There was 5 cases without intraoperative EMG monitoring, in which there was 2 cases occurred with transient numbness in one side of the thigh or inguinal region. The other 30 cases underwent real-time EMG monitoring in the working channel installation process. Once occurred abnormal evoked potential, the puncture direction immediately was changed, greatly reducing the risk of lumbosacral plexus injury in operation. However, there was one patient occurred with mild numbness in front of the thigh, the reason was EMG can only monitor the movement and cannot monitor the feeling, therefore it could not completely avoid nerve damage [19]. In addition, intraoperative EMG monitoring of XLIF may lead to false negatives, which required the doctor to pay a special attention to monitoring techniques during intraoperative EMG monitoring. Houten et al. [20] reported that there was 2 cases of lateral lumbar interbody fusion occurred postoperative motor deficits, but intraoperative electrophysiological monitoring showed no abnormalities. Our previous study have showed that, from August 2013 to October 2014, there was 46 cases with lumbar degenerative disease received XLIF in our hospital using real-time EMG monitoring, and there is nerve damage critical state or injury in 17 cases, including 3 cases of monitoring negative (false negative). Therefore, the surgeons are required to be familiar with the anatomical structures in the approach, observe the tissue similar to the nerve in the field carefully under the direct vision, operate carefully, and minimize the excessive traction of the psoas muscles and the compression of the surrounding soft tissue. The work channel was installed not too far back, as much as possible at the 1/3 junction of the vertebral body. Moreover, Rodgers et al. [21] reported that intravenous administration of 10 mg dexamethasone preoperatively could prevent the occurrence of nerve injury and significantly reduce the incidence of transient motor nerve injury.

Conclusion
Direct lateral channel assisted approach can be used to perform resection and bone grafting and internal fixation, and it can be an effective and safe method for thoracolumbar tuberculotic spondylitis with the advantages of rapid recovery and less trauma.

Acknowledgements
This study was funded by the Guangxi Science and Technology Project (AD17129017).

Authors' contributions
HT put forward the concept of the study and designed the study. FG prepared the experiments, contributed to the statistical analysis and edited the manuscript. JJ and ZX contributed to the data acquisition. SH and YL contributed to the quality control of data and algorithms. GC analyzed the data and interpretation. All authors read and approved the final manuscript.

Competing interest
The authors declared that they have no competing interest.

References
1. Liu HC, Deng JP, Dong HY, Xiao TQ, Zhao XQ, Zhang ZD, Jiang Y, Liu ZG, Li Q, Wan KL. Molecular typing characteristic and drug susceptibility analysis of Mycobacterium tuberculosis isolates from Zigong, China. Biomed Res Int. 2016;2016(4):1–7.
2. Tang MX, Zhang HQ, Wang YX, Guo CF, Liu JY. Treatment of spinal tuberculosis by debridement, interbody fusion and internal fixation via posterior approach only. Orthop Surg. 2016;8(1):89.
3. DeVivo MJ, Krause JS, Lammertse DP. Recent trends in mortality and causes of death among persons with spinal cord injury. Arch Phys Med Rehabil. 1999;80(11):1411–9.
4. Reinhold M, Knop C, Beisse R, Audige L, Kandziora F, Pizanis A, Pranzl R, Gercek E, Schultheiss M, Weckbach A, et al. Operative treatment of 733 patients with acute thoracolumbar spinal injuries: comprehensive results from the second, prospective, internet-based multicenter study of the spine study Group of the German Association of trauma surgery. Eur Spine J. 2010;19(10):1657–76.
5. Jain AK. Tuberculosis of the spine: a fresh look at an old disease. J Bone Joint Surg Br Vol. 2010;92(7):905.
6. Zhang Z, Fei L, Qiang Z, Fei D, Dong S, Xu J: The outcomes of chemotherapy only treatment on mild spinal tuberculosis. J Orthop Surg Res 2016, 11(1):1–8.
7. Faciszewski T, Winter RB, Lonstein JE, Denis F, Johnson L. The surgical and medical perioperative complications of anterior spinal fusion surgery in the thoracic and lumbar spine in adults. A review of 1223 procedures. Spine. 1995;20(14):1592–9.
8. Klöckner C, Valencia R. Sagittal alignment after anterior debridement and fusion with or without additional posterior instrumentation in the treatment of pyogenic and tuberculous spondylodiscitis. Spine. 2003;28(10):1036.
9. Moon MS, Woo YK, Lee KS, Ha KY, Kim SS, Sun DH. Posterior instrumentation and anterior interbody fusion for tuberculous kyphosis of dorsal and lumbar spines. Spine. 1996;21(15):1840–1.

10. Xi-feng Zhang MD, Yan WM, Shong-hua Xiao MD, Zheng-sheng Liu MD, Yong-gang Zhang MD, Bao-wei Liu MD, Zhi-min Xia MD. Treatment of lumbar and lumbosacral spinal tuberculosis with minimally invasive surgery. Orthop Surg. 2010;2(1):64–70.

11. Huang TJ, Hsu RW, Chen SH, Liu HP. Video-assisted thoracoscopic surgery in managing tuberculous spondylitis. Clin Orthop Relat Res. 2000;379(379):143–53.

12. Kapoor SK, Agarwal PN, Jr JB, Kumar R. Video-assisted thoracoscopic decompression of tubercular spondylitis: clinical evaluation. Spine. 2005; 30(20):E605.

13. Singh R. Video-Assisted Thoracic Surgery for Tubercular Spondylitis[M]// Tuberculosis of the Central Nervous System. Springer International Publishing. 2017:963497.

14. Barbagallo GMV, Albanese V, Raich AL, Dettori JR, Sherry N, Balsano M. Lumbar lateral interbody fusion (LLIF): comparative effectiveness and safety versus PLIF/TLIF and predictive factors affecting LLIF outcome. Evid Based Spine Care J. 2014;05(01):028–37.

15. Phillips FM, Isaacs RE, Rodgers WB, Khajavi K, Tohmeh AG, Deviren V, Peterson MD, Hyde J, Kurd M. Adult degenerative scoliosis treated with XLIF: clinical and radiographical results of a prospective multicenter study with 24-month follow-up. Spine. 2013;38(21):1853.

16. Anand N, Rosemann R, Khalsa B, Baron EM. Mid-term to long-term clinical and functional outcomes of minimally invasive correction and fusion for adults with scoliosis. Neurosurg Focus. 2010;28(3):E6.

17. Tohmeh AG, Rodgers WB, Peterson MD. Dynamically evoked, discrete-threshold electromyography in the extreme lateral interbody fusion approach. J Neurosurg Spine. 2011;14(1):31–7.

18. Uribe JS, Vale FL, Dakwar E. Electromyographic monitoring and its anatomical implications in minimally invasive spine surgery. Spine. 2010; 35(26 Suppl):S368.

19. Knight RQ, Schwaegler P, Hanscom D, Roh J. Direct lateral lumbar interbody fusion for degenerative conditions: early complication profile. J Spinal Disord Tech. 2009;22(1):34–7.

20. Houten JK, Alexandre LC, Nasser R, Wollowick AL. Nerve injury during the transpsoas approach for lumbar fusion. J Neurosurg Spine. 2011;15(3):280.

21. Rodgers WB, Gerber EJ, Patterson J. Intraoperative and early postoperative complications in extreme lateral interbody fusion: an analysis of 600 cases. Spine. 2011;36(1):26.

4

Annular closure device for disc herniation: meta-analysis of clinical outcome and complications

Wen Jie Choy[1,2] (iD), Kevin Phan[1,2,3], Ashish D. Diwan[4], Chon Sum Ong[5] and Ralph J. Mobbs[1,2,3]*

Abstract

Background: Lumbar intervertebral disc herniation is a common cause of lower back and leg pain, with surgical intervention (e.g. discectomy to remove the herniated disc) recommended after an appropriate period of conservative management, however the existing or increased breach of the annulus fibrosus persists with the potential of reherniation. Several prosthesis and techniques to reduce re-herniation have been proposed including implantation of an annular closure device (ACD) – Barricaid™ and an annular tissue repair system (AR) – Anulex-Xclose™. The aim of this meta-analysis is to assist surgeons determine a potential approach to reduce incidences of recurrent lumbar disc herniation and assess the current devices regarding their outcomes and complications.

Methods: Four electronic full-text databases were systematically searched through September 2017. Data including outcomes of annular closure device/annular repair were extracted. All results were pooled utilising meta-analysis with weighted mean difference and odds ratio as summary statistics.

Results: Four studies met inclusion criteria. Three studies reported the use of Barricaid (ACD) while one study reported the use of Anulex (AR). A total of 24 symptomatic reherniation were reported among 811 discectomies with ACD/AR as compared to 51 out of 645 in the control group (OR: 0.34; 95% CI: 0.20,0.56; $I^2 = 0\%$; $P < 0.0001$). Durotomies were lower among the ACD/AR patients with only 3 reported cases compared to 7 in the control group (OR: 0.54; 95% CI: 0.13, 2.23; $I^2 = 11\%$; $P = 0.39$). Similar outcomes for post-operative Oswestry Disability Index and visual analogue scale were obtained when both groups were compared.

Conclusion: Early results showed the use of Barricaid and Anulex devices are beneficial for short term outcomes demonstrating reduction in symptomatic disc reherniation with low post-operative complication rates. Long-term studies are required to further investigate the efficacy of such devices.

Keywords: Annular closure device, Annular repair, Recurrent disc herniation, Microdiscectomy, Barricaid, Anulex, Xclose, Lumbar intervertebral disc, Disc herniation, Meta-analysis

Background

Situated between vertebral bodies of the spine, the intervertebral discs (IVDs) or discs are important in maintaining a deformable space between each vertebra, assisting in flexibility and playing a role in shock absorption simultaneously [1]. Three structures make up the IVD: centrally the nucleus pulposus (NP) is surrounded by a ring of annulus fibrosus (AF) and sandwiched between two cartilaginous endplates (CEP) superiorly and inferiorly [1, 2]. A common cause of lower back and leg pain, is lumbar disc herniation (LDH) [3]. When simple measures fail to resolve patient symptoms a discectomy using various surgical approaches (e.g. open discectomy, endoscopic and microdiscectomy) are used to remove the herniated IVD and decompress the symptomatic nerve [4, 5].

In randomised controlled studies, patients with LDH who undergo discectomy have been shown to have significantly better outcomes compared to those managed

* Correspondence: r.mobbs@unsw.edu.au
[1]Faculty of Medicine, University of New South Wales (UNSW), Sydney, Australia
[2]NeuroSpine Surgery Research Group (NSURG), Prince of Wales Private Hospital, Sydney, Australia
Full list of author information is available at the end of the article

conservatively [6–8]. However, 48% of LDH patients in a large spinal registry, responding to an outcome question at 1 year after surgery expressed unhappiness with the level of pain [9]. Further, 7-year survivorship analysis of large administrative databases indicates that 18% of patients undergo either a revision discectomy or spinal reconstruction following a discectomy [10]. Most likely, nerve root decompression and removal of the symptomatic disc sequestration with microdiscectomy may further weaken the AF, and exacerbate progressive dehydration of the NP which may lead to further loss of disc height. The weakened AF may also result in potential reherniation in about 0.5–25% of cases [11–14] and the loss of disc height may cause further nerve compression and radiculopathy, either in the short or long term post-surgery [15]. Such consequences can result in worsening pain which may subject the patient to seek additional surgeries, for instance fusion (i.e.: ALIF, PLIF, etc.) or artificial disc replacement, with fibrosis and inevitable consequences of the previous surgeries [15–21]. Currently, there are no definite guidelines or studies that recommend a certain approach or preventative measure towards recurrent LDH (RDH).

Symptomatic RDH is associated with higher hospital and surgical costs, repeated recovery and rehabilitation expenses, delayed return to work, and poorer outcomes as compared with the primary intervention. Expenses incurred include diagnostic and imaging testing, healthcare visits, epidural steroid injections, and revision surgeries with an estimated cost of $39,836 to $49,431 per patient [18, 22]. In addition to healthcare costs, RDH is associated with recurrent back and leg pain, affected function, loss of work days and quality of life, and increased narcotic usage and dependency [18, 23].

Various measures have been trialled to prevent RDH including aggressive removal of the NP, packing the IVD space with cellulose and other materials post-tissue-removal, sequestrectomy and fusion, but were associated with variable outcomes [24–27]. Recently, several prosthesis and techniques have been proposed to prevent the incidence of RDH which include implantation of an annular closure device (ACD) – Barricaid™ (Intrinsic Therapeutics, Inc., Woburn, MA, USA), and the use of an annular tissue repair system (AR) – Anulex-Xclose (Anulex Technologies, Minnetonka, MN) [28–31]. The Barricaid device comprises of a titanium anchor portion which is implanted into the adjacent vertebral body and a polymer mesh potion that is inserted into the affected disc, blocking the defect opening with the expectation of reducing the chance of reherniation from the same defect [30–32]; whereas the Anulex device comprises of tension band(s) each with 2 tissue anchors placed on either side of the annular defect / annular incision on the IVD to repair the defect

opening in a single band or multiple band pattern which in theory repairs the defect [28]. In order to evaluate the clinical outcomes of each intervention, we conducted a meta-analysis based on the available studies to assist surgeons in evaluating the available literature, and therefore a potential approach to reduce the incidences of RDH.

Methods
Literature search strategy
Literature search was carried out based on PRISMA guidelines [33] and recommendations [34]. Electronic databases used include Ovid Medline, Embase, Web of Science and PubMed. To achieve the highest possible sensitivity, the search terms used were a combination of "annular device", "annular repair", "annulus device", "disc herniation" and "recurrent disc herniation". The search was performed on 13th September 2017. Further review of the reference list of all related articles was performed to identify potential studies. All relevant articles were assessed systematically utilising the inclusion and exclusion criteria.

Selection criteria
Eligible articles for this systematic review and meta-analysis include: (1) articles discussing ACD or alternative methods to reduce rate of re-herniation, (2) articles that provide a comparison study between a population that underwent the additional procedure compared to a control group and (3) articles that provide data regarding re-herniation rates. When articles that reported the same study population were identified, those which provide the most complete data set were used. Abstracts, case reports/series and conference presentations were excluded. There were no review articles that matched our study criteria.

Data extraction and critical appraisal
All data (text, figures and tables) were extracted from available full text reports utilising a standard proforma. Data extracted from the articles include: (1) study characteristics which covers study period, institution and country of study, average length of follow up, study size and vertebra level involved; (2) patients' baseline traits covering age, weight or BMI and gender; (3) mean pre- and post-operation Oswestry Disability Index (ODI); (4) mean pre- and post-operation visual analogue scale (VAS) for back and legs; (5) outcome of surgery focusing on symptomatic disc re-herniation; and (6) post-operation complications including durotomy, wound complication and epidural hematoma. Estimated data from graphs were used for studies which did not report the exact mean and standard deviation for post-operative ODI or VAS. The articles were appraised according to

the Dutch Cochrane Centre critical review checklist proposed by MOOSE [35].

Statistical analysis

The weighted mean difference (WMD) and odds ratio (OR) were used as summary statistics. Both fixed- and random-effect models were tested. In the fixed-effects model, it was assumed that treatment effect in each study was the same, whereas in a random-effects model, it was assumed that there were variations between studies. χ^2 tests were used to study heterogeneity between trials. I^2 statistic was used to estimate the percentage of total variation across studies, owing to heterogeneity rather than chance, with values greater than 50% considered as substantial heterogeneity. I^2 can be calculated as: $I^2 = 100\% \times (Q - df)/Q$, with Q defined as Cochrane's heterogeneity statistics and df defined as degree of freedom. In the present meta-analysis, the results using the random-effects model were presented to take into account the possible clinical diversity and methodological variation between studies. Specific analyses considering confounding factors were not possible because raw data

were not available. All P values were 2-sided. All statistical analysis was conducted with Review Manager Version 5.3.2 (Cochrane Collaboration, Software Update, Oxford, United Kingdom).

Pooled analyses were portrayed via forest plots for rates of symptomatic re-herniations, durotomies and wound complications; while meta-regression was used for ODI and VAS back and leg pain.

Results

A total of 405 references were identified. Four studies [28, 30, 36, 37] met the inclusion criteria and were selected for analysis (Fig. 1). A summary of the study characteristics is shown in Table 1. The included studies were assessed for their quality and a summary is provided in Table 2. Eight hundred eleven patients underwent discectomy with an ACD or Annular Repair (ACD/AR) in these 4 studies compared to 645 patients who underwent discectomy only. All 4 studies were prospective studies with 2 of these being randomised controlled trials [28, 36]; whilst the other 2 being non-randomised comparative cohort studies [30, 37].

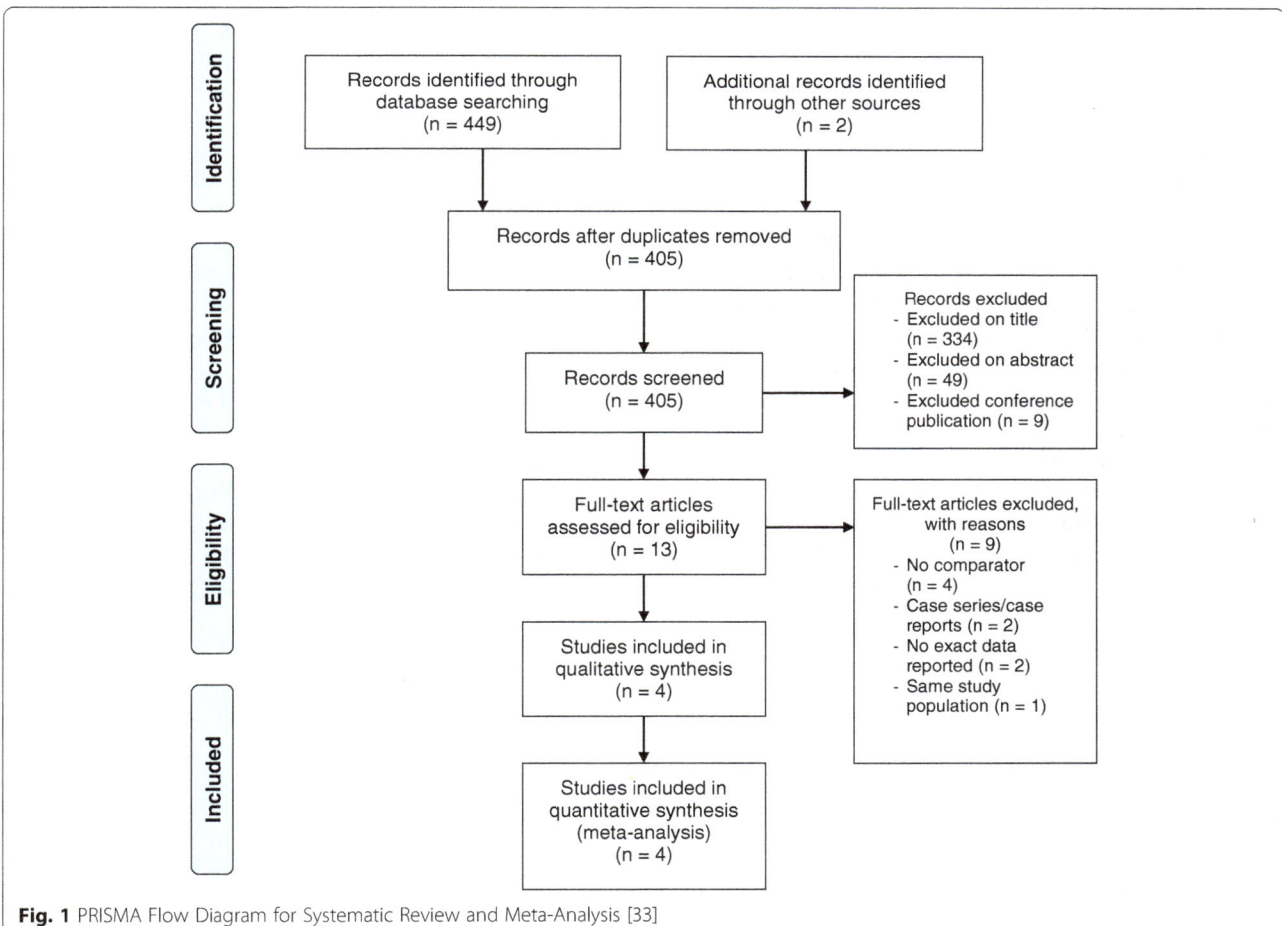

Fig. 1 PRISMA Flow Diagram for Systematic Review and Meta-Analysis [33]

Table 1 Summary of study characteristics

Reference:	Institution	Country	Study type	Lumbar Discectomy		Average Follow up
				With ACD/AR	Without ACD/AR	
Bailey et al. [28]	34 Medical Centres	United States	P, R	478	249	24 months
Klassen et al. [36]	21 Medical Centres	Europe	P, R	272	278	90 days
Parker et al. [30]	2 Universities Medical Institution	United States	P, NR	31	46	24 months
Vukas et al. [37]	Dubrava University Hospital and Rijeka University Hospital Centre	Croatia	P, NR	30	72	24 months

P prospective, *R* randomised, *NR* non-randomised

Patient characteristics

Overall, the age range of the patients were between 18 and 70 years. The reported mean age among patients who received an ACD/AR was 41.76 (range 39.92–43.60) years in 3 reported studies compared to 42.52 (range 40.72–44.31) years in the control group [28, 30, 36]. Baseline characteristics such as gender, weight, height, smoking status, diabetes or other co-morbidities were not adequately reported with only 3 studies reporting patients' gender [28, 36, 37] and 2 reporting their BMI [28, 36].

Clinical outcomes

Out of the total 811 lumbar discectomies with ACD/AR, there were 24 reported symptomatic disc reherniation as compared to 51 out of 645 incidences of symptomatic reherniation among the control group (OR: 0.34; 95% CI: 0.20,0.56; $I^2 = 0\%$; $P < 0.0001$) (Fig. 2a). Incidence of durotomy was 3 out of 811 in the ACD/AR cohort compared to 7 out of 645 in the control group (OR:0.54; 95% CI: 0.13, 2.23; $I^2 = 11\%$; $P = 0.39$) (Fig. 2b). Two studies reported 4 incidences of wound complication in 750 of the ACD/AR group compared to 7 out of 527 in the control group whereas no patients had an epidural hematoma in the ACD/AR group compared to 3 out of 527 having an incidence of post-operative hematoma [28, 36] (Fig. 2c and d).

Meta-regressions comparing improvements in ODI and VAS pain scores (both back and legs) for ACD/AR cohort showed similar outcomes when the ACD/AR cohort was compared to the control cohort. The results were statistically insignificant without any group being superior to the other [28, 30, 37] (Fig. 3).

Discussion

Our results demonstrated that the use of an ACD/AR was associated with a significant reduction in symptomatic disc re-herniation [28, 30, 36, 37] compared to patients without ACD/AR, without increased risk of durotomy, wound complication or epidural hematoma [28, 36]. There was no difference in the clinical outcome scores in follow-up ODI and VAS score for both back and leg at 90 days and 2 years when the ACD/AR group is compared to the control group [28, 30, 37].

The present study is constrained by several limitations. Firstly, there is only limited data available in the literature for this new technology, with only 4 studies included for analysis. Further studies with larger sample sizes and prospective follow-up are required to confirm the presented results. The lack of available studies also resulted in shorter outcomes (90 day results) being included in our pool analysis. The lack of blinding in the studies can result in unaccounted bias. There was considerable heterogeneity in terms of ACD technology used as well as baseline characteristics, which has been shown to be an influencing factor in disc herniations. For example, A meta-analysis carried out by Huang et al. has shown statistical correlation between patients who smoke; or have disc protrusion(s); or diabetes to have an increased risk of RDH [38]. Hence future studies investigating ACD/AR among these patient population should also be carried out to evaluate the efficacy of such devices among these patients. Future randomised

Table 2 Quality Assessment of the Included Studies

	Bailey et al.	Klassen et al.	Parker et al.	Vukas et al.
Clear definition of study population	Yes	Yes	Yes	Yes
Clear description of outcomes and outcome assessments	Yes	Yes	Yes	Yes
Independent assessment of outcome parameters	No[a]	No[a]	No[a]	No[a]
Sufficient follow-up duration	Yes	No[b]	Yes	Yes
No selective loss of follow-up	No[c]	No[c]	Yes	Yes
Identification of confounders and prognostic factors	Yes	Yes	No[d]	No[d]

[a], lack of blinding; [b], 90 days [c], patients fail to attend follow-up; [d], limitations poorly reported

A: Symptomatic disc reherniation

Study or Subgroup	ACD Events	ACD Total	no ACD Events	no ACD Total	Weight	Odds Ratio M-H, Random, 95% CI
Bailey 2013	18	478	24	249	64.6%	0.37 [0.20, 0.69]
Klassen 2017	6	272	19	278	29.6%	0.31 [0.12, 0.78]
Parker 2016	0	31	3	46	2.9%	0.20 [0.01, 3.96]
Vukas 2013	0	30	5	72	3.0%	0.20 [0.01, 3.75]
Total (95% CI)		811		645	100.0%	0.34 [0.20, 0.56]
Total events	24		51			

Heterogeneity: Tau² = 0.00; Chi² = 0.36, df = 3 (P = 0.95); I² = 0%
Test for overall effect: Z = 4.21 (P < 0.0001)

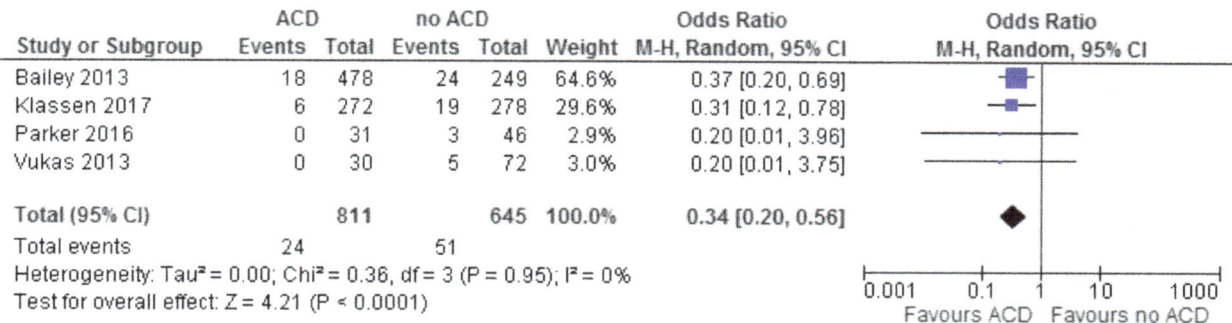

Odds Ratio M-H, Random, 95% CI — Favours ACD   Favours no ACD

B: Durotomy

Study or Subgroup	ACD Events	ACD Total	no ACD Events	no ACD Total	Weight	Odds Ratio M-H, Random, 95% CI
Bailey 2013	1	478	4	249	35.5%	0.13 [0.01, 1.16]
Klassen 2017	0	272	1	278	18.2%	0.34 [0.01, 8.37]
Parker 2016	1	31	1	46	23.1%	1.50 [0.09, 24.92]
Vukas 2013	1	30	1	72	23.2%	2.45 [0.15, 40.47]
Total (95% CI)		811		645	100.0%	0.54 [0.13, 2.23]
Total events	3		7			

Heterogeneity: Tau² = 0.24; Chi² = 3.37, df = 3 (P = 0.34); I² = 11%
Test for overall effect: Z = 0.86 (P = 0.39)

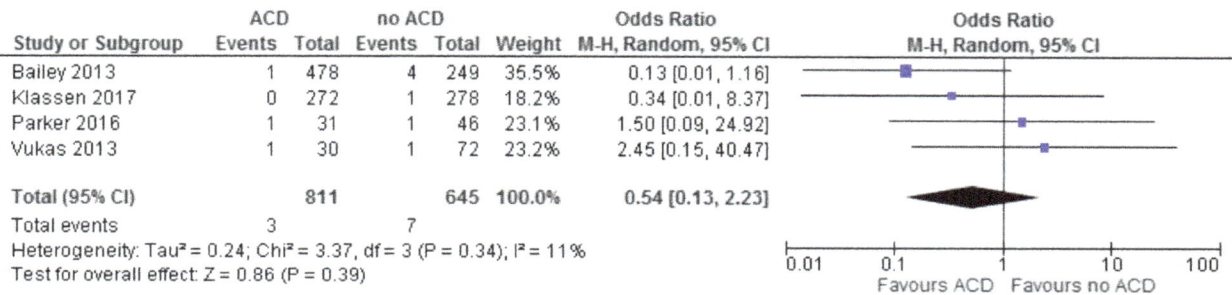

Odds Ratio M-H, Random, 95% CI — Favours ACD   Favours no ACD

C: Wound complication

Study or Subgroup	ACD Events	ACD Total	no ACD Events	no ACD Total	Weight	Odds Ratio M-H, Random, 95% CI
Bailey 2013	2	478	1	249	30.9%	1.04 [0.09, 11.55]
Klassen 2017	2	272	6	278	69.1%	0.34 [0.07, 1.68]
Total (95% CI)		750		527	100.0%	0.48 [0.13, 1.82]
Total events	4		7			

Heterogeneity: Tau² = 0.00; Chi² = 0.59, df = 1 (P = 0.44); I² = 0%
Test for overall effect: Z = 1.09 (P = 0.28)

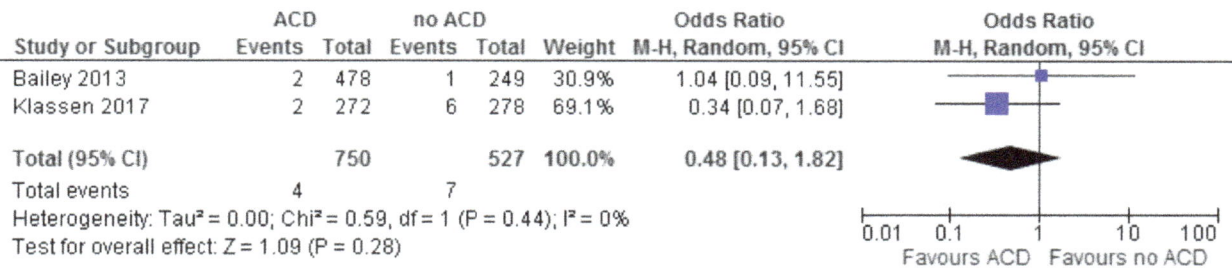

Odds Ratio M-H, Random, 95% CI — Favours ACD   Favours no ACD

D: Epidural hematoma

Study or Subgroup	ACD Events	ACD Total	no ACD Events	no ACD Total	Weight	Odds Ratio M-H, Random, 95% CI
Bailey 2013	0	478	1	249	47.4%	0.17 [0.01, 4.27]
Klassen 2017	0	272	2	278	52.6%	0.20 [0.01, 4.25]
Total (95% CI)		750		527	100.0%	0.19 [0.02, 1.71]
Total events	0		3			

Heterogeneity: Tau² = 0.00; Chi² = 0.01, df = 1 (P = 0.94); I² = 0%
Test for overall effect: Z = 1.48 (P = 0.14)

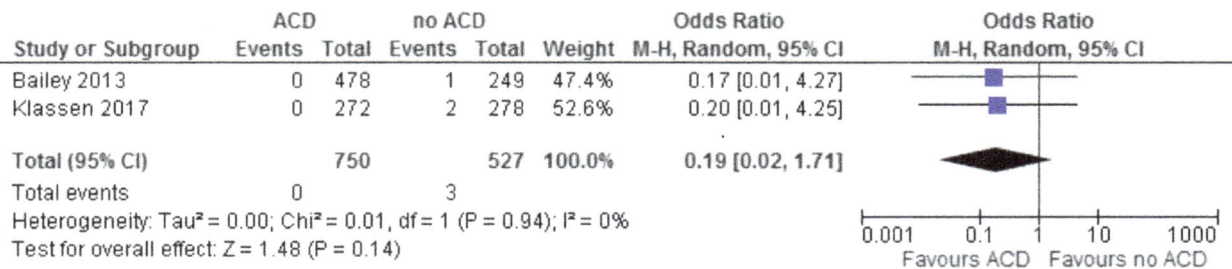

Odds Ratio M-H, Random, 95% CI — Favours ACD   Favours no ACD

Fig. 2 Comparison between ACD/AR group to no ACD/AR group. **a** Symptomatic disc reherniation; **b** Durotomy; **c** Wound complication; **d** Epidural hematoma

controlled trials (RCTs) or studies to use a similar framework of evaluation to assist more conclusive studies to be carried out in the future. Certain important aspects such as: i) patients' baseline traits (age, weight, height and gender); ii) preoperative and postoperative ODI, VAS scores and disc height; iii) the amount of disc removed; iv) post-operative complications (durotomy and wound complications); and v) long-term symptomatic

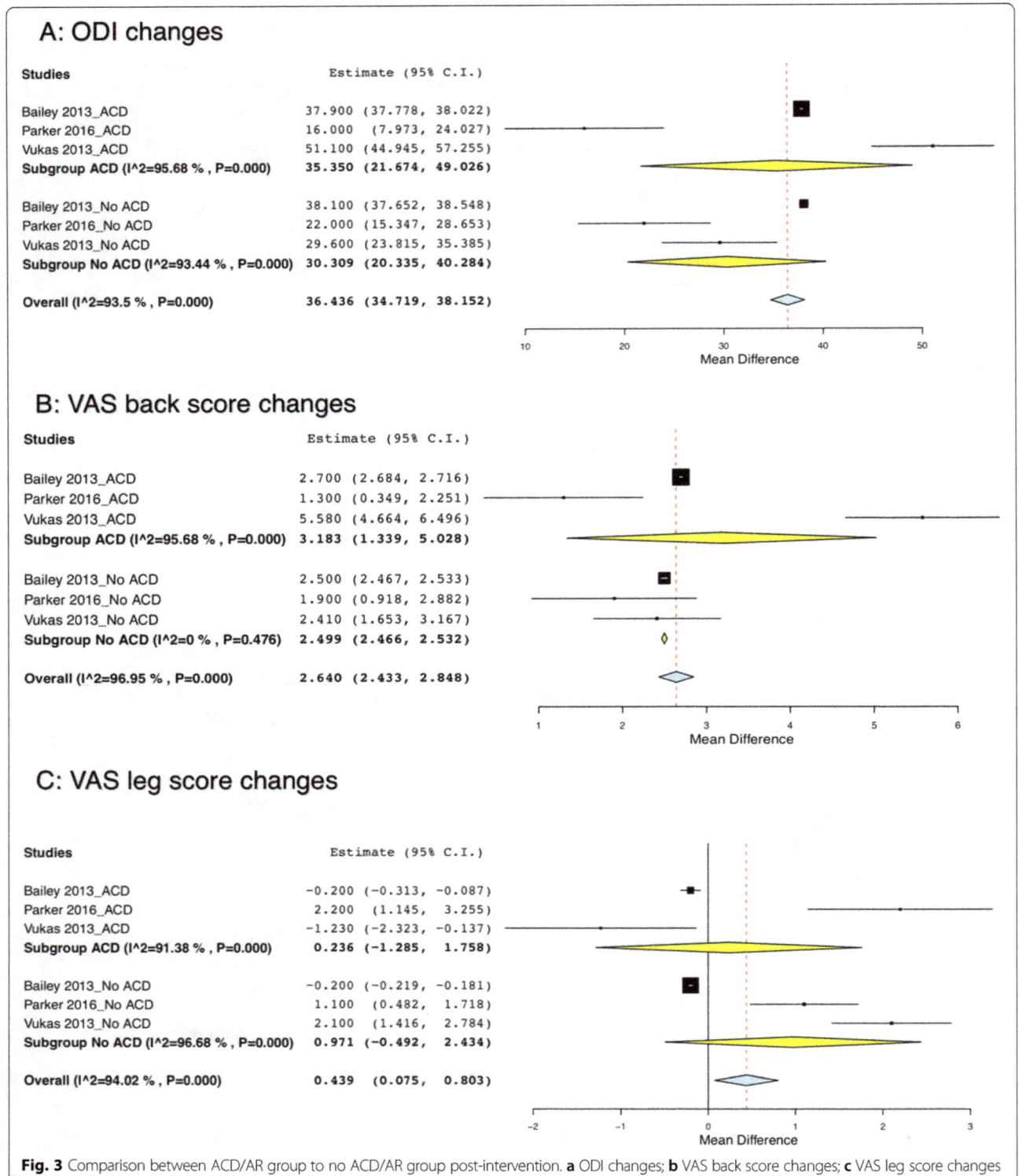

A: ODI changes

Studies	Estimate (95% C.I.)
Bailey 2013_ACD	37.900 (37.778, 38.022)
Parker 2016_ACD	16.000 (7.973, 24.027)
Vukas 2013_ACD	51.100 (44.945, 57.255)
Subgroup ACD (I^2=95.68 % , P=0.000)	35.350 (21.674, 49.026)
Bailey 2013_No ACD	38.100 (37.652, 38.548)
Parker 2016_No ACD	22.000 (15.347, 28.653)
Vukas 2013_No ACD	29.600 (23.815, 35.385)
Subgroup No ACD (I^2=93.44 % , P=0.000)	30.309 (20.335, 40.284)
Overall (I^2=93.5 % , P=0.000)	36.436 (34.719, 38.152)

B: VAS back score changes

Studies	Estimate (95% C.I.)
Bailey 2013_ACD	2.700 (2.684, 2.716)
Parker 2016_ACD	1.300 (0.349, 2.251)
Vukas 2013_ACD	5.580 (4.664, 6.496)
Subgroup ACD (I^2=95.68 % , P=0.000)	3.183 (1.339, 5.028)
Bailey 2013_No ACD	2.500 (2.467, 2.533)
Parker 2016_No ACD	1.900 (0.918, 2.882)
Vukas 2013_No ACD	2.410 (1.653, 3.167)
Subgroup No ACD (I^2=0 % , P=0.476)	2.499 (2.466, 2.532)
Overall (I^2=96.95 % , P=0.000)	2.640 (2.433, 2.848)

C: VAS leg score changes

Studies	Estimate (95% C.I.)
Bailey 2013_ACD	-0.200 (-0.313, -0.087)
Parker 2016_ACD	2.200 (1.145, 3.255)
Vukas 2013_ACD	-1.230 (-2.323, -0.137)
Subgroup ACD (I^2=91.38 % , P=0.000)	0.236 (-1.285, 1.758)
Bailey 2013_No ACD	-0.200 (-0.219, -0.181)
Parker 2016_No ACD	1.100 (0.482, 1.718)
Vukas 2013_No ACD	2.100 (1.416, 2.784)
Subgroup No ACD (I^2=96.68 % , P=0.000)	0.971 (-0.492, 2.434)
Overall (I^2=94.02 % , P=0.000)	0.439 (0.075, 0.803)

Fig. 3 Comparison between ACD/AR group to no ACD/AR group post-intervention. **a** ODI changes; **b** VAS back score changes; **c** VAS leg score changes

re-herniation to be included in the study. In order for proper comparison and efficacy of the ACD/AR to be evaluated, the study population should be compared to a control group as well.

While not part of the study in search for answers in support of the novel and potentially beneficial strategy we reviewed several publications that have shown that implantation of an ACD has other potential benefits apart from reducing the risk of symptomatic disc reherniation: i. Lequin et al. reported significant improvements in back and leg pain following the implantation of an ACD (Barricaid) post discectomy in 44 patients in a multicentre prospective study with one symptomatic and another asymptomatic reherniation [39]; ii. Trummer et al. carried out a prospective non-randomised trial comparing 64 ACD implantations to 137 controls and concluded that implantation of an ACD is beneficial in terms of maintaining disc space and reducing the risk of facet joint degeneration [31]; and iii. Bouma et al. reported significant reduction in symptomatic disc reherniation among their prospective non-randomised trial of 75 patients with 74 ACD implantations compared to literature [40]. Parker et al. reported that the use of ACD could potentially reduce the healthcare cost by roughly $220,000 per 100 discectomy procedures [41]. In addition, there are other case reports/ series reporting similar outcomes in terms of reducing the rate of symptomatic disc reherniation and pain improvement when implantation of an ACD is used [29, 42].

However, there are limitations to the use of an ACD/ AR. For instance, the Barricaid has a fixed size and has 2 parts that require implantation into both the affected IVD and the adjacent vertebral body. Should there be a significant loss of disc material, or the surface area of the herniation is too large, implantation of the Barricaid ACD would not be suitable [29, 30]. The same applies to the Anulex AR device, in which adequate disc height, and reasonable defect area will be necessary for implantation [28], hence both ARD/AR devices are only suitable to a limited group of patients. Bailey et al. proposed that 85% of patients were reported to be suitable intra-operatively for implantation of the Anulex AR device however further studies involving larger and various patient populations are needed to validate this finding [28]. Moreover, one inclusion criteria for the Barricaid ACD group was the defect has to be less than 6 mm in height and 10 mm in width [36, 37] thus making proper evaluation of the device even harder. Bouma et al. reported that only 15% of their patient population met this criterion and were eligible in their study [40]. Additionally, these devices are not suitable for patients with other spinal deformities such as spondylolisthesis as the implantation will be affected. A case report by Krukto et al. reported an incidence of aseptic instability of the ACD without signs of flora growth upon culturing as well which suggest there is still a chance of failure post-implantation [42]. Potential effects such as structural breakdown from scarring due to the surgical procedure may further weakened the surrounding structure which in turn can lead to long term poor outcomes of the ACD/AR such as implant migration.

Overall, proper efficacy of the application of ACD/AR post-discectomy could not be evaluated completely. There is only one study reporting exact data on the loss of disc height [30], in which how much disc material can be preserved with the application of these devices could not be proper gauged. Additionally, due to the limited number of RCTs carried out, we cannot conclude whether the results could be repeated. The small ACD/AR population size could also result in the small number of reported complications. Implantation of an ACD/AR will increase procedural time. Coupled with the introduction of an additional device implanted in the spine, it would undoubtedly increase the risk of durotomy or complication [28, 30, 36, 37], however this has not been borne out with the available studies to date. The results are suggestive of otherwise, in which the authors thought that the only possible explanation is surgeons are more careful when carrying out the additional procedure thus reducing post-operative complications. This is therefore a potential performance bias which can interfere with the actual data.

Our analysis leads us to the conclusion that the use of an ACD/AR is still in the early stages. There are also new methods being developed in recent times such as the application of a "Jetting Suture" technique to reduce the rate of reherniation [43]. Moreover, with recent advancement of three-dimensional printing (3DP) for patient specific implants (PSIs) in spine surgery [44–47], we believe there could be a possibility in the near future that patients with high risk of RDH be identified and receive a nucleus, or other PSI replacement to prevent RDH post-discectomy.

Conclusion

Early results demonstrate that the use of an ACD – Barricaid and AR using Anulex post-discectomy has at least equivalent efficacy to without implantation of preventative devices without differences in pain scores and perioperative complications. Additionally, both ACD and AR are beneficial for short term outcomes (up to 2 years) for the patients demonstrating significant reduction in symptomatic disc re-herniation rates associated with low post-operative complication risk. However, given the limited amount of studies and data, we could not determine the superiority of either Barricaid or Anulex over the other. This outcome requires further studies and investigations especially with appropriate and detailed data on annular defect sizes compared with risk of recurrence. Long term follow-up is paramount to determine any potential delayed or late complications of these devices, especially the Barricaid with respects to further interventions such as fusion or disc replacement as the device may hinder operative exposure and technique. Other potential studies investigating sub groups of patients who could potentially benefit from these devices should be carried out. Future projects researching whether annular repairs will assist with regenerative technologies in maintaining mesenchymal stem cells or hydro-gel composites to stay in position post discectomy are recommended.

Abbreviations
3DP: Three-dimensional printing; ACD: Annular closure device; AF: Annulus fibrosus; AR: Annular tissue repair system; CEP: Cartilaginous endplates; IVD: Intervertebral disc; LDH: Lumbar disc herniation; NP: Nucleus pulposus; ODI: Oswestry disability index; OR: Odds ratio; PSI: Patient specific implant; RCT: Randomised controlled trials; RDH: Recurrent lumbar disc herniation; VAS: Visual analogue scale; WMD: Weighted mean difference

Authors' contributions
WJC performed the literature search, collected the data and written most of the manuscript. KP checked the literature search and performed statistical analysis. AD revised the manuscript. CSO assisted in data collection. RM assisted in writing and revised the manuscript. All authors read and approved the final manuscript.

Competing interests
The authors declare that they have no competing interests.

Author details
[1]Faculty of Medicine, University of New South Wales (UNSW), Sydney, Australia. [2]NeuroSpine Surgery Research Group (NSURG), Prince of Wales Private Hospital, Sydney, Australia. [3]Department of Neurosurgery, Prince of Wales Private Hospital, Sydney, Australia. [4]Spine Service, Department of Orthopaedic Surgery, St. George & Sutherland Clinical School, University of New South Wales, Kogarah 2217, New South Wales, Australia. [5]Newcastle University Medicine Malaysia (NUMed), Johor, Malaysia.

References
1. Humzah MD, Soames RW. Human intervertebral disc: structure and function. Anat Rec. 1988;220:337–56.
2. Schroeder GD, Guyre CA, Vaccaro AR. The epidemiology and pathophysiology of lumbar disc herniations. Seminars Spine Surg. 2016;28: 2–7.
3. Koes BW, van Tulder MW, Peul WC. Diagnosis and treatment of sciatica. BMJ. 2007;334:1313–7.
4. Phan K, Dunn AE, Rao PJ, Mobbs RJ. Far lateral microdiscectomy: a minimally-invasive surgical technique for the treatment of far lateral lumbar disc herniation. J Spine Surg. 2016;2:59–63.
5. Yokosuka J, Oshima Y, Kaneko T, Takano Y, Inanami H, Koga H. Advantages and disadvantages of posterolateral approach for percutaneous endoscopic lumbar discectomy. J Spine Surg. 2016;2:158–66.
6. Weinstein JN, Lurie JD, Tosteson TD, et al. Surgical vs nonoperative treatment for lumbar disk herniation: the spine patient outcomes research trial (SPORT) observational cohort. JAMA. 2006;296:2451–9.
7. Lurie JD, Tosteson TD, Tosteson ANA, et al. Surgical versus non-operative treatment for lumbar disc herniation: eight-year results for the spine patient outcomes research trial (SPORT). Spine. 2014;39:3–16.
8. Weinstein JN, Lurie JD, Tosteson TD, et al. Surgical versus non-operative treatment for lumbar disc herniation: four-year results for the spine patient outcomes research trial (SPORT). Spine. 2008;33:2789–800.
9. Fekete TF, Haschtmann D, Kleinstück FS, Porchet F, Jeszenszky D, Mannion AF. What level of pain are patients happy to live with after surgery for lumbar degenerative disorders? Spine J. 2016;16:S12–S8.
10. Virk SS, Diwan A, Phillips FM, Sandhu H, Khan SN. What is the Rate of Revision Discectomies After Primary Discectomy on a National Scale? Clin Orthop Relat Res. 2017;475:2752–62.
11. Aizawa T, Ozawa H, Kusakabe T, et al. Reoperation for recurrent lumbar disc herniation: a study over a 20-year period in a Japanese population. J Orthop Sci. 2012;17:107–13.
12. Berjano P, Pejrona M, Damilano M. Microdiscectomy for recurrent L5–S1 disc herniation. Eur Spine J. 2013;22:2915–7.
13. Lebow RL, Adogwa O, Parker SL, Sharma A, Cheng J, McGirt MJ. Asymptomatic same-site recurrent disc herniation after lumbar discectomy: results of a prospective longitudinal study with 2-year serial imaging. Spine (Phila Pa 1976). 2011;36:2147–51.
14. Swartz KR, Trost GR. Recurrent lumbar disc herniation. Neurosurg Focus. 2003;15:1–4.
15. Drazin D, Ugiliweneza B, Al-Khouja L, et al. Treatment of recurrent disc herniation: a systematic review. Cureus. 2016;8:e622.
16. Vialle LR, Vialle EN, Suárez Henao JE, Giraldo G. LUMBAR DISC HERNIATION. Rev Bras Ortop (English Edition). 2010;45:17–22.
17. Liu C, Zhou Y. Percutaneous endoscopic lumbar diskectomy and minimally invasive transforaminal lumbar interbody fusion for recurrent lumbar disk herniation. World Neurosurg. 2017;98:14–20.
18. Adogwa O, Parker SL, Shau DN, et al. Cost per quality-adjusted life year gained of revision neural decompression and instrumented fusion for same-level recurrent lumbar stenosis: defining the value of surgical intervention. J Neurosurg Spine. 2012;16:135–40.
19. Mroz TE, Lubelski D, Williams SK, et al. Differences in the surgical treatment of recurrent lumbar disc herniation among spine surgeons in the United States. Spine J. 2014;14:2334–43.
20. Mobbs RJ, Phan K, Malham G, Seex K, Rao PJ. Lumbar interbody fusion: techniques, indications and comparison of interbody fusion options including PLIF, TLIF, MI-TLIF, OLIF/ATP, LLIF and ALIF. J Spine Surg. 2015;1:2–18.
21. Phan K, Lackey A, Chang N, et al. Anterior lumbar interbody fusion (ALIF) as an option for recurrent disc herniations: a systematic review and meta-analysis. J Spine Surg. 2017;3:587–95.
22. Ambrossi GLG, McGirt MJ, Sciubba DM, et al. Recurrent lumbar disc herniation after single-level lumbar discectomy: incidence and health care cost analysis. Neurosurgery. 2009;65:574–8.
23. O'Donnell JA, Anderson JT, Haas AR, et al. Treatment of recurrent lumbar disc herniation with or without fusion in workers' compensation subjects. Spine. 2017;42:E864–E70.
24. Mastronardi L, Puzzilli F. Packing of intervertebral spaces with oxidized regenerated cellulose to prevent the recurrence of lumbar disc herniation. Neurosurgery. 2003;52:1106–9.
25. McGirt MJ, Ambrossi GL, Datoo G, et al. Recurrent disc herniation and long-term back pain after primary lumbar discectomy: review of outcomes reported for limited versus aggressive disc removal. Neurosurgery. 2009;64: 338–44.
26. Thome C, Barth M, Scharf J, Schmiedek P. Outcome after lumbar sequestrectomy compared with microdiscectomy: a prospective randomized study. J Neurosurg Spine. 2005;2:271–8.
27. Dower A, Chatterji R, Swart A, Winder MJ. Surgical management of recurrent lumbar disc herniation and the role of fusion. J. Clin. Neurosci. 2016;23:44–50.
28. Bailey A, Araghi A, Blumenthal S, Huffmon GV. Prospective, multicenter, randomized, controlled study of anular repair in lumbar discectomy: two-year follow-up. Spine (Phila Pa 1976). 2013;38:1161–9.
29. Hahn BS, Ji GY, Moon B, et al. Use of annular closure device (Barricaid(R)) for preventing lumbar disc reherniation: one-year results of three cases. Korean J Neurotrauma. 2014;10:119–22.
30. Parker SL, Grahovac G, Vukas D, et al. Effect of an annular closure device (Barricaid) on same-level recurrent disk herniation and disk height loss after primary lumbar discectomy: two-year results of a multicenter prospective cohort study. Clin Spine Surg. 2016;29:454–60.
31. Trummer M, Eustacchio S, Barth M, Klassen PD, Stein S. Protecting facet joints post-lumbar discectomy: Barricaid annular closure device reduces risk of facet degeneration. Clin Neurol Neurosurg. 2013;115:1440–5.
32. Klassen PD, Hes R, Bouma GJ, et al. A multicenter, prospective, randomized study protocol to demonstrate the superiority of a bone-anchored prosthesis for anular closure used in conjunction with limited discectomy to limited discectomy alone for primary lumbar disc herniation. Int J Clin Trials. 2016;3:120–31.
33. Moher D, Liberati A, Tetzlaff J, Altman DG. Preferred reporting items for systematic reviews and meta-analyses: the PRISMA statement. BMJ. 2009; 339:b2535.

34. Phan K, Mobbs RJ. Systematic reviews and meta-analyses in spine surgery, neurosurgery and orthopedics: guidelines for the surgeon scientist. J Spine Surg. 2015;1:19–27.

35. Stroup DF, Berlin JA, Morton SC, et al. Meta-analysis of observational studies in epidemiology: a proposal for reporting. Meta-analysis of observational studies in epidemiology (MOOSE) group. JAMA. 2000;283:2008–12.

36. Klassen PD, Bernstein DT, Köhler H-P, et al. Bone-anchored annular closure following lumbar discectomy reduces risk of complications and reoperations within 90 days of discharge. J Pain Res. 2017;10:2047–55.

37. Vukas D, Ledic D, Grahovac G, Kolic Z, Rotim K, Vilendecic M. Clinical outcomes in patients after lumbar disk surgery with annular reinforcement device: two-year follow up. Acta Clin Croat. 2013;52:87–91.

38. Huang W, Han Z, Liu J, Yu L, Yu X. Risk factors for recurrent lumbar disc herniation: a systematic review and meta-analysis. Medicine. 2016;95:e2378.

39. Lequin MB, Barth M, Thome C, Bouma GJ. Primary limited lumbar discectomy with an annulus closure device: one-year clinical and radiographic results from a prospective, multi-center study. Korean J Spine. 2012;9:340–7.

40. Bouma GJ, Barth M, Ledic D, Vilendecic M. The high-risk discectomy patient: prevention of reherniation in patients with large anular defects using an anular closure device. Eur Spine J. 2013;22:1030–6.

41. Parker SL, Grahovac G, Vukas D, Ledic D, Vilendecic M, McGirt MJ. Cost savings associated with prevention of recurrent lumbar disc herniation with a novel annular closure device: a multicenter prospective cohort study. J Neurol Surg A Cent Eur Neurosurg. 2013;74:285–9.

42. Krutko AV, Baykov ES, Sadovoy MA. Reoperation after microdiscectomy of lumbar herniation: case report. Int J Surg Case Rep. 2016;24:119–23.

43. Qi L, Li M, Si H, et al. The clinical application of "jetting suture" technique in annular repair under microendoscopic discectomy: a prospective single-cohort observational study. Medicine (Baltimore). 2016;95:e4503.

44. Choy WJ, Mobbs RJ, Wilcox B, Phan S, Phan K, Sutterlin CE 3rd. Reconstruction of Thoracic Spine Using a Personalized 3D-Printed Vertebral Body in Adolescent with T9 Primary Bone Tumor. World Neurosurg. 2017; 105:1032.e13–7.

45. Mobbs RJ, Coughlan M, Thompson R, Sutterlin CE 3rd, Phan K. The utility of 3D printing for surgical planning and patient-specific implant design for complex spinal pathologies: case report. J Neurosurg Spine. 2017;26:513–8.

46. Phan K, Sgro A, Maharaj MM, D'Urso P, Mobbs RJ. Application of a 3D custom printed patient specific spinal implant for C1/2 arthrodesis. J Spine Surg. 2016;2:314–8.

47. Wilcox B, Mobbs RJ, Wu A-M, Phan K. Systematic review of 3D printing in spinal surgery: the current state of play. J Spine Surg. 2017;3:433–43.

5

Nutrient foramen location on the laminae provides a landmark for pedicle screw entry: a cadaveric study

Masahito Oshina[1][*], Yasushi Oshima[1], Yoshitaka Matsubayashi[1], Yuki Taniguchi[1], Hirotaka Chikuda[1], Kiehyun Daniel Riew[2] and Sakae Tanaka[1]

Abstract

Background: Nutrient foramina are often encountered around the entry point of pedicle screws. Further, while probing the pedicle for pedicle screw insertion around the nutrient foramen, bleeding from the probe insertion hole is often observed. The purpose of this study was to investigate the frequency of occurrence of nutrient foramina, the association between the nutrient foramen and pedicle, and the safety and accuracy of cervical and thoracic pedicle screw placement using the nutrient foramen as the entry point.

Methods: We identified the location of the nutrient foramina for the dorsal branches of the segmental artery and their anatomical association to the pedicles and bony landmarks in the vertebrae for C3–T12 in seven cadavers. We also determined the frequency with which the nutrient foramina were present in 119 cadaveric vertebrae. We identified the pedicle location, base of the superior articular facet, and lateral border of laminae with respect to the nutrient foramen.

Results: The overall presence of the nutrient foramina was 63% (150/238) in the specimens, with 60% (42/70) and 64% (108/168) identifiable in the cervical and thoracic vertebrae, respectively. In the cervical vertebrae, the nutrient foramen was located on the outer wall of the pedicle and was positioned between the cephalad and caudal walls. In the thoracic spine, 98% (106/108) nutrient foramina were located inside the pedicle walls.

Conclusions: Our study findings confirm that the location of the nutrient foramen can be used for identifying the entry point for pedicle screws. In the cervical vertebrae, the nutrient foramina are located lateral to pedicle but within the cranial and caudal margins. In the thoracic vertebrae, the nutrient foramina are located in the medial and caudal regions of the pedicle. Thus, to decrease the risk of overshoot, the entry point for thoracic pedicle screws should be positioned a few millimeters cephalad and lateral to the nutrient foramen.

Keywords: Nutrient foramen, Laminae, Pedicle screw, Entry point, Cervical spine, Thoracic spine

Background

Pedicle screws have been used since Boucher [1] reported this technique for the lumbar spine in 1959. Several entry points for pedicle screws have been described, but the risk of neural, vascular, or visceral injury remains [2–8]. The safety of screw placement can be improved if intraoperative fluoroscopy and computed tomography (CT) and image-assisted navigation are employed [9–12]. However,

these techniques do not completely eliminate the risk of injury. Therefore, obtaining information that can help in improving the accuracy of pedicle screw placement is desirable.

Nutrient foramina are often encountered around the entry point of pedicle screws. Further, while probing the pedicle for pedicle screw insertion around the nutrient foramen, bleeding from the probe insertion hole is often observed. These nutrient foramina are considered to be the entry points for the dorsal branch of segmental arteries, and they have a predictable location on the laminae [13]. A previous study described the details of

* Correspondence: masahito04031979@yahoo.co.jp
[1]Department of Orthopaedic Surgery, The University of Tokyo Hospital, 7-3-1, Hongo, Bunkyo-Ku, Tokyo 113-8655, Japan
Full list of author information is available at the end of the article

intravertebral vasculature following radiopaque dye injection [14], but the positional association of the vasculature to the pedicles has not yet been reported. This study was performed to determine the frequency of occurrence of nutrient foramina, the association between the nutrient foramen location and pedicle and other bony landmarks, and the safety and accuracy of cervical and thoracic pedicle screw placement using nutrient foramina as the entry point.

Methods

We used seven cadavers (four male and three female) for this study. The mean age of the cadavers at the time of death was 87.9 years. The cadavers were provided by the Department of Anatomy (The University of Tokyo, Japan). In total, 238 pedicles and nutrient foramina of the dorsal branches of segmental arteries between the C3 and T12 were evaluated manually. The cadavers were placed in the prone position with the neck in the neutral position. Soft tissue was removed to expose the laminae, facet joints, and transverse processes.

We manually examined each cadaver for the presence of nutrient foramina for the dorsal branches of the segmental artery around the superior articular facet and transverse processes. The presence of a nutrient foramen was confirmed by the identification of a circular depression with a lack of cortical continuity (Fig. 1).

If a nutrient foramen was present, the distance from the lateral border of the lamina and the bottom of the superior articular facet was measured (Fig. 2). The nutrient foramina were found to be usually located just caudal to the superior articular facet and medial to the base of the transverse process on the border of the laminae and

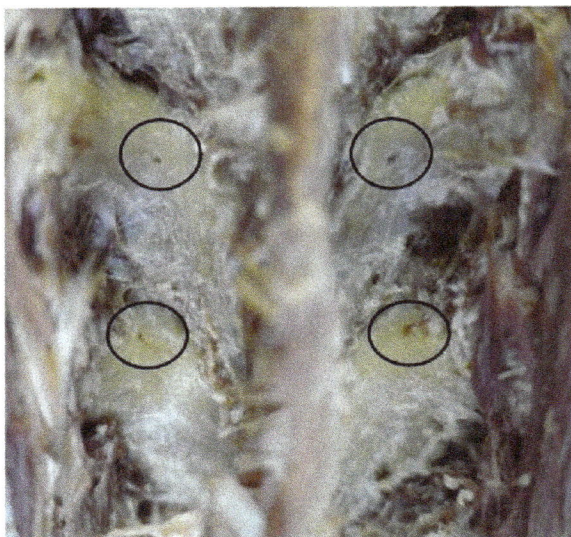

Fig. 2 Nutrient foramina in the studied area and distance from the nutrient foramen to the bottom of superior articular facet and the lateral border of laminae

cranial to the inferior margin of the transverse process. If two nutrient foramina were present in this area, the larger one was evaluated. Nutrient foramina in other areas were excluded (Fig. 2).

A Kirschner wire measuring 1.2 mm in diameter (TACT MEDICAL INC., Tokyo, Japan) was orthogonally inserted through the nutrient foramen toward the vertebral body without changing direction in the sagittal and axial planes. The Kirschner wire was used instead of a pedicle screw so that the nutrient foramen and the canal remained intact. After the nutrient foramen was marked, the lamina was cut using a chisel. To inspect the inside of intact pedicles, some nutrient foramina were evaluated by cutting the pedicle with a chisel at the foramen without Kirschner wire insertion. The association between the nutrient foramen and pedicle positions was examined on the C3–T12 laminae.

All measurements were made using an electronic digital caliper (precision 0.01 mm; PLATA, Osaka, Japan). We manually measured four anatomic parameters related to the mouth of the dorsal branch of the segmental artery on the C3–T12 laminae. The same caliper was used to measure the distance between the nutrient foramina and various structures. The following parameters were assessed:

1. Percentage of occurrence of nutrient foramina. The area of evaluation was determined using definite bony landmarks.
2. Caudally directed distance from the bottom of the superior articular facet.
3. Medially directed distance from the lateral border of the lamina.
4. Assessment of whether the orthogonal line of lamina at a nutrient foramen was located inside or

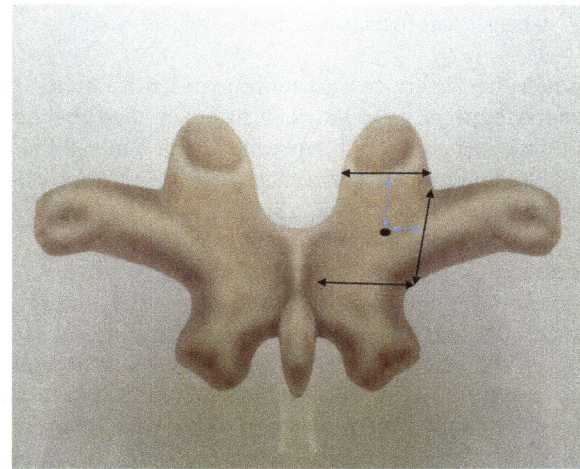

Fig. 1 Nutrient foramen on laminae

outside the pedicle, with the location determined when it was located inside the pedicle wall.

When there were two or more exposed foramina, the distance between the nutrient foramen and the bony landmark was compared between the left and right sides using Student's *t*-test. Differences with *P* values of < 0.05 were considered statistically significant.

Results

Nutrient foramina were present within the evaluation area in 60% (42/70) of cervical vertebrae and 64% (108/168) of thoracic vertebrae. Overall, nutrient foramina were present in 63% of vertebrae (150/238; Fig. 1 and Tables 1 and 2). There were no significant differences bilaterally in the distance between the nutrient foramen and bony landmarks.

Association between the superior articular facet and the nutrient foramen

When making calculations, we excluded the nutrient foramina on the superior articular facet and those located caudally to the transverse process (Tables 1 and 2). The distance from the base of the superior articular facet to the nutrient foramen had a range of 1.28–4.98 mm in the cervical vertebrae and 2.22–6.50 mm in the thoracic vertebrae. The distance from the base of the superior articular facet to the nutrient foramen was similar between the cervical and thoracic vertebrae.

Association between the base of the transverse process and the nutrient foramen

The distance from the lateral laminar border and base of the transverse process to the nutrient foramen was 3.14–7.25 mm in the cervical vertebrae and 2.01–7.32 mm in the thoracic vertebrae. The distance tended to be similar between the cervical and thoracic vertebrae (Tables 1 and 2).

In the cervical vertebrae, the nutrient foramen was usually located inside the vertebral laminar notch. In the thoracic vertebrae, no nutrient foramen was located medial to the inflection point, where the lamina meets the transverse process. At the T11 and T12 levels, nutrient foramina were located just inside the accessory

process and tended to be close to the lateral laminar border. It may be considered that the nutrient foramen position on the laminae moves caudally at this level, probably because laminae are narrower.

Association between the pedicle and nutrient foramen

In the cervical spine, almost all Kirschner wires inserted into the nutrient foramen reached the outer aspect of the pedicle and were located immediately above the course of the vertebral artery. However, at the C7 level, the wires reached beyond the outer aspect of the vertebral artery. In the cervical spine, two nutrient foramina in C3 vertebra deviated vertically from the pedicle axis to the caudal direction, whereas the others were located in the cephalad and caudal margins.

In the thoracic spine, two nutrient foramina in T2 vertebra deviated from the pedicle axis to the caudal direction. However, the deviated nutrient foramina were located within the pedicle width, and no nutrient foramen was observed to perforate the medial pedicle wall. The remaining nutrient foramina were all located on the medial and caudal sides of the pedicle (Fig. 3). Some nutrient foramina were observed in the inner aspect of pedicles after laminae were cut (Fig. 4).

In total, 98% (106/108) of thoracic nutrient foramina were located within the margins of the pedicle walls. In addition, some nutrient foramina located on the superior articular facet were also within the margins of the pedicle wall. However, they were excluded because the location was out of the investigational range. The nutrient foramina situated below the transverse process were outside the margins of the pedicle walls.

Discussion

The segmental artery gives rise to smaller branches that supply the vertebral body in its proximal portion. Three types of branches exist: ventral, dorsal, and spinal. The course of the dorsal branch is sub-laminar before it perforates the muscles [14, 15]. The nutrient foramina for the dorsal branches of the segmental artery were evaluated in this study. We found that the foramina were located close to the entry point for pedicle screws in almost all specimens, and we investigated the frequency of its presence and its positional association to the

Table 1 Number of exposed nutrient foramina and mean distance from foramina to the bony landmark

	Exposure (/14)	Lt (/7)	Rt (/7)	Lt. superior articular facet (mm)	Lt. border of the laminae (mm)	Rt. superior articular facet (mm)	Rt. border of the laminae (mm)
C3	9	4	5	2.51 ± 1.18	4.70 ± 1.33	2.96 ± 0.76	4.12 ± 1.92
C4	6	2	4	2.84 ± 5.57	3.74 ± 0.07	2.57 ± 0.38	3.82 ± 0.48
C5	9	6	3	3.08 ± 1.27	5.28 ± 1.73	3.79 ± 1.52	6.27 ± 1.35
C6	10	4	6	2.76 ± 0.37	4.82 ± 1.28	3.04 ± 0.61	4.86 ± 1.00
C7	8	4	4	2.93 ± 0.45	6.81 ± 0.86	3.63 ± 0.43	6.67 ± 0.67

Table 2 Number of exposed foramina and mean distance from the foramina to the bony landmark

	Exposure (/14)	Lt (/7)	Rt (/7)	Lt. superior articular facet (mm)	Lt. border of the laminae (mm)	Rt. superior articular facet (mm)	Rt. border of the laminae (mm)
T1	12	6	6	4.09 ± 0.52	3.64 ± 0.63	4.09 ± 0.71	3.75 ± 0.68
T2	11	5	6	4.44 ± 1.55	3.99 ± 0.86	4.30 ± 1.24	4.24 ± 1.02
T3	8	4	4	4.71 ± 1.01	3.99 ± 0.46	4.69 ± 0.89	4.27 ± 0.24
T4	8	4	4	4.07 ± 1.21	4.07 ± 0.53	3.62 ± 1.48	3.91 ± 0.42
T5	4	3	1	3.67 ± 0.26	3.61 ± 0.72	5.74	4.40
T6	8	5	3	4.44 ± 1.23	4.02 ± 0.36	4.44 ± 1.21	3.80 ± 0.60
T7	7	4	3	3.54 ± 0.45	4.23 ± 0.17	3.49 ± 0.28	3.90 ± 0.53
T8	10	5	5	3.55 ± 0.54	4.49 ± 1.25	3.38 ± 0.71	4.18 ± 0.89
T9	8	4	4	3.80 ± 0.90	4.64 ± 1.80	4.11 ± 0.79	4.08 ± 0.49
T10	12	5	7	4.20 ± 0.81	4.08 ± 0.43	3.64 ± 0.95	4.27 ± 0.35
T11	8	4	4	4.03 ± 0.23	3.28 ± 1.19	3.56 ± 0.92	3.67 ± 1.13
T12	12	6	6	4.65 ± 1.37	2.67 ± 0.58	4.28 ± 1.54	2.84 ± 0.53

pedicle. When the nutrient foramen was cut, we were able to observe the path of the vessel, which went through the cortical bone into the pedicle, continuously on the outer aspect of the laminae [14] (Fig. 4). Although obvious pathways are depicted in Fig. 4, it is unclear whether all nutrient foramina pass through the pedicle. This is because the smaller pathways could have been destroyed and compressed when we cut the bone using the chisel. In addition, when nutrient foramina and vessel pathways are small, it may be difficult to identify them. In this study, we visually identified the presence and location of nutrient foramina on the laminae by careful examination. Another method for identifying the nutrient foramina is CT [16]. Nutrient foramina can often be confirmed using three-dimensional CT (3DCT), but the confirmation depends on the size of the nutrient foramen and whether it was captured on a slice.

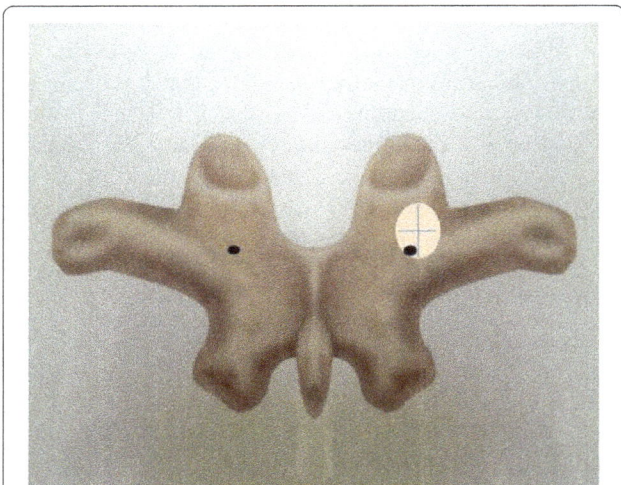

Fig. 3 In most cases, nutrient foramina existed in the medial caudal side of pedicle

Therefore, this technique cannot assess the presence of a nutrient foramen with sufficient detail and accuracy, without very fine slice CT scans. Thus, the confirmation of screw insertion into a nutrient foramen via CT or navigation system can only be performed when CT is able to accurately visualize the foramina. However, with very fine slice CT scans, one can validate the technique that we used in this study. We are currently in the process of conducting such a study.

In the cervical spine

With regard to the rate of nutrient foramen occurrence and its association to bony landmarks, if facet joint hypertrophy is relatively severe, the identification of the nutrient foramen becomes difficult because the foramen gets closer to the enlarged facet and is covered by an overlapping osteophyte. This issue is particularly the case in the cervical spine. In such cases, the nutrient foramen can still be used as a landmark for the entry point for pedicle screws, but the direction of insertion should be medially directed. For example, when we determine the trajectory of the pedicle screw, this entry point should be selected considering the medially inclined pedicle axis, as reported previously [2, 17]; this is because the nutrient foramen is located immediately above the vertebral artery. In the sagittal plane, the trajectory should be orthogonal to the dorsal spine curvature; thus, the C3 insertion trajectory is expected to deviate caudally. Rao et al. [18] reported that sagittal pedicle angulation was directed cranially at C3 (13.9°) and C4 (7.3°). As noted in previous studies [18, 19], accuracy may be enhanced if the cephalad direction is used at the C3 and C4 vertebrae.

In the thoracic spine

With regard to the rate of nutrient foramen exposure, in contrast to the cervical vertebra, the thoracic vertebrae

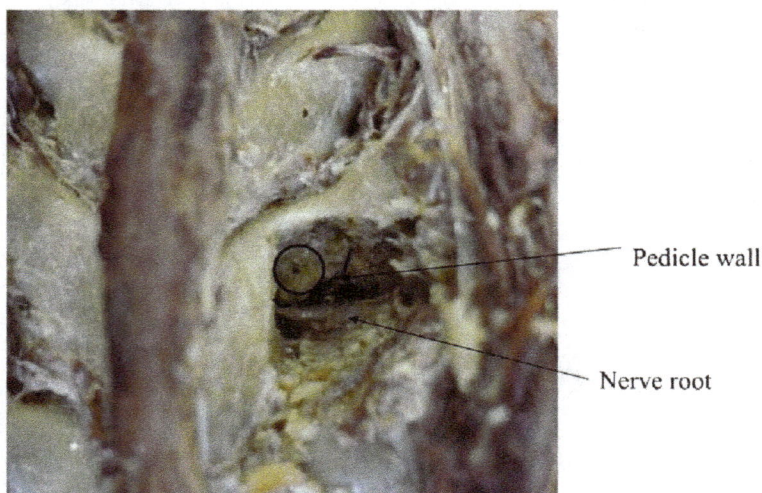

Fig. 4 Nutrient foramen penetrating deep into the pedicle

were less degenerative, and the thoracic nutrient foramina were consistently identifiable. Nutrient foramina were almost at the inflection point between the lamina and transverse process. Nutrient foramina tended to be present in a more cranial position at T7 and T8, suggesting that the pedicles are also positioned more cranially, which is similar to that previously reported [18–20]. Nutrient foramina located within the margins of the pedicle (106/108) were located in the medial and caudal portion of the pedicle. Therefore, thoracic pedicle screw entry points should be positioned a few millimeters cephalad and lateral to the nutrient foramen. Mid-thoracic pedicles are usually vertical and do not require an extreme medial angulation.

Our study has several limitations. The number of cadavers included was small, making it difficult to compare the location of the nutrient foramen at each level by statistical analysis. Increasing the number of cadavers should increase the accuracy of the assessments. Similar to our study, Yang, et al. [21] have reported that nutrient foramina were present in 63% from T4 to T8 vertebrae. The difference of presentation among other ethnicities and Asian is remains unclear because their study did not take into account the race of the cadavers. However, as a pilot study for identifying 42 cervical and 108 thoracic nutrient foramina, we believe that we have adequate data to demonstrate the association between the nutrient foramina and pedicles in the cervical and thoracic vertebrae. Another limitation is that one cannot rely on the nutrient foramina as a guide for placing pedicle screws in isolation. To date, no foolproof technique has been identified for placing cervical and thoracic pedicle screws. We believe that the greatest utility of the nutrient foramina is that when present and when identified on a 3DCT image, one has a perfect intraoperative landmark to use as a guide for inserting the pedicle screws. One can use a preoperative navigation software to determine the ideal starting point, in addition to using the nutrient foramen as an intra-operatively identifiable landmark.

Conclusion

Our study results indicate that the nutrient foramen is identifiable in the majority of cervical and thoracic vertebrae and that it is in close proximity or within the margins of the pedicle walls. The location of the nutrient foramen was consistent, especially in the thoracic spine. The cervical nutrient foramina were located lateral to pedicle, but within the cranial and caudal margins. The thoracic nutrient foramen is most commonly located inside of the pedicle wall, and it is positioned in the medial and caudal aspect of the pedicle. Thus, to provide a smaller overshoot risk, although prior confirmation by CT is needed, the thoracic pedicle screw entry point should be positioned a few millimeters cephalad and lateral to the nutrient foramen. Most importantly, we believe that if the nutrient foramen can be identified on a 3DCT image, it can be used, along with a navigation software or freehand technique, to pre-operatively plan the starting point and trajectory of a pedicle screw using the nutrient foramen as a reference point.

Abbreviations
3DCT: Three-dimensional computed tomography; CT: Computed tomography

Acknowledgements
We would like to thank Enago for providing editorial assistance.

Authors' contributions
MO contributed to the conception, design, and data acquisition. MO and YO analyzed and interpreted the data. MO and KR drafted the manuscript. YM, YT, YO, HC, ST, and KR critically reviewed the manuscript. All authors have read and approved the final manuscript.

Competing interests

All authors have declared the following potential conflicts of interest: MO, none. YO, none. YT, none. YM, none. HC, none.

ST, Endowments: Astellas Pharma Inc., Ayumi Pharmaceutical Corporation, Pfizer Japan Inc., Bristol-Myers Squibb, Daiichi Sankyo Company, Limited, Chugai Pharmaceutical Co., Ltd., Grants: The Japan Agency for Medical Research and Development, Grant-in-Aid for Scientific Research (A), Grant-in-Aid for Exploratory Research, Expert testimony: Amgen Inc., Amgen Inc. Asahi Kasei Pharma, Asahi Corporation, Amgen Astellas BioPharma K.K., Ono Pharmaceutical CO., LTD., Kyocera Medical Corporation, Daiichi Sankyo Company, Limited, Eli Lilly Japan K.K., Pfizer Japan Inc.

KR, Second opinion: Advanced Medical.

Consultation: Medtronic, Zeiss, Zimmer, Biomet.

Speaker: Grand Rounds, Medtronic, Zeiss, Zimmer, Biomet.

Stocks: Osprey, Expanding Orthopedics, Spineology, Spinal Kinetics, Nexgen Spine.

Author details

[1]Department of Orthopaedic Surgery, The University of Tokyo Hospital, 7-3-1, Hongo, Bunkyo-Ku, Tokyo 113-8655, Japan. [2]Department of Orthopedic Surgery, Columbia University, New York, NY, USA.

References

1. Boucher HH. A method of spinal fusion. J Bone Joint Surg Br. 1959;41:248–59.
2. Abumi K, Itoh H, Taneichi H, Kaneda K. Transpedicular screw fixation for traumatic lesions of the middle and lower cervical spine: description of the techniques and preliminary report. J Spinal Disord. 1994;7:19–28.
3. Cinotti G, Gumina S, Ripani M, Postacchini F. Pedicle instrumentation in the thoracic spine. A morphometric and cadaveric study for placement of screws. Spine. 1999;24:114–9.
4. Kim YJ, Lenke LG, Bridwell KH, Cho YS, Riew KD. Free hand pedicle screw placement in the thoracic spine: is it safe? Spine. 2004;29:333–42.
5. Zheng X, Chaudhari R, Wu C, Mehbod AA, Transfeldt EE. Subaxial cervical pedicle screw insertion with newly defined entry point and trajectory: accuracy evaluation in cadavers. Eur Spine J. 2010;19:105–12.
6. Parker SL, McGirt MJ, Farber SH, Amin AG, Rick AM, Suk I, et al. Accuracy of free-hand pedicle screws in the thoracic and lumbar spine: analysis 6816 consecutive screws. Neurosurgery. 2011;68:170–8.
7. Karaikovic EE, Kunakornsawat S, Daubs MD, Madsen RW, Gaines RW Jr. Surgical anatomy of the cervical pedicles: landmarks for posterior cervical pedicle entrance localization. J Spinal Disord. 2000;13:63–72.
8. Park JH, Jeon SR, Roh SW, Kim JH, Rhim SC. The safety and accuracy of freehand pedicle screw placement in the subaxial cervical spine: a series of 45 consecutive patients. Spine. 2014;39:280–5.
9. Nooh A, Aoude A, Fortin M, Aldebeyan S, Abduljabbar FH, et al. Use of computer assistance in lumbar fusion surgery: analysis of 15 222 patients in the ACS-NSQIP database. Global Spine J. 2017;7:617–23.
10. Nooh A, Lubov J, Aoude A, Aldebeyan S, Jarzem P, Ouellet J, et al. Differences between manufacturers of computed tomography-based computer-assisted surgery systems do exist: a systematic literature review. Global Spine J. 2017;7:83–94. https://doi.org/10.1055/s-0036-1583942. Epub 2017 Feb 1
11. Al-Habib AF, Al-Akkad S. Segmental surface referencing during intraoperative three-dimensional image-guided spine navigation: an early validation with comparison to automated referencing. Global Spine J. 2016;6:765–70.
12. Cordemans V, Kaminski L, Banse X, Francq BG, Cartiaux O. Accuracy of a new intraoperative cone beam CT imaging technique (Artis zeego II) compared to postoperative CT scan for assessment of pedicle screws placement and breaches detection. Eur Spine J. 2017;26:2906–16.
13. Liu JM, Jiang J, Liu ZL, Long XH, Chen WZ, Zhou Y, et al. A new entrance technique for C2 pedicle screw placement and the use in patients with atlantoaxial instability. Clin Spine Surg. 2017;30:E573–7.
14. Ratcliffe JF. The arterial anatomy of the adult human lumbar vertebral body: a microarteriographic study. J Anat. 1980;131:57–79.
15. Lazorthes G, Gouaze A, Zadeh JO, Santini JJ, Lazorthes Y, Burdin P. Arterial vascularization of the spinal cord: recent studies of the anastomotic substitution pathways. J Neurosurg. 1971;35:253–62.
16. Cunningham CA, Black SM. The vascular collar of the ilium: three-dimensional evaluation of the dominant nutrient foramen. Clin Anat. 2013;26:502–8.
17. Sakamoto T, Neo M, Nakamura T. Transpedicular screw placement evaluated by axial computed tomography of the cervical pedicle. Spine. 2004;29:2510–4.
18. Rao RD, Marawar SV, Stemper BD, Yoganandan N, Shender BS. Computerized tomographic morphometric analysis of subaxial cervical spine pedicles in young asymptomatic volunteers. J Bone Joint Surg Am. 2008;90:1914–21.
19. Kanna PR, Shetty AP, Rajasekaran S. Anatomical feasibility of pediatric cervical pedicle screw insertion by computed tomographic morphometric evaluation of 376 pediatric cervical pedicles. Spine. 2001;36:1297–304.
20. McCormack BM, Benzel EC, Adams MS, Baldwin NG, Rupp FW, Maher DJ. Anatomy of the thoracic pedicle. Neurosurgery. 1995;37:303–8.
21. Yang JY, Lenke LG. Usefulness of the nutrient foramen of lamina for insertion of thoracic pedicle screws. J Spinal Disord Tech. 2008;21:205–8.

6

Radiocarpal fusion and midcarpal resection interposition arthroplasty: long-term results in severely destroyed rheumatoid wrists

Christoph Biehl[1]*[iD], Thomas Braun[1], Ulrich Thormann[1], Amir Oda[2], Gabor Szalay[1] and Stefan Rehart[3]

Abstract

Background: The aim of this retrospective study is to evaluate distal resection interposition arthroplasty of the wrist as a tool to restore mobility as well as to restore stability in severely destroyed wrist joints.

Methods: Thirty-four wrists in 28 rheumatoid arthritis patients were included. The mean follow-up time was 9 years after surgical treatment with clinical and radiological examination. The results were accessed based on a modification of Clayton´s scoring system as well as a functional questionnaire.

Results: 71% patients were satisfied with pain, function and activities of daily life. Better results were reported by patients with a young age, early surgical intervention, a shorter duration of the disease, and lesser involvement of other joints.

Conclusions: The results for radiocarpal arthrodesis were comparable to those of synovectomy or arthrodesis of the wrist. The results after total wrist joint arthroplasty varies probably as the result of different patient groups, implant types and evolution of prosthetic designs, and are not comparable with the present study.

Keywords: Rheumatoid arthritis, Partial wrist arthrodesis, Wrist fusion, Rheumatoid wrist, Functional outcome

Background

Patients with progressive rheumatoid arthritis are severely handicapped in many ways. In more than 90% of patients, the wrist is affected. Any wrist involvement can lead to excessive pain, malfunction and conceivably to a progression of deformation of the fingers, which are usually already compromised in patients with rheumatoid arthritis [1–3]. The wrist is the key joint for an overall treatment strategy for hand and finger deformities and for loss of function [4, 5].

The role of surgical treatment remains a subject of controversy in the clinical management of rheumatoid patients associated with advanced hand dysfunction and destruction (Larsen stage 3–5). In the literature, especially in Anglo-American papers, total wrist arthroplasty (TWA) and total wrist fusion (TWF) appear to be the only solution for rheumatoid wrists, ignoring detailed stage-adapted therapies such as those of the Scandinavian, German and Japanese tradition of rheumatoid surgeons [6–8]. If surgery is indicated in Larsen-stage III-IV, a proximal wrist fusion will ensure stability. In addition, mobilization of the distal row protects limited mobility of the wrist [9].

Correct indication and good clinical results will lead to an alternative to complete arthrodesis or wrist prosthesis. In cases of severely destroyed proximal and distal rows of the carpus, resection interposition arthroplasty (RIAP) provides stability based on radiocarpal fusion, preserving an acceptable range of motion provided by the resection interposition arthroplasty of the midcarpal joint; this, in summary, is advantageous for daily activities [10–12].

In 1981, Tillmann and Thabe modified the proximal resection arthroplasty because of persistent instability to arthrodesis of the proximal row with interposition of the dorsal capsule into the distal joint line for severely destroyed wrists (Larsen IV and V) [13, 14]. The purpose of this retrospective study was to evaluate the clinical and radiological outcomes of 34 distal resection interposition arthroplasty.

* Correspondence: christoph.biehl@chiru.med.uni-giessen.de
[1]Klinik und Poliklinik für Unfall-, Hand- und Wiederherstellungschirurgie - Operative Notaufnahme, UKGM Gießen, Rudolf-Buchheim-Str. 7, 35392 Giessen, Germany
Full list of author information is available at the end of the article

Methods

Indication

In cases of midcarpal joint involvement, according to the progressive stages of Larsen, Dale and Eek (LDE)-classification, total wrist fusion (TWF) was the most common treatment in severely destroyed wrists for more than 70% (Figs. 1 and 2).

At times the decision as to the best surgical treatment was difficult, as in cases of severely destroyed wrist joints in rheumatoid arthritis patients. On the one hand, wrist arthrodesis causes a total loss of flexion and extension, causing difficulties for personal hygiene, the most frequent complaint following arthrodesis. On the other hand, endoprosthetic reconstruction carries the risk of loosening and infection [15]. Neither arthrodesis nor endoprosthetic treatment are completely satisfactory and safe solutions. In an effort to combine the best features of both techniques, radiocarpal fusion can be performed in combination with resection interposition arthroplasty between the lunate and capitate with unacceptable destruction of the capitate head [3, 16].

There are a number of prerequisites for distal resection-interposition-arthroplasty (RIAP) of the wrist joint. The opportunity for this operation depends on destruction-type II or III according to Simmen/Huber, the

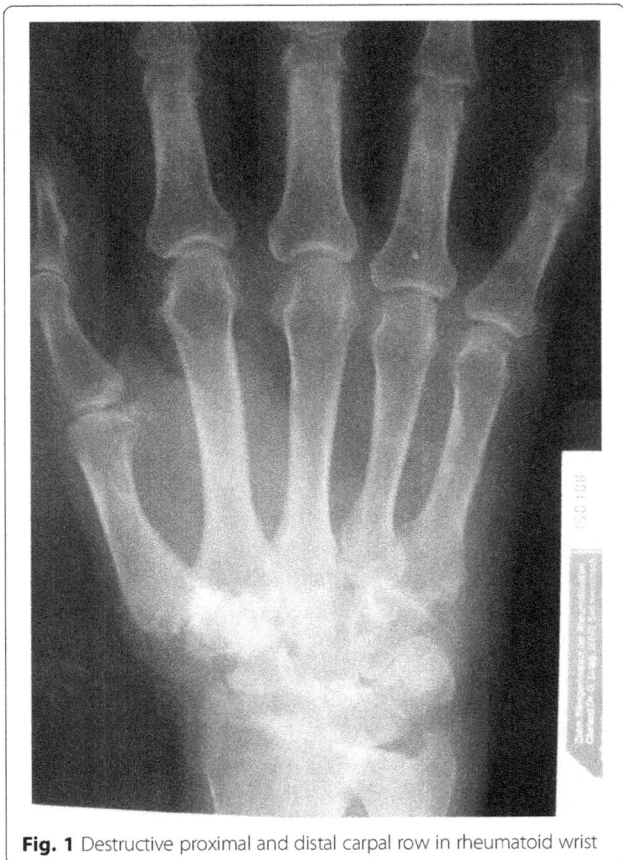

Fig. 1 Destructive proximal and distal carpal row in rheumatoid wrist

possibility for soft tissue balancing (tendon transfer), a nearly intact carpal bone height (> 80% of normal high) and an adequate outpatient supply [12, 17]. Four-corner-fusion was the former treatment option, as it was preferred in osteoarthritis patients, but with poor results in rheumatoid arthritic wrists. These were caused by fundamentally different pathologies and primary false transfers from these cases with severe problems of wrist balancing in rheumatoid arthritis patients.

Surgical procedure [3, 5, 18]

The operation use a dorsal approach. After synovectomy of the extensor tendons denervation of the posterior interosseous nerve is performed, and in cases of ulnar instability, an excision of the distal 2 cm of the ulna is performed.

The arthrodesis of the proximal row (radiolunate and radioscaphoid) is achieved using staples (Fig. 3) [5, 14], cannulated screws or angular stable plates. Subsequently, approximately 5 mm of the destroyed articular surface of capitate and hamate is resected to rebuild the articular line. A flap of the dorsal capsule or extensor retinaculum is prepared and fixed by interpositioning in the proximal row [5, 18].

Ligament balancing is easier this way for destructive rheumatoid wrists than for carpal arthrodesis, as in four-corner-fusion.

The extensor carpi ulnaris tendon is captured by Swanson's slope (special prepared retinacula flap) on top of the dorsal ulna [2] or by distal ulna stabilization. Postoperative a special Vainio finger bandage and a volar plaster slab for the wrist should be worn for 6 nights [19]. For more detailed information and figures see the supplementary file "operation technique" (Additional file 1).

Assessment of the method

Between 1989 and 2002, 28 patients with 34 wrists were treated with distal resection interposition arthroplasty of the wrist at the department of rheumaorthopedic surgery. The average age was 60.6 years. Of these, 78.6% were female, and the dominant hand was affected in 50%. The duration of rheumatoid arthritis ranged from 9 to 54 years with a mean of 18.2 years. The time of follow-up after surgery ranged from 2 to 25 years with an average follow-up of 9.3 years. The interval between the onset of the disease and the operation was an average of approximately 9.1 years.

All patients were examined according to a special protocol. Basic information was recorded, including age, gender, affected side, duration of the disease and date of operation. They were further asked about pain, swelling and certain daily activities. The daily activities were evaluated according to a specially designed questionnaire (modified PROMs) that identified difficulties with common daily activities that could be affected by rheumatoid arthritis (functional questionnaire score, Additional file 2). The score is equal to the

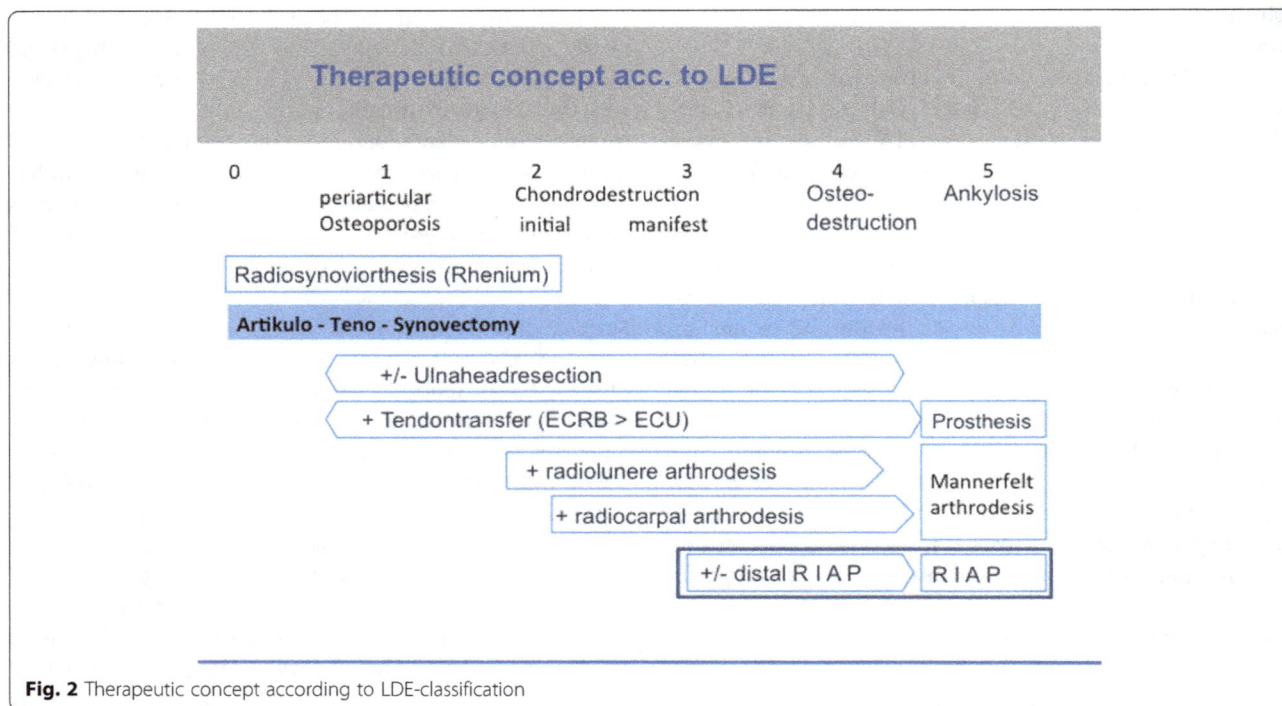

Therapeutic concept acc. to LDE

0	1	2		3	4	5
	periarticular Osteoporosis	Chondrodestruction initial	manifest		Osteo-destruction	Ankylosis

Radiosynoviorthesis (Rhenium)

Artikulo - Teno - Synovectomy

+/- Ulnaheadresection

+ Tendontransfer (ECRB > ECU)   Prosthesis

+ radiolunere arthrodesis

+ radiocarpal arthrodesis   Mannerfelt arthrodesis

+/- distal R I A P   R I A P

Fig. 2 Therapeutic concept according to LDE-classification

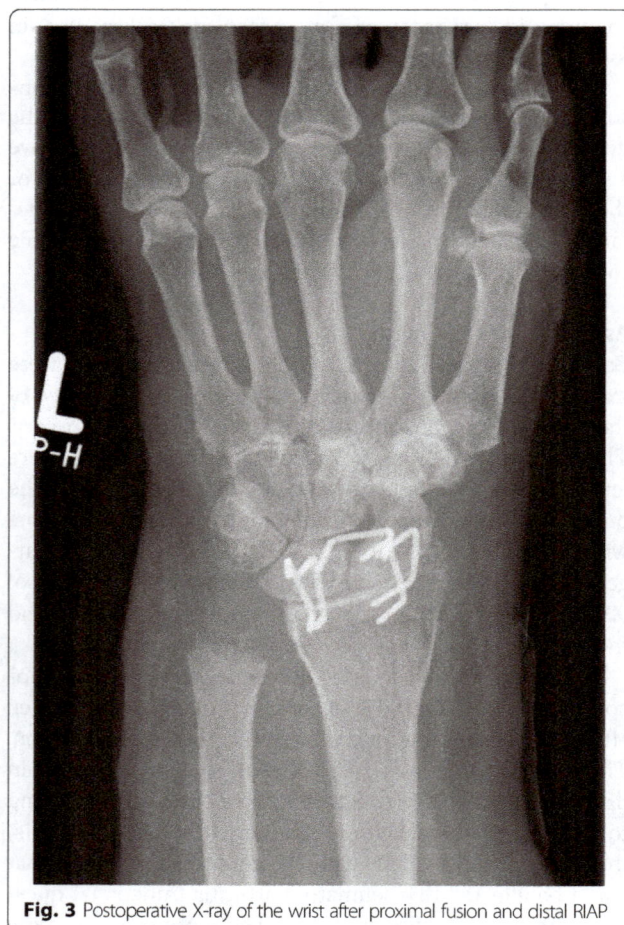

Fig. 3 Postoperative X-ray of the wrist after proximal fusion and distal RIAP

Quick-DASH-Score, using the same questions about daily life (Using a knife and fork for eating, hygiene, hair styling, using scissors, elevation of a hat, picking up coins, writing, lying down over the hand, using the keys and opening a bottle). A careful clinical and radiological examination was done to evaluate the degree of joint destruction according to the Larsen-Dale-Eek [20] and Simmen and Huber [17] classifications. The carpal height index and ulnar translation index [21] were also measured.

The results were assessed clinically and radiologically. Radiological examination was routinely performed 6 weeks postoperative. In cases of prolonged bone healing, there was another examination 4 weeks later. In addition, there was another radiological examination if patients reported new or prolonged problems at the time of clinical examination. The clinical assessment was based on a modified Clayton score system [22], as well as a functional questionnaire score, FFbH (4-point Likert-Scale with 30 points for 10 questions) [23]. A score of 30 was the best, and zero was the worst in terms of assessment of patient satisfaction. The clinical score according to the modified 100-point Clayton score was either excellent (90–100 points), good (70–89 points), fair (60–69 points) or poor (< 60 points). At the time of examination of rheumatoid patients in the mid-80s, the DASH-score and other comparable scores had not yet been established. In other studies from this department, we showed that the results of DASH-score and functional questionnaires for activities of daily living were statistically comparable [24].

The statistical analysis of the final results in terms of scores and age, as well as duration from the beginning of the disease to operation were assessed with a two-way ANOVA test and a Mann-Whitney-U-test for non-parametric samples. P-values of post hoc tests were adjusted for multiple comparisons. The level of significance was set at < 0.05 for all analyses.

Results

According to the Clayton score, 10 wrists (29.4%) showed excellent results, 14 wrists (41.2%) were good, 4 wrists (11.8%) were fair, and 6 wrists (17.6%) were poor (Table 1a). The Clayton score includes the parameters balance, mobility, pain reduction and extensor-strength. The fair results were compared to the preoperative data but were devaluated due to handicaps of the other joints. If we combined the categories excellent and good as satisfactory results and the fair plus poor categories as unsatisfactory results, then satisfactory results were found in 24 wrists (70.6%; $p = 0.00$), and unsatisfactory results were found in 10 wrists (29.4%, Additional file 3, Table 1a). The relationship between patient satisfaction and results at follow-up according to Clayton score were statistically significant (Additional file 3, Table 1b). Comparing the Clayton score with the functional questionnaire score, the correlation was also significant.

The pain details decreases from preoperative 6.3 pts. at the visual analog scale (V A S) to 2.6 pts. at time of follow-up. Most patients changed at time of follow-up from severe pain to mild or no pain. There were differences seen in pain intensity between satisfied patient

and these who were not satisfied with the results of the operation. These differences were statistically significant ($p = 0.058$).

Young patients as well as females showed better results, but with no statistical significance. The final results were inversely proportional to the age of the patients. Satisfactory results in young patients (mean age 58 years) were seen in 19 wrists against 15 wrists in older patients (mean age 63.7 years) ($p = 0.227$). From these 24 satisfactory wrists 19 were female wrists (79.2%) and 5 male wrists (20.8%). Unsatisfactory results were measured 6 times in female (60%) and 4 times in male wrists (40%) ($p = 0.248$).

The results were clearer with shorter duration of the disease and with shorter duration between the beginning of the disease and the operation (Additional file 4). This correlation was significant ($p = 0.049$) (Additional file 4). Furthermore, a statistically significant correlation was seen between the time of operation and the final result ($p = 0.026$). In all tests, the correlation was negative and widespread with a Spearman-correlation coefficient of – 0.5.

The operated wrists showed good range of motion especially among patients with satisfactory results (Additional file 3, Table 1c). A slight loss of motion was seen at time of follow-up, even more in patient with unsatisfactory results.

Regarding grip power after operation, we observed better results in 22 wrists, 5 wrists showed no power difference, and 7 wrists had diminished power after the operation. The correlation between wrist power and the final results was statistically significant at follow-up ($p = 0.028$) (Additional file 4). Concurrent problems in shoulder, elbow and fingers negatively affected the power of the wrist joint in these patients. In addition the grip strength was dissected in pinch, weight, extension strength and grip average tests. Except the key pinch all other results showed a positive correlation to the satisfactory subgroup (Additional file 4: Table S7ff).

As part of the score evaluation, patients were examined for shoulder, elbow and finger function. They were asked about pain and problems in daily life and were clinically examined. Patients with mild or no concurrent shoulder, elbow or finger problems showed better final wrist scores than patients with moderate or severe problems. Additionally the subjective results of the upper extremity joints were correlated to different results of the wrists. Next to Clayton-score the relation to grip power were pointed out (Additional file 4: Table S13ff.). Most problems were reported in finger joints in dissatisfied operations (70% severe or poor results with unsatisfactory wrists; $p = 0.084$), followed by shoulder problems (30%; $p = 0.961$) and at last elbow involvement (24%; $p = 0.566$). However, this difference was not statistically significant.

Table 1 a) overall results operated wrists; b) relation between patient satisfaction and functional questionnaire score [27]; c) range of motion and final results at follow-up

	Satisfactory	Unsatisfactory
a) Wrist (Grade)	24 (70.59%)	10 (29.41%)
Excellent	10 (29.4%)	
Good	14 (41.18%)	
Fair		4 (11.76%)
Poor		6 (17.65%)
b) Daily Score		
Minimum – Mean – Maximum	2.00–18.25 – 29.00	0.00–8.30–15.00
Std. Deviation	8.79353	4.73873
t	5.291	
p	.002	
c) Range of motion		
Flexion/Extension	15.97–0 – 22.5	11–0 – 1 .6
Ab–/Adduction	7.2–0 – 13	4.5–0 – 8.7
Pro-/Supination	73.75–0 – 47.9	63–0 – 43.5

Radiographic analysis

Hand function, including gripping force, depends primarily on the reconstruction of the carpal height. Only extensive reconstruction permits the physiological bias of the subsequent joints and tendons of the long finger, preventing further destruction or deformity of the carpus. The CHI (carpal height index, standard value: 0.54 +/- 0.03) was used here as a measuring method. In our cohort, this index was 0.4 after reconstruction and bone healing and statistically not significant ($p = 0.689$). This is slightly lower than in that of comparable studies [15: CHI: 0.48]. However, patients were treated surgically with a more advanced LDE stage in our study compared with other studies (LDE IV-V vs. III-IV). This difference was due to the preparation by fusion of the proximal row, and the destruction of the midcarpal row.

The radiological results showed a fusion rate of 94% (32/34 wrists), equal to that of other studies [9, 25].

Two wrists required revision with secondary total arthrodesis after 2 years.

Discussion

For the operative management of advanced rheumatoid hand destruction, total wrist arthrodesis is the most popular operation for most hand surgeons. Knowledge regarding the rheumatoid wrist, the long-term complex changes in these chronic diseases and the various therapies for these wrists is not widespread [1, 10]. For destroyed wrists of Larsen-stage III to IV, there are some alternative options, including proximal fusion with distal resection interposition arthroplasty. The advantage for total wrist fusion (TWF) is its simplicity, its general predictability and its predictable outcome. Moreover, arthroplasty has a high rate of aseptic loosening and other major complications such as dislocation or progressive instability [15, 26, 27]. For mobility and pain-free activities of daily living, arthroplasty is a highly rewarding procedure in certain conditions. However, operation numbers have decreased in recent years [14].

Most daily activities require combined movement of the wrist at the radiodorsal level, as well as in the ulnopalmar direction [28, 29]. Many kinematic studies have shown that the midcarpal joint is essential for common daily activities [28, 30]. Personal hygiene requires an active extension-flexion arc of 25 degrees, but other activities including eating, drinking, using the telephone or even reading a book require an active range of motion of approximately 40 degrees [16, 28]. Therefore, surgeons need to try to preserve midcarpal function as much as possible [31]. An almost adequate range of motion can be achieved after an appropriately aligned radiolunate or radioscapholunate fusion. Many patients, especially women, prefer the opportunity to have stable joints and acceptable motion, even if it is less [32]. This is because many patients have less pain and become accustomed to

the restriction [33]. Tillmann and Thabe also found that natural fusion of carpal joints to an os carpale preserved moderate mobility in combination with less pain [13].

Long-term results of more than 10 years after radiolunate arthrodesis showed sufficient residual mobility [34]. In mutilated wrists, midcarpal instability will persist with collapse of the carpus and lower CHI [30]. These joints could be transferred from an unstable to a stable secondary osteoarthritis form by this procedure [25, 35, 36]. Taleisnik reported that partial arthrodesis/fusion in patients with rheumatoid arthritis was an excellent procedure (up to Larsen III and mild IV) whether performed alone or in association with distal arthroplasty [3]. In our series, the combination of fusion of the proximal row with distal resection interposition arthroplasty offered required stability combined with a sufficient range of motion for coping with most daily activities.

Previous studies by various authors showed that radiocarpal arthrodesis within the first 5 years allowed patients painless movement with a stable proximal joint [3]. In these situations, similar results to those with the isolated proximal arthrodesis could be achieved [3, 37].

In addition to maintaining mobility in the wrist, the achievement of everyday pain relief is of crucial importance. Overall, most studies showed high numbers of pain free wrists (> 85%) with restrictions in joint-projected pain originating mostly from additional affected joints such as elbows or shoulders (34, 36).

Most follow-up studies of TWA report an average mobility of 40° to 50°, comparable with our results [25, 38]. Study results in posttraumatic arthritis were similar to results in rheumatoid patients [39, 40].

Persistent swelling is the main indicator of the activity of rheumatoid arthritis. Synovectomy has a direct impact on the postoperative result, as data have shown [34]. Patients with persistent swelling showed power loss and poor results that were associated with the progression of the rheumatoid disease and not with the operation itself.

Radiocarpal rather than midcarpal fusion is therefore recommended to preserve midcarpal function if the cartilage in the midcarpal joint is intact.

Murphy et al. reported a flexion-extension arc of approximately 76 degrees, a radio-ulnar deviation of 28 degrees and pronation-supination of 168 degrees after wrist arthroplasty, more than we reported in our series after RIAP [27]. Nevertheless, we believe that the stability from radiocarpal arthrodesis combined with a sufficient range of motion from distal RIAP in rheumatoid wrists offers the requirements necessary for the demands of daily activity.

Functional analysis of wrists with arthrodesis of the proximal row showed an oblique plane motion [29]. In addition, the wrist moved almost completely along either the sagittal or coronal plane, as long as forearm function was intact [21]. In affected rheumatoid wrists, the range of motion remained in the same plane but was smaller than in normal wrists.

Grip power

Stable and pain-free function of the wrist is a prerequisite for postoperatively increasing grip power. In the literature, better grip power, or at least 75% of the normal power in comparison with the opposite side, has been reported [36, 37].

In our series, the postoperative grip power in comparison with the preoperative status increased subjectively: 64% of the wrists had better power postoperatively, and only 20.5% had worse power ($p = 0.016$).

These results were influenced by the progressive destructive nature of rheumatoid arthritis, especially in the fingers and extensor tendons after long-standing rheumatoid disease. In our series, the duration prior to operation ranged from 9 to 54 years. Patients with no or mild finger problems showed significantly better grip power than patients with moderate or severe hand and finger problems.

In our study, we showed satisfactory results in more than 70% of patients after radiocarpal arthrodesis and distal RIAP of the midcarpal joint. In our cases with additional involvement of the midcarpal joint, distal RIAP restored the function of the joint and showed results close to those of an intact midcarpal joint. The mean value of the carpal height index was 0.4, with no significant correlation to the final results according Clayton score. The same applied for the ulnar translation index that had a mean of 0.28 and no significant correlation to the final Clayton score.

In comparison with other studies (also from our department), patient satisfaction showed comparable results to those of patients undergoing synovectomy or total wrist fusion (TWF) [36, 39]. Patient satisfaction with the operation and the outcome depended on finger and grip function [34]. The highest scores were seen in patients with early synovectomy and TWF.

Conclusion

The distal RIAP [5, 18] is a good alternative treatment for rheumatoid wrists with radiocarpal as well as midcarpal involvement [19, 37], as it provides the stability and satisfactory range of motion that is necessary for daily activities [22]. Revision and conversion to total arthrodesis in cases of unsatisfactory results is a salvage procedure without crucial loss of carpal height. The results of surgical intervention were better in early radiocarpal destructions and we suggest a more active approach than "wait and see" in rheumatic radiocarpal and midcarpal involvement.

Abbreviations
APW: Anatomical physiological wrist-prosthesis; ATS: Articulo-teno-synovectomy; CHI: Carpal-High-index; ECU: Extensor carpi ulnaris tendon; FFbH: Funktions-Fragebogen Hannover; LDE - Classification: Larsen, Dale and Eek – classification; MPW: Modular physiological wrist-prosthesis; PROMs: Patient reported outcome measures; RIAP: Resection-interposition-arthroplasty

Acknowledgements
We thank Christian Heiss, Prof., Chairman of the Clinic for trauma-, hand- and reconstructive surgery, Justus-Liebig-University Giessen for comments that greatly improved the manuscript.
We would like to thank Prof. Thabe for the opportunity to give his experience in the medical care of rheumatoid patients to us. He is and remains a great teacher for us.

Authors' contributions
CB and AO designed the retrospective cohort study and were responsible for data collection. CB, AO and SR were responsible for the patient reported outcomes component of the study. CB, AO and SR performed the statistical analysis and drafted the manuscript. UT and TB corrected the manuscript to improve the quality of the written English. GS made substantial contributions to analysis and interpretation of data. All authors read and approved the final manuscript.

Competing interests
The authors declare that they have no competing interests.

Author details
Klinik und Poliklinik für Unfall-, Hand- und Wiederherstellungschirurgie - Operative Notaufnahme, UKGM Gießen, Rudolf-Buchheim-Str. 7, 35392 Giessen, Germany. ²Klinik für orthopädische Chirurgie der unteren Extremitäten und Endoprothetik, Krankenhaus Rummelsberg GmbH, Rummelsberg 71, 90592, Schwarzenbruck, Germany. ³Klinik für Orthopädie und Unfallchirurgie, AGAPLESION MARKUS KRANKENHAUS, Chefarzt Prof. Dr. med. Stefan Rehart, Wilhelm–Epstein–Straße 4, D-60431 Frankfurt am Main, Germany.

References
1. Dinges H, Furst M, Ruther H, Schill S. Operative differential therapy of rheumatic wrists. Z Rheumatol. 2007;66:388–94.
2. Swanson AB, de Groot Swanson G, Maupin BK. Flexible implant arthroplasty of the radiocarpal joint. Surgical technique and long-term study. Clin Orthop Relat Res. 1984;(187):94–106.
3. Taleisnik J. Combined radiocarpal arthrodesis and midcarpal (lunocapitate) arthroplasty for treatment of rheumatoid arthritis of the wrist. J Hand Surg. 1987;12:1–8.
4. Malahias M, Gardner H, Hindocha S, Juma A, Khan W. The future of rheumatoid arthritis and hand surgery - combining evolutionary pharmacology and surgical technique. Open Orthopaedics J. 2012;6(1):88–94.
5. Thabe H. Das Handgelenk. In: Thabe H and Brackertz D. (eds.) *Praktische Rheumaorthopädie*, Chapman and Hall, 1997.
6. Bhamra J, Bhamra K, Hindocha S, Khan W. The role of wrist fusion and wrist arthroplasty in rheumatoid arthritis. Curr Rheumatol Rev. 2017;13(1):23–8.
7. Kane PM, Stull JD, Culp RW. Concomitant Total wrist and Total elbow arthroplasty in a rheumatoid patient. J Wrist Surg. 2016;5(2):137–42.
8. Wei DH, Feldon P. Total wrist arthrodesis: indications and clinical outcomes. J Am Acad Orthop Surg. 2017;25(1):3–11.
9. Meier R, Lanz U, Krimmer H. Partial fusion of the wrist - an alternative procedure to the total wrist arthrodesis. Unfallchirurg. 2002;105:762–74.
10. Clayton ML, Ferlic DA et al. Arthroplasty of the wrist. In: Simmen B.R, Hagena, F-W (eds). *The wrist in rheumatoid arthritis*. 1st edition, Basel, Karger 1992, 17: 186–197.
11. Ghattas L, Mascella F, Pomponio G. Hand surgery in rheumatoid arthritis: state of the art and suggestions for research. Rheumatology (Oxford). 2005;44:834–45.
12. Raven EEJ, van den Bekerom MPJ, Beumer A, van Dijk CN. Radiocarpal and Midcarpal instability in rheumatoid patients: a systematic review. Open Orthopaedics J. 2015;9:246–54.
13. Tillmann K, Thabe H. Technique and results of resection and interposition arthroplasty of the wrist in rheumatoid arthritis. Reconstr Surg Traumatol. 1981;18:84–91.

14. Gordon LH, King D. Partial wrist arthrodesis for old un-united fractures of the carpal navicular. Am J Surg. 1961;102:460–4.
15. Harlingen D, Heesterbeek PJ, JdV M. High rate of complications and radiographic loosening of the biaxial total wrist arthroplasty in rheumatoid arthritis: 32 wrists followed for 6 (5-8) years. Acta Orthop. 2011;82(6):721–6.
16. Brumfield RH, Champoux JA. A biomechanical study of normal functional wrist motion. Clin Orthop Relat Res. 1984;(187):23–5.
17. Simmen BR, Huber H. The wrist joint in chronic polyarthritis--a new classification based on the type of destruction in relation to the natural course and the consequences for surgical therapy. Handchir Mikrochir Plast Chir. 1994;26:182–9.
18. Thabe H. Endoprosthetic replacement of the rheumatoid wrist. Z Rheumatol. 2011;70:395–9.
19. Carlsen BT, Shin AY. Wrist instability. Scand J Surg. 2008;97:324–32.
20. Larsen A, Dale K, Eek M. Radiographic evaluation of rheumatoid arthritis and related conditions by standard reference films. Acta Radiol Diagn. 1977;18:481–91.
21. Youme Y, McMurthy RY, Flatt AE, Gillespie TE. Kinematics of the wrist. I. An experimental study of radial-ulnar deviation and flexion-extension. J Bone Joint Surg Am Vol. 1978;60:423–31.
22. Clayton ML. Surgery of the rheumatoid hand. Clin Orthop. 1964;36:47–59.
23. Raspe H, Hagedorn U, Kohlmann T, Matussek S. Funktionsfragebogen ffbh. Ein Instrument zur Funktionsdiagnostik bei polyartikulären Erkrankungen. In: Sigrist j (hrsg) wohnortnahe Betreuung Rheumakranker. In: Rheumatologie DG (eds.) Qualitätssicherung in der Rheumatologie. Stuttgart, New York, Steinkopff, 1990 / 2008.
24. Biehl C, Stoll M, Jung J. The MPH-wrist prosthesis in rheumatoid patients, long-term results. London: EFORT; 2014.
25. Kilgus M, Weishaupt D, Kunzi W, Meyer VE. Radioscapholunate fusion: long-term results. Handchir Mikrochir Plast Chir. 2003;35:317–22.
26. Cavaliere CM, Chung KC. Total wrist arthroplasty and total wrist arthrodesis in rheumatoid arthritis: a decision analysis from the hand surgeons' perspective. J Hand Surg. 2008;33(10):1744–55.
27. Murphy DM, Khoury JG, Imbriglia JE, Adams BD. Comparison of arthroplasty and arthrodesis for the rheumatoid wrist. J Hand Surg Am. 2003;28:570–6.
28. Saffar P, Seumaan I. The study of the biomechanics of wrist movements in an oblique plane. In: Schvind FA, An KN, Cooney WP, Garcia-Elias M, editors. Advances in the biomechanics of the hand and wrist. New York: Plenum Press; 1994. p. 305–11.
29. Werner FW, Green JK, Short WH, Masaoka S. Scaphoid and lunate motion during a wrist dart throw motion. J Hand Surg Am. 2004;29:418–22.
30. Goto A, Moritomo H, Murase T, et al. In vivo three-dimensional wrist motion analysis using magnetic resonance imaging and volume-based registration. J Orthop Res. 2005;23:750–6.
31. Moritomo H, Murase T, Goto A, Oka K, Sugamoto K, Yoshikawa H. Capitate-based kinematics of the midcarpal joint during wrist radioulnar deviation: an in vivo three-dimensional motion analysis. J Hand Surg. 2004;29:668–75.
32. Melamed E, Marascalchi B, Hinds RM, Rizzo M, Capo JT. Trends in the utilization of Total wrist arthroplasty versus wrist fusion for treatment of advanced wrist arthritis. J Wrist Surg. 2016;5(3):211–6.
33. Chung KC, Kotsis SV. Outcomes of hand surgery in the patient with rheumatoid arthritis. Curr Opin Rheumatol. 2010;22(3):336–41.
34. Schill S, Luhr T, Thabe H. Radiolunate arthrodesis of the rheumatoid wrist - mid- and long-term results. Z Rheumatol. 2002;61:551–9.
35. Borisch N, Haussmann P. The rheumatoid wrist. Pathobiomechanics and therapy. Der Orthopade. 2002;31:1159–67.
36. Ishikawa H, Murasawa A, Nakazono K. Long-term follow-up study of radiocarpal arthrodesis for the rheumatoid wrist. J Hand Surg. 2005;30:658–66.
37. Honkanen PB, Makela S, Konttinen YT, Lehto MU. Radiocarpal arthrodesis in the treatment of the rheumatoid wrist. A prospective midterm follow-up. J Hand Surg Eur Vol. 2007;32:368–76.
38. Kuhlmann JN, Fahrer M, Kapandji IA, Tubiana R. Stability of the normal wrist In: Tubiana R. The hand, Saunders, 1998.
39. Boeckstyns ME, Herzberg G, Merser S. Favorable results after total wrist arthroplasty: 65 wrists in 60 patients followed for 5-9 years. Acta Orthop. 2013;84(4):415–9.
40. Lautenbach M, Millrose M, Langner I, Eisenschenk A. Results of Mannerfelt wrist arthrodesis for rheumatoid arthritis in relation to the position of the fused wrist. Int Orthop. 2013;37(12):2409–13.

7

Validation of the Liverpool Elbow Score for evaluation of elbow stiffness

Ziyang Sun[1] and Cunyi Fan[1,2]*

Abstract

Background: The Liverpool Elbow Score (LES) has been widely used to assess the outcomes of total elbow replacement in various conditions. However, there have been no published validation studies on LES for patients with stiff elbows undergoing arthrolysis. The purpose of this study was to find out whether LES could be equally applied to evaluate joint function in patients with elbow stiffness.

Methods: A total of 63 patients with elbow stiffness were included in this retrospective validation study. The LES combines a nine-item patient-answered questionnaire (PAQ) and a six-item clinical assessment score (CAS), and can also be divided to evaluate two different parameters: elbow motion capacity (EMC) and elbow-related symptoms (ERS). Construct validity was assessed by correlating LES with previously validated scoring systems, and Spearman correlation coefficients (SCCs) were calculated. Effect size (ES) and standardized response mean (SRM) were calculated to determine responsiveness.

Results: There were no ceiling or floor effects in the target population. Good-to-excellent validity was determined based on total score (0.45–0.89), PAQ (0.42–0.88), CAS (0.35–0.60), EMC (0.46–0.86), and ERS (0.36–0.59). High responsiveness (ES/SRM) was observed in total score (2.80/2.24), PAQ (2.34/1.78), CAS (2.90/2.34), EMC (2.92/2.35), and ERS (0.55/0.52).

Conclusion: Our results suggest that the LES is a valid elbow-specific scoring system that can be used to evaluate joint function in patients with elbow stiffness, though some items included had some weakness either.

Keywords: Liverpool elbow score, Elbow stiffness, Scoring systems, Validation, Validity, Responsiveness

Background

Elbow stiffness is a well-recognized disabling condition that causes functional impairment in the upper limb and interferes with daily activities. It is a very common complication after injuries or secondary to arthropathy, as both bony and soft tissue factors are the most important aetiologies [1–3]. Patients with limited elbow motion usually complain of difficulties in work, leisure activities, and even basic activities of daily living. Sometimes they are troubled with symptoms like pain, numbness, weakness, and instability. Clinical scoring systems are the most popular functional measurements used in the evaluation of orthopaedic patients. These systems are used to estimate the severity of dysfunction, evaluate treatment effectiveness, and compare different treatment methods [4, 5].

The Liverpool Elbow Score (LES, Fig. 1) was first introduced in 2004 as an elbow-specific outcome score to be completed by both the clinicians and patients. The LES combines a nine-item patient-answered questionnaire (PAQ, P1-P9) and a six-item clinical assessment score (CAS, C1-C6) [6]. The CAS comprises items that evaluate range of motion (C1-C4), muscle strength (C5), and ulnar nerve function (C6), whereas the PAQ assesses function and the ability to perform activities of daily living (P1-P7), levels of pain (P8), and participation in sporting and recreational activities (P9). The components of the LES, similar to most other elbow-related scoring systems, could also be divided into 2 parts comprising elbow motion capacities (EMC, C1-C4 and P1-P7 and P9) and elbow-related symptoms (ERS, C5-C6 and P8). ERS covers the items pertaining to muscle strength (C5) and ulnar nerve function (C6) from

* Correspondence: cyfan@sjtu.edu.cn
[1]Department of Orthopaedics, Shanghai Jiao Tong University Affiliated Sixth People's Hospital, 600 Yishan Road, Shanghai 200233, People's Republic of China
[2]Department of Orthopaedics, Shanghai Sixth People's Hospital East Affiliated to Shanghai University of Medicine & Health Sciences, Shanghai, People's Republic of China

	Score 4	Score 3	Score 2	Score 1	Score 0
Clinical assessment					
C1 Flexion	–	>135°	120–135°	90–120°	<90°
C2 Extension	–	None	<20	20–30°	>30°
C3 Pronation (add 1 to score if wrist/forearm pathology)		–	>50°	50–20°	<20°
C4 Supination (add 1 to score if wrist/forearm pathology)		–	>50°	50–20°	<20°
C5 Strength: average of flexion, extension, pronation and supination	Apparently normal	Complete motion against gravity and some resistance	Complete motion against gravity	Complete motion with gravity eliminated	Absent
C6 Ulnar nerve	–	None	Sensory	Motor: no disability	Motor: with disability
Patient-answered questions: *During the past four weeks:*					
P1 How often have you had to use your other arm to do things normally done by the affected arm?	Never	Once or twice	Sometimes	Many times	Every time
P2 Has your elbow problem caused you any difficulty in combing your hair?	None	Little	Moderate	Severe	Unable to do
P3 Has your elbow problem caused you any difficulty in washing yourself?	None	Little	Moderate	Severe	Unable to do
P4 Has your elbow problem caused you any difficulty in feeding yourself?	None	Little	Moderate	Severe	Unable to do
P5 Has your elbow problem caused you any difficulty in dressing yourself?	None	Little	Moderate	Severe	Unable to do
P6 Has your elbow problem caused you any difficulty in trying to do household activities?	None	Little	Moderate	Severe	Unable to do
P7 Has your elbow problem caused you any difficulty in lifting, e.g. a kettle, a milk bottle, groceries?	None	Little	Moderate	Severe	Unable to do
P8 How would you describe the pain from this elbow?	None	Little	Moderate	Severe	Unbearable
P9 Has your elbow problem affected your sport and leisure activities?	None	Little	Moderate	Severe	Unable to do

Fig. 1 The components of the Liverpool Elbow Score

the CAS and pain (P8) from the PAQ. The remaining items form the EMC (C1-C4, P1-P7 and P9). In the original study, all items were measured on a scale from 0 to 10 and transformed in the calculation of the final score. The final scores were calculated as "final scores (LES) = (2/9) * (C1 + C2 + C3 + C4 + C6) + (1/6) * (C5 + P1 + P2 + P3 + P4 + P5 + P6 + P7 + P8 + P9)", with values ranging from 0 to 10. The lower scores represented greater symptom and functional severity. Detailed item distributions in each of the different parts along with the individual score calculations and score ranges are shown in Table 1.

After being demonstrated to be a reliable, valid and responsive outcome tool, the LES began to be used to assess outcomes after total elbow replacement in the management of rheumatoid arthritis [7, 8], posttraumatic arthritis [8–10], olecranon fractures [10] and distal humeral fractures [11, 12]. However, there have been no published validation studies of LES for patients with stiff elbows undergoing arthrolysis. Additionally, a well-established validation study might not be applicable to different populations, which means that a previously validated tool might have to be re-validated to justify its use in different populations [13]. Therefore, the purpose of this study was to determine whether the LES can be equally applied in different populations to evaluate joint function in patients with elbow stiffness.

Methods
Translation procedure
All the scoring systems (LES: Liverpool Elbow Score; DASH: Disability of arm, shoulder and hand questionnaire; OES: Oxford Elbow Score; MEPS: Mayo Elbow Performance Score; SF-36: Short Form-36) used in this

Table 1 Items distribution, scores calculation and score ranges of LES and different parts

Part	Items distribution	Scores calculation	Score ranges	
			Best	Worst
LES (total)	C1-C6, P1-P9	(2/9)* (C1 + C2 + C3 + C4 + C6) + (1/6)* (C5 + P1 + P2 + P3 + P4 + P5 + P6 + P7 + P8 + P9)	10	0
PAQ	P1-P9	(1/6)* (P1 + P2 + P3 + P4 + P5 + P6 + P7 + P8 + P9)	6	0
CAS	C1-C6	(2/9)* (C1 + C2 + C3 + C4 + C6) + (1/6)* (C5)	4	0
EMC	C1-C4, P1-P7, P9	(2/9)* (C1 + C2 + C3 + C4) + (1/6)* (P1 + P2 + P3 + P4 + P5 + P6 + P7 + P9)	8	0
ERS	C5-C6, P8	(2/9)* (C6) + (1/6)* (C5 + P8)	2	0

LES Liverpool Elbow Score, *PAQ* patient-answered questionnaire part, *CAS* clinical assessment score part, *EMC* elbow motion capacity, *ERS* elbow-related symptoms

study were translated into Simplified Chinese (Mainland) versions prior to having patients complete the questionnaires. Among these, MEPS has been widely used in China to evaluate elbow function, and validations of DASH and SF-36 have been performed in China [14, 15]. For LES and OES, however, there have been no other validation studies for these two scores in Simplified Chinese (Mainland) versions to this point.

Therefore, a 6-step method was used that included translation, synthesis, back-translation, expert committee review, pre-testing, and submission for appraisal, according to the guidelines of the cross-cultural adaptation process provided by Guillemin et al. [16, 17]. Briefly, the English versions of the LES and OES were translated separately by two native Chinese translators. A synthesized Simplified Chinese (Mainland) translation version was established after uniform agreement was reached between the two translators. The translated versions which was back-translated by two native English bilingual speakers who were blinded to the original English version. Then the four translators and two orthopaedic surgeons composed an expert committee that was established to compare the Chinese version to the original and back-translated versions. After an agreement on the semantic, idiomatic, experiential, and conceptual equivalence between the original and the target versions, and with an absence of language issues when the final version was pretested in 15 Chinese patients with elbow stiffness, the expert committee reached a consensus on the final version.

Patients and study design

This was a retrospective validation study of patients who presented to our institution for elbow arthrolysis secondary to elbow stiffness between September 2016 and December 2016. Exclusion criteria were (1) unwillingness to participate or cooperate with follow-up; (2) illiteracy or an inability to comprehend the contents of the questionnaires; and (3) mental illness. All the patients underwent open arthrolysis by the same surgeon (C. F.) [18]. During the study period, 81 patients underwent surgery for elbow stiffness at our institution. Of these, 68 met the inclusion criteria. However, 5 of the 68 were excluded because of refusal or loss to follow up. The remaining 63 included patients were 45 men and 18 women, with a mean age of 35 years and a mean follow-up time of 13 months (other demographics and characteristics are shown in Table 2). The sample size of the respondents for validation of a scoring system was assumed to exceed three times the number of items in the system [19]. Therefore, with a total of 15 items, a total sample size of 63 was considered sufficient. All patients were asked to complete the patient-rated parts of LES, DASH, OES and SF-36. The physician-rated parts of

Table 2 Demographics and clinical characteristics of patients

Characteristics	
No. of patients	63
Male	45 (71)
Age, years	35 ± 13 (11–62)
Height, cm	169 ± 9, (143–188)
Weight, Kg	66 ± 13, (32–105)
BMI, kg/m2	23.1 ± 3.4 (15.7–32.2)
Dominant arm	34 (54)
Follow-up time[a], months	13 ± 1 (12–15)

Categorical variables are presented as number (%)
Continuous variables presented as mean ± standard deviation, (range)
BMI body mass index
[a]follow-up time means month post-operation from elbow release

LES and MEPS were assessed following a written protocol so that all the patients were examined using the same method.

Testing and evaluation of measurement qualities

Floor and ceiling effects, reliability, construct validity, and responsiveness were required for a full validation of the scoring system [20, 21].

Reliability

Reliability measures whether the scores of the same patient show differences when implemented at different times or by different doctors (test-retest reliability), and whether the items in a domain have measured the same concept (internal consistency). However, this could not be measured due to the retrospective nature of our study.

Construct validity

Construct validity is defined as the degree to which the scores of a particular instrument are related to a gold standard test. Unfortunately, no gold standard test has been established to reflect pre- and post-arthrolysis status. The DASH can be used to measure disability in any region of the upper limb and has been shown to be valid and responsive compared to other joint-specific measures of the upper extremity, and comprises 2 parts (Disability and Symptoms) [22]. The OES was reported to be a valid, reliable, and responsive self-administered instrument that can be used for several types of elbow function measurements, and it comprise 3 parts (Pain, Elbow Function and Social-psychological) [23]. The DASH and OES have been shown to correlate to general health measures such as the SF-36 [23, 24]. Consisting of physician-rated pain, ROM, stability, and a patient-rated daily function, MEPS [25] was the most widely used elbow function assessment, according to a systematic review including 980 studies and exploring trends and distributions of clinical rating systems in elbow research [26]. Construct validity was assessed by correlating LES to DASH, OES, MEPS, and SF-36 (PCS and MCS) in total scores (TOTAL), PAQ, CAS, EMC and ERS. Spearman's correlation coefficients (SCCs) were calculated. In this study, the Disability portion of DASH, the Elbow Function portion of OES, and the range of motion and daily activity function portion of MEPS comprised the EMC. The symptom portion of DASH, the pain portion of OES, and the pain and stability portions of MEPS comprised the ERS. The TOTAL, PAQ, and CAS portions of the LES were correlated with the TOTAL portions of DASH, OES, MEPS, and SF-36 (PCS and MCS). EMC and ERS portions of the LES were correlated with EMC and the ERS portions of DASH, OES and MEPS, as well as the TOTAL part of SF-36 (PCS and MCS).

Responsiveness

Responsiveness measures the sensitivity in changes in preoperative and follow-up results. In our study, the effect size (ES) and standardized response mean (SRM) were calculated for the TOTAL part of LES, DASH, OES, MEPS, and SF-36 (PCS and MCS) and the EMC and ERS parts of LES, DASH, OES, MEPS, as well as CAS and PAQ parts of LES. The ES was calculated as the mean difference between the baseline scores and the follow-up scores divided by the standard deviation of the baseline scores [27]. The SRM was calculated as the mean change in the scores divided by the standard deviation of the change in scores [28].

Statistical analyses

All statistical analyses were performed using IBM SPSS, Version 22.0 (IBM Corp, Armonk, NY, USA). Categorical data are presented as numbers (percentages). Continuous data are presented as means ± standard deviations (range). P values of less than 0.05 were considered statistically significant. Floor or ceiling effects existed when more than 15% of the patient collective achieved the highest or lowest possible score on the LES [29].SCC was considered strong for construct validity if the value was greater than 0.5, moderate if the value was between 0.5 and 0.35, and weak if the value was less than 0.35 [30]. An ES of 0.2 to 0.5 reflected small responsiveness, 0.5 to 0.8, moderate responsiveness, and greater than 0.8, large responsiveness, as well as SRM [31].

Results

All patients completed the PAQ with no difficulties and with no items missing or showing multiple responses. No floor or ceiling effects were found in the target population (Table 3). All of the SCCs were positive except the relationship with DASH, which was scored in a different direction (Table 4). The LES overall scores

Table 3 Floor and ceiling effects of LES

Component	LES (No.[a])		Floor effect (%[b])	Ceiling effect (%[b])
	Lower limit	Upper limit		
TOTAL	2.3 (1)	9.1 (1)	0	0
PAQ	0.8 (1)	6.0 (1)	0	0
CAS	1.1 (1)	3.1 (2)	0	1.6
EMC	0.8 (1)	7.1 (1)	0	0
ERS	1.1 (1)	2.0 (4)	0	6.4

LES Liverpool Elbow Score, *TOTAL* total scores, *PAQ* patient-answered questionnaire, *CAS* clinical assessment score part, *EMC* elbow motion capacity, *ERS* elbow-related symptoms
[a]Number of patients showing the lowest or highest values in various parts;
[b]Percent of patients achieving the lowest or highest values in various parts

correlated well with all the compared total scores ($p < 0.001$ for all), as DASH ($r = 0.89$ preoperatively and 0.86 post-operatively), OES ($r = 0.83$ and 0.79), MEPS ($r = 0.66$ and 0.49), SF-36 (PCS, $r = 0.65$ and 0.64; MCS, $r = 0.45$ and 0.68), as well as with the PAQ and CAS parts of LES. The EMC and ERS parts of LES correlated either strongly or moderately with similar parts of DASH, OES, and MEPS as well as with SF-36/PCS and SF-36/MCS preoperatively and postoperatively. All in all, the different LES parts also correlated well with DASH, OES, MEPS, and SF-36, with either high or moderate correlations in TOTAL (0.45–0.89), PAQ (0.42–0.88), CAS (0.35–0.60), EMC (0.46–0.86), and ERS (0.36–0.59).

The LES was found to be more responsive (change from preoperative to follow up) than all the compared scores: DASH, OES, MEPS and SF-36 scores (Table 5).

Table 4 Construct validity. Spearman Correlation Coefficients (SCCs) between LES and DASH, OES, MEPS and SF-36

	TOTAL	PAQ	CAS	EMC	ERS
Preoperative data					
DASH	0.89***	0.88***	0.44***	0.86***	0.54***
OES	0.83***	0.82***	0.45***	0.82***	0.51***
MEPS	0.66***	0.65***	0.38**	0.67***	0.36**
SF-36/PCS	0.65***	0.63***	0.42**	0.60***	0.45***
SF-36/MCS	0.45***	0.42**	0.35**	0.50***	0.41**
Follow-up data					
DASH	0.86***	0.87***	0.57***	0.72***	0.59***
OES	0.79***	0.87***	0.46***	0.69***	0.54***
MEPS	0.49***	0.53***	0.35**	0.46***	0.43***
SF-36/PCS	0.64***	0.50***	0.52***	0.52***	0.50***
SF-36/MCS	0.68***	0.50***	0.60***	0.60***	0.50***

LES Liverpool Elbow Score, *TOTAL* total scores, *PAQ* patient-answered questionnaire, *CAS* clinical assessment score, *EMC* elbow motion capacity, *ERS* elbow-related symptoms, *DASH* Disability of arm, shoulder and hand questionnaire, *OES* Oxford Elbow Score, *MEPS* Mayo Elbow Performance Score, *SF-36/PCS* physical component summary part of Short Form-36, *SF-36/MCS* mental component summary part of Short Form-36, *SCCs* Spearman Correlation Coefficients
**$P < 0.01$, ***$P < 0.001$

Table 5 Responsiveness of LES compared with DASH, OES, MEPS and SF-36

Questionnaires	Mean (SD)			P value	ES	SRM
	Preoperative	Follow-up	Change			
LES						
TOTAL	5.7 (1.3)	8.8 (0.8)	3.1 (1.4)	< 0.001	2.80 (L)	2.24 (L)
PAQ	3.4 (1.1)	5.5 (0.5)	2.1 (1.2)	< 0.001	2.34 (L)	1.78 (L)
CAS	2.3 (0.4)	3.3 (0.3)	1.0 (0.4)	< 0.001	2.90 (L)	2.34 (L)
EMC	3.9 (1.2)	6.9 (0.7)	3.0 (1.3)	< 0.001	2.92 (L)	2.35 (L)
ERS	1.8 (0.2)	1.9 (0.2)	0.1 (0.2)	0.001	0.55 (M)	0.52 (M)
DASH						
TOTAL	35 (18)	8 (9)	27 (18)	< 0.001	1.96 (L)	1.51 (L)
EMC	27 (15)	5 (8)	22 (15)	< 0.001	1.90 (L)	1.48 (L)
ERS	7 (4)	3 (2)	4 (4)	< 0.001	1.41 (L)	1.04 (L)
OES						
TOTAL	61 (16)	88 (9)	27 (17)	< 0.001	2.12 (L)	1.65 (L)
EMC	65 (19)	95 (11)	30 (19)	< 0.001	1.99 (L)	1.61 (L)
ERS	74 (19)	86 (11)	13 (20)	< 0.001	0.81 (L)	0.63 (M)
MEPS						
TOTAL	65 (12)	88 (7)	23 (14)	< 0.001	2.32 (L)	1.72 (L)
EMC	23 (10)	44 (2)	22 (10)	< 0.001	2.87 (L)	2.11 (L)
ERS	42 (8)	44 (6)	2 (8)	0.064	0.26 (S)	0.21 (S)
SF-36						
PCS	60 (17)	82 (17)	22 (26)	< 0.001	1.28 (L)	0.83 (L)
MCS	53 (20)	78 (18)	24 (25)	< 0.001	1.28 (L)	0.98 (L)

LES Liverpool Elbow Score, *TOTAL* total scores, *PAQ* patient-answered questionnaire, *CAS* clinical assessment score, *EMC* elbow motion capacity, *ERS* elbow-related symptoms, *DASH* Disability of arm, shoulder and hand questionnaire, *OES* Oxford Elbow Score, *MEPS* Mayo Elbow Performance Score, *PCS* physical component summary part, *MCS* mental component summary part, *SD* standard deviation, *ES* effect size, *SRM* standardized response mean
(L) a large responsiveness, ES of greater than 0.8; (M) a moderate responsiveness, ES of 0.5 to 0.8; and (S) a small responsiveness, ES of less than 0.5; as well as SRM

LES showed a large (ES/SRM > 0.8/0.8) responsiveness for TOTAL (2.80/2.24, $p < .001$), and all parts of the PAQ, CAS, and EMC (except for ERS with a moderate responsiveness of 0.55/0.52, $p = .001$). This analysis also showed that LES was more responsive than DASH with an ES/SRM of 1.96/1.51 ($p < .001$), OES of 2.12/1.65 ($p < .001$), MEPS of 2.32/1.72 ($p < .001$) and SF-36 (PCS, 1.28/0.83, $p < .001$ and MCS, 1.28/0.98, $p < .001$).

Discussion

The most important finding of this study was that the LES was a valid elbow-specific scoring system to evaluate joint functions in patients with elbow stiffness, and contains both subjective and objective parameters. It is based on a 15-item tool with a scale ranging from 0 to 10 points, with higher scores indicating better function.

The LES was simple enough to be rapidly administered in clinics and there were no ceiling or floor effects in our study, which demonstrated that the distribution of LES was satisfactory. Regrettably, reliability could not be measured due to the retrospective study design. Construct validity and responsiveness were assessed for validation. Because

no gold standard measurement had been established for comparison of the construct validity between elbow scores, correlations (SCCs) of LES with previously validated scoring systems were determined by 0.44–0.89 for DASH and 0.35–0.67 for MEPS. In fact, validity was shown by good correlations with DASH ($r = 0.79$; $r = 0.89$ preoperatively and 0.86 postoperatively in our study) and NHP (Nottingham Health Profile, $r = 0.54$) in the original publication study for arthritis [6]. Additionally, a good correlation (SCC, 0.84; 0.66 in this study) was also shown with MEPS for patients undergoing total elbow arthroplasty [8]. Currently, the method of choice to determine responsiveness remains unknown, though various statistics are available [32]. The determination of the effective size (ES) and standardized response mean (SRM) in addition to the Global Perceived Effect (GPE) Score was considered to be an appropriate improvement to assess responsiveness [33]. Due to the retrospective nature of the study, ES and SRM were calculated and a large responsiveness was found in LES, which were larger than DASH, OES, MEPS, and SF-36 in our study. The responsiveness of LES was found to correlate well with DASH (r = 0.45; 0.85 in our study) and NHP (r = 0.42) in the original study [6]. LES was also found to have large ES (1.64; 2.80 in our study), SRM (1.25; 2.24 in our study) and GRR (Guyatt responsiveness ratio, 1.69) during the follow-up period for patients undergoing elbow arthroplasty [32]. Interestingly, we found a lower responsiveness in ERS compared to DASH and OES. Our explanation for this difference was that there were extra stiffness items and quality of life items in the ERS of DASH, and the ERS of OES contains only items for pain, which would contribute to the bias of the comparison.

Recently, self-assessment scores in outcome studies are becoming more and more popular due to their financial and logistic advantages [34]. However, leaving objective parameters out might miss important aspects of elbow pathology that are important in symptom assessment and are impossible to evaluate by only using a self-assessment score. These aspects include elbow instability, reduced muscle strength, and nerve dysfunction. In fact, functions and symptoms in an individual joint may not be evaluated accurately by subjective questionnaires alone [35]. The questions presented to patients are also sometimes lengthy and not relevant to specific problems [36]. Objective parameters alone have been also found to have no correlation with patient's satisfaction [37], life background, since expectations and satisfaction are different for different individuals. Therefore, it is preferable for the LES to be used to evaluate the joint functions of patients with elbow stiffness by using self-assessment questionnaires in addition to physician-assessment parameters.

However, there are also some weaknesses that need to be realized when using the LES to evaluate joint function in patients with elbow stiffness. The researchers that invented the LES decided to remove the instability test from the objective parameters as they thought it was associated with a rare elbow problem. When presented, it would have such a massive impact on elbow function that it would be easily detected [6]. However, according to our clinical experience, we believe that elbow instability is a perfect sign of collateral ligament dysfunction, which is a common complication in elbow trauma, and an indication for surgical therapeutic options and postoperative rehabilitation. Therefore, it would be better if instability was considered. For measuring strength as an elbow specific function, the MRC scale was used in most systems, as was the LES, which is a subjective qualitative assessment made by the surgeons. However, L Shahgholi. found that half of the patients clinically assessed as having normal (5/5) elbow flexion strength on manual muscle testing exhibited less than 42% of their age-expected strength on quantitative testing, as well as elbow extension strength testing. They concluded that even when performed by experienced clinicians, manual muscle testing may be more misleading than expected for subjects graded as having normal (5/5) strength [38, 39].

Therefore, measuring strength with a dynamometer would be a more objective and responsive measure than measuring strength with the MRC scale, and it could be measured over time and compared to normative data. Strength associated with grip, elbow and wrist motion are all necessary in assessing elbow function, especially in patients planning for elbow arthrolysis surgery, as reduced muscle strength is a common complication after arthrolysis [40]. Additionally, pain has a strong impact on elbow function and health status measures [41]. Due to the strong influence of psychological and sociological factors on the experience of pain, the expression of pain should probably be evaluated separately from objective parameters in physician-rated domains [42]. Though the expression of pain is obtained from the PAQ portion of the LES, it comprises only 1/9 ($\sim$ 11%) of the PAQ and 1/15 ($\sim$ 7%) of the whole scores, which is in contrast to most of other scoring systems, in which pain is weighted as 30–50% of the total score [4, 5]. In fact, a five-level Likert scale could not fully generalize the expression of pain from patients and detect its changes from pre- to post-operation. We believe that these limitations may also contribute to its moderate responsiveness in the ERS. Finally, according to the International Classification of Functioning, Disability and Health (ICF), health and disability would be better measured in three domains: physician-rated body functions and structures, patient-rated activities and participation, and patient-rated quality of life [43]. Unfortunately, LES does not include items inquiring about patients' qualities of life.

This study has some weaknesses. The biggest limitation of this study was that the test-retest reliability and internal consistency could not be validated due to the retrospective nature of the study, which is an important step (i.e. reliability) in evaluating a scoring system. The retrospective study could contribute to the bias in the validated results. Another limitation is that as it was a single-centre study, and it could not be said with certainty that these results could be applied to other centres. Therefore, further prospective research with a larger population from multiple clinical centres is needed.

Conclusion

Based on the present data, our results suggested that the LES is a valid elbow-specific scoring system and is applicable to evaluate joint functions of patients with elbow stiffness, although some items included had some weakness either. Further prospective research using a larger population from multiple clinical centres is required in future.

Abbreviations

CAS: Clinical assessment score; DASH: Disability of arm, shoulder and hand questionnaire; EMC: Elbow motion capacity; ERS: Elbow-related symptoms; ES: Effect size; LES: Liverpool Elbow Score; MEPS: Mayo Elbow Performance Score; OES: Oxford Elbow Score; PAQ: Patient-answered questionnaire; SCC: Spearman correlation coefficients; SF-36: Short Form-36; SF-36/MCS: Mental component summary part of Short Form-36; SF-36/PCS: Physical component summary part of Short Form-36; SRM: Standardized response mean

Acknowledgements

This study was supported by the Department of Orthopaedics from Shanghai Sixth People's Hospital East Affiliated to Shanghai University of Medicine & Health Sciences. The authors would like to thank the personnel from the elbow stiffness clinical team leading by prof. FCY for participating in the patient and data collection.

Authors' contributions

SZY conceived and designed this study, performed the literature searches, extracted the data, performed the statistical analyses, interpreted the data and drafted the manuscript. FCY revised the manuscript and acted as guarantor for the paper. The guarantors accept full responsibility for the conduct of the study, had access to the data, and controlled the decision to publish. Both authors approved the final manuscript.

Competing interests

The authors declare that they have no competing interests.

References

1. Ranganathan K, Loder S, Agarwal S, Wong VW, Forsberg J, Davis TA, Wang S, James AW, Levi B. Heterotopic ossification: basic-science principles and clinical correlates. J Bone Joint Surg Am. 2015;97(13):1101–11.
2. Hildebrand KA, Zhang M, Befus AD, Salo PT, Hart DA. A myofibroblast-mast cell-neuropeptide axis of fibrosis in post-traumatic joint contractures: an in vitro analysis of mechanistic components. J Orthop Res. 2014;32(10):1290–6.
3. Doornberg JN, Bosse T, Cohen MS, Jupiter JB, Ring D, Kloen P. Temporary presence of myofibroblasts in human elbow capsule after trauma. J Bone Joint Surg Am. 2014;96(5):e36.
4. Longo UG, Franceschi F, Loppini M, Maffulli N, Denaro V. Rating systems for evaluation of the elbow. Br Med Bull. 2008;87:131–61.
5. Smith MV, Calfee RP, Baumgarten KM, Brophy RH, Wright RW. Upper extremity-specific measures of disability and outcomes in orthopaedic surgery. J Bone Joint Surg Am. 2012;94(3):277–85.
6. Sathyamoorthy P, Kemp GJ, Rawal A, Rayner V, Frostick SP. Development and validation of an elbow score. Rheumatology (Oxford, England). 2004;43(11):1434–40.
7. Dawson J, Doll H, Boller I, Fitzpatrick R, Little C, Rees J, Carr A. Comparative responsiveness and minimal change for the Oxford elbow score following surgery. Qual Life Res Int J Qual Life Asp Treat Care Rehab. 2008;17(10):1257–67.
8. Ashmore AM, Gozzard C, Blewitt N. Use of the Liverpool elbow score as a postal questionnaire for the assessment of outcome after total elbow arthroplasty. J Shoulder Elb Surg. 2007;16(3 Suppl):S55–8.
9. Amirfeyz R, Blewitt N. Mid-term outcome of GSB-III total elbow arthroplasty in patients with rheumatoid arthritis and patients with post-traumatic arthritis. Arch Orthop Trauma Surg. 2009;129(11):1505–10.
10. Munoz-Mahamud E, Fernandez-Valencia JA, Riba J. Plate osteosynthesis for severe olecranon fractures. J Orthop Surg (Hong Kong). 2010;18(1):80–4.
11. Reising K, Hauschild O, Strohm PC, Suedkamp NP. Stabilisation of articular fractures of the distal humerus: early experience with a novel perpendicular plate system. Injury. 2009;40(6):611–7.
12. Kalogrianitis S, Sinopidis C, El Meligy M, Rawal A, Frostick SP. Unlinked elbow arthroplasty as primary treatment for fractures of the distal humerus. J Shoulder Elb Surg. 2008;17(2):287–92.
13. Beirer M, Friese H, Lenich A, Cronlein M, Sandmann GH, Biberthaler P, Kirchhoff C, Siebenlist S. The elbow self-assessment score (ESAS): development and validation of a new patient-reported outcome measurement tool for elbow disorders. Knee Surg, Sports Traumatol, Arthrosc. 2017;25(7):2230–6.
14. Chen H, Ji X, Zhang W, Zhang Y, Zhang L, Tang P. Validation of the simplified Chinese (mainland) version of the disability of the arm, shoulder, and hand questionnaire (DASH-CHNPLAGH). J Orthop Surg Res. 2015;10:76.
15. Li L, Wang HM, Shen Y. Chinese SF-36 health survey: translation, cultural adaptation, validation, and normalisation. J Epidemiol Community Health. 2003;57(4):259–63.
16. Guillemin F. Cross-cultural adaptation and validation of health status measures. Scand J Rheumatol. 1995;24(2):61–3.
17. Guillemin F, Bombardier C, Beaton D. Cross-cultural adaptation of health-related quality of life measures: literature review and proposed guidelines. J Clin Epidemiol. 1993;46(12):1417–32.
18. Yu S, Chen M, Fan C. Team Approach: Elbow Contracture Due to Heterotopic Ossification. JBJS reviews. 2017;5(1) https://doi.org/10.2106/JBJS.RVW.16.00008.
19. Barrett P, Kline P. The Observation to Variable Ratio in Factor Analysis, vol. 1; 1981.
20. Terwee CB, Bot SD, de Boer MR, van der Windt DA, Knol DL, Dekker J, Bouter LM, de Vet HC. Quality criteria were proposed for measurement properties of health status questionnaires. J Clin Epidemiol. 2007;60(1):34–42.
21. The B, Reininga IH, El Moumni M, Eygendaal D. Elbow-specific clinical rating systems: extent of established validity, reliability, and responsiveness. J Shoulder Elb Surg. 2013;22(10):1380–94.
22. Beaton DE, Katz JN, Fossel AH, Wright JG, Tarasuk V, Bombardier C. Measuring the whole or the parts? Validity, reliability, and responsiveness of the disabilities of the arm, shoulder and hand outcome measure in different regions of the upper extremity. J Hand Ther. 2001;14(2):128–46.
23. Dawson J, Doll H, Boller I, Fitzpatrick R, Little C, Rees J, Jenkinson C, Carr AJ. The development and validation of a patient-reported questionnaire to assess outcomes of elbow surgery. J Bone Joint Surg Br Vol. 2008;90(4):466–73.
24. SooHoo NF, McDonald AP, Seiler JG 3rd, McGillivary GR. Evaluation of the construct validity of the DASH questionnaire by correlation to the SF-36. J Hand Surg. 2002;27(3):537–41.
25. Morrey BF, Adams RA. Semiconstrained arthroplasty for the treatment of rheumatoid arthritis of the elbow. J Bone Joint Surg Am. 1992;74(4):479–90.
26. Evans JP, Smith CD, Fine NF, Porter I, Gangannagaripalli J, Goodwin VA, Valderas JM. Clinical rating systems in elbow research-a systematic review exploring trends and distributions of use. J Shoulder Elbow Surg. 2018;27:e98–e106.
27. Kazis LE, Anderson JJ, Meenan RF. Effect sizes for interpreting changes in health status. Med Care. 1989;27(3 Suppl):S178–89.
28. Peolsson A, Vavruch L, Hedlund R. Long-term randomised comparison between a carbon fibre cage and the Cloward procedure in the cervical spine. Eur Spine J. 2007;16(2):173–8.
29. McHorney CA, Tarlov AR. Individual-patient monitoring in clinical practice: are available health status surveys adequate? Qual Life Res Int J Qual Life Asp Treat Care Rehab. 1995;4(4):293–307.
30. Kim SJ, Basur MS, Park CK, Chong S, Kang YG, Kim MJ, Jeong JS, Kim TK. Crosscultural adaptation and validation of the Korean version of the new knee society knee scoring system. Clin Orthop Relat Res. 2017;475(6):1629–39.
31. Revicki D, Hays RD, Cella D, Sloan J. Recommended methods for determining responsiveness and minimally important differences for patient-reported outcomes. J Clin Epidemiol. 2008;61(2):102–9.
32. Vishwanathan K, Alizadehkhaiyat O, Kemp GJ, Frostick SP. Responsiveness of the Liverpool elbow score in elbow arthroplasty. J Shoulder Elb Surg. 2013;22(3):312–7.
33. de Vet HC, Terwee CB, Ostelo RW, Beckerman H, Knol DL, Bouter LM. Minimal changes in health status questionnaires: distinction between minimally detectable change and minimally important change. Health Qual Life Outcomes. 2006;4:54.
34. Siemiatycki J. A comparison of mail, telephone, and home interview strategies for household health surveys. Am J Public Health. 1979;69(3):238–45.
35. Beaton DE, Richards RR. Measuring function of the shoulder. A cross-sectional comparison of five questionnaires. J Bone Joint Surg Am. 1996;78(6):882–90.
36. Patrick DL, Deyo RA. Generic and disease-specific measures in assessing health status and quality of life. Med Care. 1989;27(3 Suppl):S217–32.
37. Capuano L, Poulain S, Hardy P, Longo UG, Denaro V, Maffulli N. No correlation between physicians administered elbow rating systems and patient's satisfaction. J Sports Med Phys Fitness. 2011;51(2):255–9.
38. Shahgholi L, Bengtson KA, Bishop AT, Shin AY, Spinner RJ, Basford JR, Kaufman KR. A comparison of manual and quantitative elbow strength testing. Am J Phys Med Rehab. 2012;91(10):856–62.
39. Werle S, Goldhahn J, Drerup S, Simmen BR, Sprott H, Herren DB. Age- and gender-specific normative data of grip and pinch strength in a healthy adult Swiss population. J Hand Surg Eur Vol. 2009;34(1):76–84.

40. Cai J, Wang W, Yan H, Sun Y, Chen W, Chen S, Fan C. Complications of open elbow Arthrolysis in post-traumatic elbow stiffness: a systematic review. PLoS One. 2015;10(9):e0138547.

41. Elliott TE, Renier CM, Palcher JA. Chronic pain, depression, and quality of life: correlations and predictive value of the SF-36. Pain Med (Malden, Mass). 2003;4(4):331–9.

42. Doornberg JN, Ring D, Fabian LM, Malhotra L, Zurakowski D, Jupiter JB. Pain dominates measurements of elbow function and health status. J Bone Joint Surg Am. 2005;87(8):1725–31.

43. Organization WH. International classification of functioning, Disability and Health (ICF). In: Kirch W, ed. Encyclopedia of Public Health. Dordrecht: Springer Netherlands. 2008:217–20.

8

Low molecular weight heparin versus other anti-thrombotic agents for prevention of venous thromboembolic events after total hip or total knee replacement surgery

Xin Lu and Jin Lin*[iD]

Abstract

Background: Venous thromboembolism (VTE) is an important complication following total hip replacement (THR) and total knee replacement (TKR) surgeries. Aim of this study was to comprehensively compare the clinical outcomes of low-molecular-weight heparin (LMWH) with other anticoagulants in patients who underwent TKR or THR surgery.

Methods: Medline, Cochrane, EMBASE, and Google Scholar databases were searched for eligible randomized controlled studies (RCTs) published before June 30, 2017. Meta-analyses of odds ratios were performed along with subgroup and sensitivity analyses.

Results: Twenty-one RCTs were included. In comparison with placebo, LMWH treatment was associated with a lower risk of VTE and deep vein thrombosis (DVT) (P values < 0.001) but similar risk of pulmonary embolism (PE) (P = 0.227) in THR subjects. Compared to factor Xa inhibitors, LMWH treatment was associated with higher risk of VTE in TKR subjects (P < 0.001), and higher DVT risk (P < 0.001) but similar risk of PE and major bleeding in both THR and TKR. The risk of either VTE, DVT, PE, or major bleeding was similar between LMWH and direct thrombin inhibitors in both THR and TKR, but major bleeding was lower with LMWH in patients who underwent THR (P = 0.048).

Conclusion: In comparison with factor Xa inhibitors, LMWH may have higher risk of VTE and DVT, whereas compared to direct thrombin inhibitors, LMWH may have lower risk of major bleeding after THR or TKR.

Keywords: Low molecular weight heparin, Total knee replacement, Total hip replacement, Bleeding, Thrombosis

Background

Venous thromboembolism (VTE) is an important complication following total hip replacement (THR) and total knee replacement (TKR) surgeries. The risk of postoperative thromboembolic events was estimated to be approximately 50% for an asymptomatic event and 15% to 30% for a symptomatic event in the absence of prophylactic treatment [1, 2]. These procedures can also result in deep venous thrombosis (DVT), pulmonary embolism (PE), infection, and death [3]. Asian patients

aged ≥40 years had a significantly higher relative risk of developing DVT, proximal DVT and PE [4].

Anticoagulants are routinely used and recommended after major orthopedic surgery to prevent VTE Anticoagulants has been found to reduce the risk of thromboembolic events by approximately 50% to 80% when prescribed prophylactically [1]. Both the American College of Chest Physicians (ACCP) and American Association of Orthopedic Surgeons (AAOS) guidelines for VTE prophylaxis recommend antithrombotic prophylaxis following THR or TKR [2, 4]. However, although pharmacologic thromboprophylaxis in patients with THR or TKR may decrease the incidence of VTE and other thrombus related events, it can cause increased risk of major bleeding [2, 5]. A strong

* Correspondence: captainlx@163.com
Department of Orthopaedics, Peking Union Medical College Hospital, Chinese Academy of Medical Sciences and Peking Union Medical College, Beijing, China

relationship between major bleeding and poor outcome irrespective of the study drug used has been demonstrated [6]. Hence, the trade-offs between fewer symptomatic PE and DVT with thromboprophylaxis versus increased major bleeding should be considered [2, 7].

Current guidelines for thromboprophylaxis recommend the use of vitamin K antagonists (e.g. warfarin), low-molecular-weight heparins (LMWH), aspirin, or indirect inhibitor of factor Xa [8]. The efficacy and safety of LMWH is well established [5, 9]. It has a long half-life with good bioavailability [9] and is administered once daily subcutaneous dose without laboratory monitoring or dose adjustment. It is safe and effective for extended out-of-hospital prophylaxis after TKR or THR surgery [10]. Disadvantages associated with LMWH include parenteral administration, expense, potential thrombocytopenia, and poor patient adherence [11, 12]. In a previous meta-analysis, patients who received LMWH (e.g. enoxaparin) prophylaxis had lower incidence of DVT after knee arthroscopic surgery compared to patients who did not receive LMWH prophylaxis [13].

New generation of oral anticoagulants, such as dabigatran etexilate, ximelagatran, rivaroxaban, and apixaban, are now available for prophylaxis against VTE in patients undergoing TKR or THR surgery [14]. Factor Xa inhibitors (i.e., rivaroxaban, darexaban, and apixaban) and direct thrombin inhibitors (i.e., ximelagatran and dabigatran etexilate) have more predictable anticoagulant effects compared to LMWH which also overcome the need to monitor patients receiving short-term thromboprophylaxis [6]. However, disadvantages associated with these drugs include costs and lack of antidotes for timely reversal of bleeding [6].

Currently, there is no comprehensive review to summarize the relative effectiveness of LMWH by comparing it with placebo, factor Xa inhibitors or direct thrombin inhibitors in preventing VTE and incidence of major bleeding when used as thromboprophylaxis agent in TKR or THR surgical interventions. The aim of this meta-analysis was to assess the in-patient clinical outcomes of LMWH compared to factor Xa inhibitors and direct thrombin inhibitors in TKR or THR surgery subjects.

Methods
Search strategy
The study was performed in accordance with the PRISMA guidelines. Following databases were searched for studies published before June 30, 2017: Medline, Cochrane, EMBASE, and Google Scholar. The search term (Hip OR Knee), (replacement OR arthroplasty), (low molecular weight heparin OR enoxaparin), (Venous Thromboembolism OR Pulmonary Embolism OR Vein Thrombosis) AND (inhibitor of factor Xa OR direct thrombin inhibitor) and Randomized controlled trial (RCTs) were used.

Eligibility
Eligible studies had to have investigated patients undergoing hip or knee arthroplasty or replacement, and to have compared patients receiving LMWH (enoxaparin) with placebo, factor Xa inhibitors or direct thrombin inhibitors. Included studies had to have reported outcomes of interests (given below). Retrospective studies, one arm studies, letters, commentaries, editorials, case reports, proceedings, and personal communications were excluded. Also excluded were studies that evaluated anticoagulants other than direct thrombin and factor Xa inhibitors (e.g. aspirin or warfarin).

Quality assessment
The quality of the included studies was assessed using Quality in Prognostic Studies (QUIPS), which consists of six domains (study participation, study attrition, prognostic factor measurement, outcome measurement, confounding measurement and account, analysis) [15, 16].

Data and statistical analysis
The following information/data was extracted from studies that met the inclusion criteria: the name of the first author, year of publication, study design, number of participants in each group, participants' age and gender, and major outcomes. The outcomes of interest were the risk or odds of thrombotic events (VTE, DVT, PE, major bleeding). Basic characteristics of the included studies were summarized as mean ± standard deviations (SD), mean (range: min., max.), or median (min., max.) for age, and n (%) for gender and patient number. The outcomes were summarized as n/N (patients with events out of total number of patients) for given intervention as LMWH vs controls (placebo, or factor Xa inhibitor, or a direct thrombin inhibitor). When assessment of an outcome included ≥3 studies, an effect size odd ratio (OR) with corresponding 95% confidence intervals (95% CI) was calculated for each individual study and then overall effect size was generated . Meta-analyses was not performed when ≤2 studies reported an outcome of interest. Odds ratios > 1 implied patients with LMWH treatment had a higher rate of a given outcome than those treated with control; OR < 1 indicated patients with LMWH treatment had a lower rate of a specific outcome than patients receiving control therapy; OR = 1 suggested the rate of an outcome was similar between LMWH and control treatments.

A χ^2 test for homogeneity was conducted, and an inconsistency index (I^2) and Q statistics were determined [17]. If the I^2 statistic was > 50%, a random-effects model (Der Simonian–Laird method) was used [18]. Otherwise, a fixed-effects model (Mantel-Haenszel method) was employed. Combined effects were calculated, and a two-sided P value of < 0.05 was considered significant. Sensitivity analyses were performed using a leave-one-out approach. Publication bias was assessed as guided by the Cochrane Handbook for Systematic and summarized using Review Manager Software (Version 5.3). However, the funnel plot and Egger's test were not performed because the limitation of the study numbers (≤10 per outcome) [19]. All data were organized in Microsoft Office Excel 2007 spread sheets and all meta-analyses were performed using Comprehensive Meta-Analysis statistical software, version 2.0 (Biostat, Englewood, NJ, USA). Safety analyses were performed with Stata software (version 12, Stata Corporation, Texas, USA).

Results

Search results

A total of 184 articles were identified through database searches and nine through corroborative searches (Fig. 1). After removing duplicates and an initial screen of abstracts and titles to remove studies that did not meet the inclusion criteria, 31 studies underwent full text review. Subsequently, 10 articles were excluded due to the ineligible design (retrospective study or commentary) (*n* = 4),

being a single-arm study (*n* = 3), and not reporting outcome of interest (*n* = 3). Consequently, 21 studies were included in the systematic review and meta-analysis [10, 20–39].

Characteristics of included studies

The studies were divided into three subgroups based on the non-LMWH treatment: Group I: LMWH vs. placebo (3 studies); Group II: LMWH vs. direct thrombin inhibitors (8 studies; 4 studies with ximelagatran and 4 with dabigatran etexilate); Group III: LMWH vs. factor Xa inhibitor (10 studies; 6 with studied rivaroxaban, 3 with apixaban, and 1 with darexaban). The study of Kim et al. (2016) had two control groups: rivaroxaban group and placebo group [20]. Therefore, the data from Kim et al. [20] for LMWH vs. placebo were included in meta-analysis of Group I. Group I included 962 participants (708 for LMWH and 254 for placebo), Group II included 18,116 participants (7530 for LMWH and 10,586 for control), and Group III included 26,639 participants (12,713 for LMWH and 13,926 for control). The mean ages for most studies were in general ≥60 years, except for Kim et al. [20]

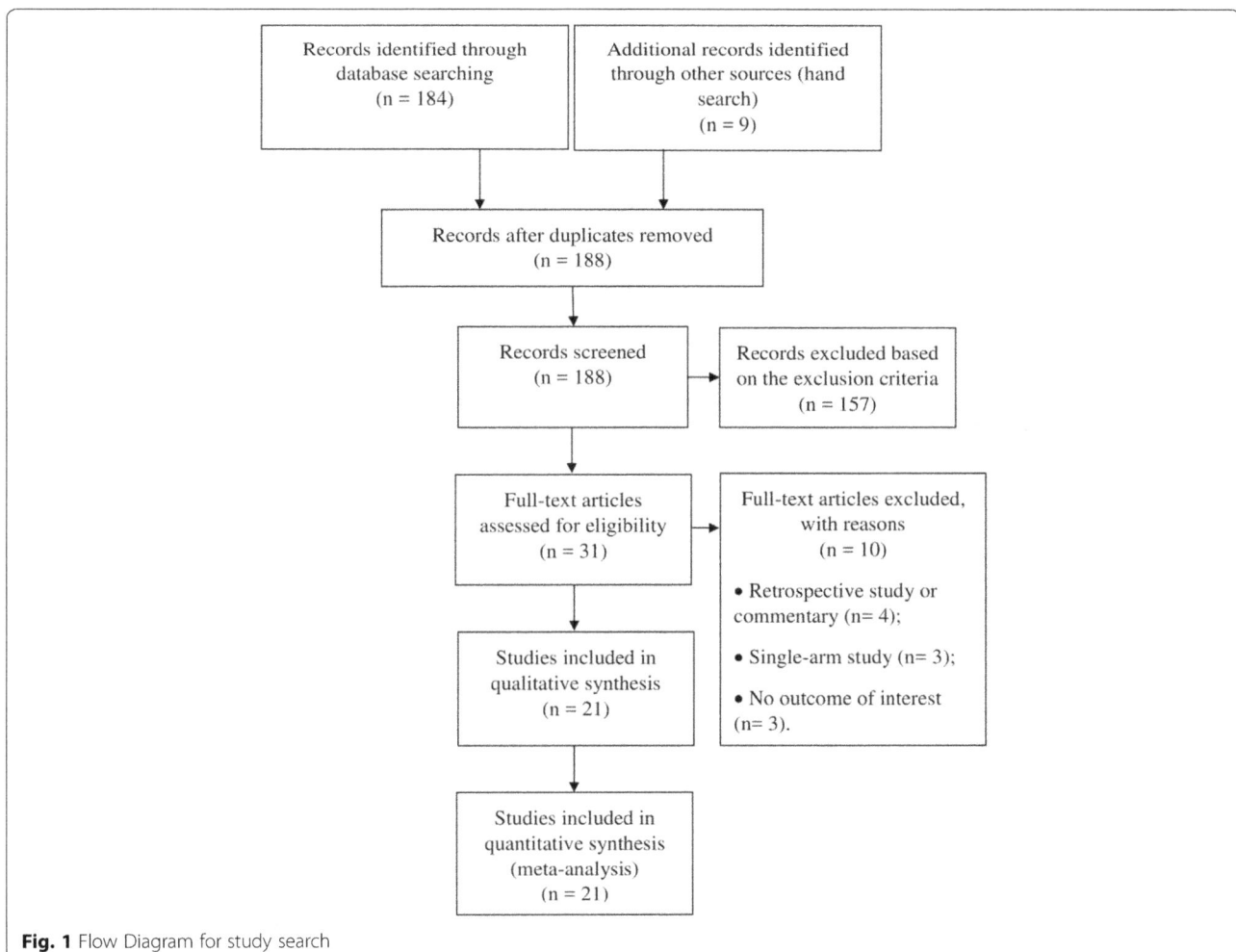

Fig. 1 Flow Diagram for study search

Table 1 Patients' characteristics among the studies

1st author (year)	Treatments	Details of treatment (dose and routes of Administration)	number of patients	Procedure (n)	Age mean ± SD years	Sex, Males (%)	BMI, kg/m²	Follow-up time (days)
I. LMWH vs. placebo (saline)								
Fuji (2008) [10]	Enoxaparin	20 mg sc qd for 14d	81	THR	63.3±10.4	10 (12.3)	23.5±3.4	90
		40 mg sc qd for 14d	80		60.6±9.9	6 (7.5)	23.5±3.7	
		20 mg sc bid for 14d	90		63.0±9.3	15 (16.7)	23.7±3.6	
	Placebo	Saline bid for 14d	86		62.0±10.3	11 (12.8)	24.0±3.4	
	Enoxaparin	20 mg sc qd for 14d	78	TKR	68.8±9.0	15 (19.2)	25.7±4.5	90
		40 mg sc qd for 14d	74		70.0±9.4	11 (14.9)	25.3±4.0	
		20 mg sc bid for 14d	84		68.3±8.7	5 (6)	24.0±4.0	
	Placebo	Saline bid for 14d	79		68.7±9.5	15 (19)	25.4±3.7	
Bergqvist (1996) [20]	Enoxaparin	40 mg (0.4 ml) sc qd	131	THR	median = 70 (range: 44–87)	56 (42.7)	median = 25.8 (range:18.6–37.9)	n/a
	Placebo	0.4 ml saline qd	131		median = 70 (range: 44–87)	57 (43.5)	median = 26.8 (range: 19.2–49.1)	
Planes (1996) [21]	Enoxaparin	40 mg sc qd for 2d	90	THR	70±9.1	47 (52.2)	25·55±3·19	21
	Placebo	Saline qd	89		68±8.2	55 (61.8)	25·85±3·49	
II. LMWH vs. inhibitor of factor Xa								
Kim (2016) [1]	Enoxaparin	40 mg sc qd for 14d	184	THR	43.9±9.4	114 (62.0)	25.4±3.8	N/A
	Rivaroxaban	10 mg qd for 14d	184		44.4±8.6	99 (53.8)	24.8±3.1	
	Placebo	1 ml saline or placebo tablet qd	185		43.4±9.9	109 (58.9)	24.3±3.4	
Zou (2014) [3]	Enoxaparin	4000 anti-Xa IU (0.4 ml) qd for 14d	112	TKR	mean = 65.7 (range:54–80)	20 (17.85)	mean = 27.0 (range:20.3–37.0)	28
	Rivaroxaban	10 mg qd for 14d	102		mean = 63.5 (range:50–82)	32 (31.37)	mean = 27.5 (range:18.0–39.5)	
	Aspirin	100 mg qd for 14d	110		mean = 62.7 (range:47–79)	28 (25.45)	mean = 27.8 (range:17.8–40.0)	
Kakkar (2008) [RECORD 2] [11]	enoxaparin	40 mg sc qd for 10–14 d (with placebo tablet for 31–39d)	1229	THR	61.6±13.7	578 (47)	27.1±5.2	n/a
	Rivaroxaban	10 mg qd 31–39 d (with placebo injection for 10–14 d)	1228		61.4±13.2	561 (45.7)	26.8±4.8	
Eriksson (2008) [RECORD 1] [12]	Enoxaparin	40 mg sc qd for 35d (range, 31–39d) (with placebo tablet)	2224	THR	median = 63.3 (range:18–93)	982 (44.2)	median = 27.9 (range:15.2–50.2)	30–42
	Rivaroxaban	10 mg qd for 35d (range, 31–39d) (with placebo injection)	2209		median = 63.1 (range:18–91)	989 (44.8)	median = 27.8 (range:16.2–53.4)	

which participants had mean age of about 43 to 44 years. Male patients ranged from 6% [29] to 62% [20]. Mean body mass index (BMI) ranged from 23.5 kg/m^2 [29] to 32.6 kg/m^2 [10]. Details are provided in Table 1.

The drug dose and routes of administration were diverse among the studies. Enoxaparin was the only LMWH used in the included studies at a dose of 40 mg once daily as subcutaneous injection in 15 studies. However, for five studies, the postoperative regimen of 30 mg of enoxaparin administered subcutaneously every 12 h (30 mg bid) was used as this regimen was approved by the Food and Drug Administration (FDA) [21, 26–28, 36]. Zou et al. [22] used enoxaparin sodium as 4000 anti-Xa activity IU (0.4 ml) once daily dose, and Fuji et al. [29] assessed the effectiveness of three different doses of enoxaparin given subcutaneously; 20 mg qd, 40 mg qd, and 20 mg bid. The length of follow-up period ranged from 12 days (Eriksson et al. [21]) to 90 days (Fuji et al. [29]).

The efficacy and safety outcomes including rate of total VTE, DVT, PE, major bleeding, and clinical relevant non-major bleeding or minor bleeding are summarized in Table 2. In placebo- controlled studies, enoxaparin (LMWH) was associated with lower incidence of major VTE and DVT for both THR and TKR than placebo. In studies in which the effectiveness of enoxaparin was compared with factor Xa inhibitors (i.e., rivaroxaban, apixaban, or darexaban), the incidence of major VTE and DVT in the enoxaparin groups, in general, was lower than in the factor Xa inhibitor groups for both THR and TKR. In studies which compared enoxaparin with direct thrombin inhibitors, enoxaparin appeared to have a higher percentage of patients with major VTE and DVT than ximelagatran but similar or a lower percentage of patients with these events compared with dabigatran etexilate. The percentage of patients with major or minor bleeding for any given treatment appeared to vary across all studies. Results of the meta-analyses are summarized in Additional file 1: Table S1.

Meta-analysis
Venous thromboembolism
In Group I (LMWH vs. placebo), three studies reported complete total VTE data for THR [29, 38, 39]. Fixed effect model was used due to low heterogeneity in the data (THR: Q value = 2.922, df = 2, P = 0.232, I-squared = 31.56%). The overall effect size showed that the LMWH treatment had significantly lower odds of VTE than the placebo group (OR = 0.481, 95% CI = 0.338–0.685, P < 0.001) (Fig. 2a; Additional file 1: Table S1).

In Group II (LMWH vs. inhibitor of factor Xa), nine studies, 5 for THR [20, 21, 28, 30, 31] and 4 for TKR [24, 25, 27, 32], reported complete total VTE data. Random effects model was considered for THR due to the presence of high heterogeneity for the THR data but low

heterogeneity for the TKR data, fixed effect model was used (THR: Q value = 37.097, df = 4, P < 0.001, I-squared = 89.22%; TKR: Q value = 0.906, df = 3, P = 0.824, I-squared = 0%). The overall effect size showed that LMWH group had higher chance of VTE rate than factor Xa inhibitor group for TKR (OR = 2.162, 95% CI = 1.513–3.089, P < 0.001) but a similar VTE risk for THR (OR = 2.023, 95% CI = 0.880–4.648, P = 0.097) (Fig. 2b; Additional file 1: Table S1).

For Group III (LMWH vs. direct thrombin inhibitor), five studies had complete total VTE data for THR [23, 34–37] and four for TKR [10, 26, 35, 37]. Because data for both THR and TKR findings was heterogenous across the studies (THR: Q-value = 24.722, df = 4, P < 0.001, I-squared = 83.82%; TKR: Q-value = 24.292, df = 3, P < 0.001, I-squared = 87.65%), hence random effect models were applied. The overall effect size showed that there was no significant difference between LMWH and direct thrombin inhibitors in the incidence of VTE for either THR (OR = 1.31, 95% CI = 0.757–2.267, P = 0.335) or TKR (OR = 1.378, 95% CI = 0.817–2.323, P = 0.229) (Fig. 2c; Additional file 1: Table S1).

Deep vein thrombosis
In Group I (LMWH vs. placebo), four studies reported complete total DVT data for THR subjects [20, 29, 38, 39]. A fixed effect model was used as little heterogeneity in the data was observed (THR: Q value = 4.060, df = 3, P = 0.255, I-squared = 26.11%). The overall effect size showed that the LMWH treatment had significantly lower incidence of DVT than placebo group. (OR = 0.464, 95% CI = 0.332–0.647, P < 0.001) (Fig. 3a).

In Group II (LMWH vs. inhibitor of factor Xa), ten studies, 5 for THR [20, 21, 28, 30, 31] and 5 for TKR) [22, 24, 25, 27, 32], had complete data for the rate of DVT. A random effects model was used for both THR and TKR due to the presence of high heterogeneity in the data (THR: Q value = 35.701, df = 4, P < 0.001, I-squared = 88.80%; TKR: Q value = 13.523, df = 4, P = 0.009, I-squared = 70.42%). The overall effect size showed that LMWH group was associated with a higher risk of DVT than factor Xa inhibitors for THR subjects (OR = 2.351, 95% CI = 1.040–5.314, P = 0.040) or TKR (OR = 1.827, 95% CI = 1.352–2.468, P < .001) (Fig. 3b; Additional file 1: Table S1).

For Group III (LMWH vs. direct thrombin inhibitor), three studies reported complete DVT data for THR [23, 36, 37] and three studies reported full data for TKR [10, 26, 37]. A random effect model was used for both THR and TKR analyses as high heterogeneity was observed in the data across studies (THR: Q-value = 13.895, df = 2, p-value = 0.001, I-squared = 85.61%; TKR: Q-value = 16.857, df = 2, P < 0.001, I-squared = 88.14%). The overall effect size showed that there was no significant difference between LMWH and direct thrombin inhibitor

Table 1 Patients' characteristics among the studies (Continued)

1st author (year)	Treatments	Details of treatment (dose and routes of Administration)	number of patients	Procedure (n)	Age mean ± SD years	Sex, Males (%)	BMI, kg/m²	Follow-up time (days)
Lassen (2008) [RECORD 3] [13]	Enoxaparin	40 mg sc qd for 10-14d	1239	TKR	median = 67.6 (range:30-90)	419 (33.7)	median = 29.8 (range:16.0-54.3)	30-35
	Rivaroxaban	10 mg qd for 10-14d	1220		median = 67.6 (range:28-91)	363 (29.8)	median = 29.5 (range:16.3-51.1)	
Turpie (2009) [RECORD 4] [8]	Enoxaparin	30 mg sc bid for 10-14d	1508	TKR	64.7 ± 9.7	541(35.9)	30.7 ± 6.0	30-35
	Rivaroxaban	10 mg qd for 10-14d	1526		64.4 ± 9.7	519 (34.0)	30.9 ± 6.2	
Lassen (2009) [ADVANCE-1] [9]	Enoxaparin	30 mg sc bid for 10-14d (with placebo tablet)	1596	TKR	mean = 65.7 (range: 33-89)	610 (38.2)	mean = 31.1 (range:17.7-57.6)	60
	Apixaban	2.5 mg bid for 10-14d (with placebo tablet)	1599		mean = 65.9 (range:26-93)	602 (37.6)	mean = 31.2 (range:18.1-57.7)	
Lassen (2010a) [ADVANCE-2] [5]	Enoxaparin	40 mg sc qd for 10-14d (with placebo tablet)	1529	TKR	median = 67 (IQR:60-73)	402 (26)	median = 29.3 (IQR:26.1-32.7)	60
	Apixaban	2.5 mg bid for 10-14d (with placebo tablet)	1528		median = 67 (IQR:59-73)	439 (29)	median = 29.1 (IQR:25.8-32.4)	
Lassen (2010b) [ADVANCE-3] [6]	Enoxaparin	40 mg sc qd for 32-38d (with placebo tablet)	2699	THR	mean = 60.6 (range: 19-93)	1248 (46.2)	mean = 28.1 (range:12.5-48.7)	65 ± 5
	Apixaban	2.5 mg bid for 32-38d (with placebo tablet)	2708		mean = 60.9 (range: 19-92)	1278 (47.2)	mean = 28.2 (range:15.4-58.5)	
Eriksson (2014) [2]	enoxaparin	40 mg sc qd, for 35 d	314/393(ITT)	THR	61.1 ± 11.79	166 (42.2)	28.4 ± 4.66	12
	Darexaban	15 mg bid for 35 d	374/269 (ITT)		60.4 ± 10.95	188 (50.3)	28.4 ± 4.97	
		30 mg qd for 35 d	383/293 (ITT)		59.5 ± 11.73	191 (49.9)	28.8 ± 5.14	
		30 mg bid for 35 d	296/387 (ITT)		59.8 ± 12.13	204 (52.7)	28.5 ± 5.22	
		60 mg qd for 35 d	274/385 (ITT)		59.5 ± 11.82	182 (47.3)	28.9 ± 5.00	

III. *LMWH vs. direct thrombin inhibitor*

1st author (year)	Treatments	Details of treatment (dose and routes of Administration)	number of patients	Procedure (n)	Age mean ± SD years	Sex, Males (%)	BMI, kg/m²	Follow-up time (days)
Heit (2001) [19]	LMWH	Enoxaparin: 30 mg sc bid for 6-12d	125	TKR	68 ± 10	48 (38)	31.8 ± 7.0	n/a
	Ximelagatran		475					
		8 mg for 6-12d	85		65 ± 10	34 (40)	32.6 ± 5.7	
		12 mg for 6-12d	134		67 ± 11	56 (42)	30.9 ± 6.0	
		18 mg for 6-12d	126		68 ± 10	45 (36)	30.9 ± 6.0	
		24 mg for 6-12d	130		67 ± 11	46 (35)	31.4 ± 5.7	
Eriksson (2003); METHRO III study [18]	Enoxaparin	40 mg sc qd started 12 h before surgery for 8-10d	1389	THR (957) TKR (432)	mean = 65.8 (range: 26-93)	549 (40)		n/a
	Ximelagatran	24 mg bid for 8-10d beginning the next day of surgery for 8-10d	1399	THR (966) TKR (433)	mean = 66.4 (range:25-93)	515 (37)		

Table 1 Patients' characteristics among the studies *(Continued)*

1st author (year)	Treatments	Details of treatment (dose and routes of Administration)	number of patients	Procedure (n)	Age mean ± SD years	Sex, Males (%)	BMI, kg/m^2	Follow-up time (days)
Colwell (2003) [17]	Enoxaparin	30 mg sc bid for 7-12d	910	THR	64.0 ± 13.1 (n = 775)	377 (48.6)	28.3 ± 5.3	n/a
	Ximelagatran	24 mg bid for 7-12d	906		64.5 ± 12.8 (n = 782)	372 (47.6)	28.4 ± 5.3	
Eriksson (2003); EXPRESS study [16]	Enoxaparin	40 mg sc qd started 12 h before surgery for 8-10d	1387 (ITT)	THR (942) TKR (445)	median = 67 (range:20-89)	542 (39.1)		n/a
	Ximelagatran	24 mg bid for 8-10d beginning the next day of surgery for 8-10d	1377 (ITT)	THR (914) TKR (463)	median = 67 (range:24-88)	509 (37.0)		
RE-MOBILIZE (2009) [7]	Enoxaparin	30 mg sc bid for 12-15d	868	TKR	66.3 ± 9.6	4364 (1.9)		n/a
	Dabigatran Etexilate	220 mg qd for 12-15d	857		66.2 ± 9.5	371 (43.3)		
		150 mg qd for 12-15d	871		65.9 ± 9.5	364 (41.8)		
Eriksson (2007) a [RE-MODEL] [14]	Enoxaparin	40 mg sc qd for 6-10d	694	TKR	68 ± 9	216 (31)		6-10
	Dabigatran etexilate	220 mg qd for 6-10d	679		67 ± 9	238 (35)		
		150 mg qd for 6-10d	703		68 ± 9	252 (36)		
Eriksson (2007) b [RE-NOVATE; Patients from Europe, Australia, and South Africa] [15]	Enoxaparin	40 mg sc qd for 28-35d	1154	THR	64 ± 11	503 (44)		28-35
	Dabigatran etexilate	220 mg qd for 28-35d	1146		65 ± 10	510 (44)		
		150 mg qd for 28-35d	1163		63 ± 11	496 (43)		
Eriksson (2011) [RE-NOVATE II; Patients from North America] [4]	Enoxaparin	40 mg sc qd for 28-35d (with placebo tablet for 28-35d)	1003	THR	62 ± 11	501 (50)	27.8 ± 4.8	28-35
	Dabigatran etexilate	220 mg qd for 28-35d (with placebo injection for 28-35d)	1010		62 ± 12	541 (53.6)	27.8 ± 4.8	

Abbreviations: bid, twice daily; qd, once daily; INR international normalized ratio; IQR inter-quartile range; ITT intent-to-treat, IU international unit, sc subcutaneously, SD standard deviation, THA total hip arthroplasty, THR total hip replacement, TKA total knee arthroplasty, TKR total knee replacement

Table 2 Summary of the efficacy and safety outcomes among the studies

1st author (year)	Treatments	number of patients	Procedure	Efficacy[b]				Safety[b]	
				Death during follow-up	Major VTE (DVT + PE)[a]	DVT	PE	Major bleeding	Minor or non-major bleeding
I. LMWH vs. placebo (saline)									
Fuji (2008) [29]	Enoxaparin	251	THR		66/251	66/251	0/251	6/306	12/306
	20 mg qd	81			21/81	21/81	–	1/100	1/100
	40 mg qd	80			27/80	27/80	–	2/102	7/102
	20 mg bid	90			18/90	18/90	–	3/104	4/104
	Placebo	86			36/86	36/86	0/86	0/101	2/101
	Enoxaparin	236	TKR		86/236	84/236	2/236	4/275	21/275
	20 mg qd	78			35/78	34/78	1/78	0/89	5/89
	40 mg qd	74			26/74	25/74	1/74	1/91	6/91
	20 mg bid	84			25/84	25/84	0/84	3/95	10/95
	Placebo	79			48/79	48/79	0/79	4/89	4/89
Bergqvist (1996) [38]	Enoxaparin, 40 mg	131	THR	0	21/117	21/117	0/117		
	Placebo	131	THR	0	45/116	45/116	0/116		
Planes (1996) [39]	Enoxaparin, 40 mg	90	THR	0		6/85			
	Placebo	89	THR	0		17/88			
Kim (2016) [20]	Enoxaparin	184	THR	0	11/184	11/184	0/184		
	Rivaroxaban	184		0	11/184	10/184	1/184		
	Placebo	185		0	13/185	12/185	1/185		
Zou (2014) [22]	LMWH	112	TKA			14/112			
	Rivaroxaban	102				3/102			
	Aspirin	110				18/110			
Kakkar (2008) [RECORD 2] [30]	enoxaparin	1229	THR	6/869	75/869	71/869	4/869	1/1229	
	Rivaroxaban	1228	THR	2/864	15/864	14/864	1/864	1/1228	
Eriksson (2008) [RECORD 1] [31]	Enoxaparin	2224	THR	0/1558	33/1678	53/1558	1/1558	2/2224	129/2224
	Rivaroxaban	2209		1/1598	4/1686	12/1598	4/1598	6/2209	128/2209
Lassen (2008) [RECORD 3] [32]	Enoxaparin	1239	TKR	4/1217	24/925	160/878	4/878	6/1239	54/1239
	Rivaroxaban	1220		0/1201	9/908	79/824	0/824	7/1220	53/1220
Turpie (2009) [RECORD 4] [27]	Enoxaparin	1564	TKR	3/1508	22/1112	86/959	8/1508	4/1508	138/1508
	Rivaroxaban	1584		4/1526	13/1122	61/965	4/1526	10/1526	155/1526

Table 2 Summary of the efficacy and safety outcomes among the studies (Continued)

1st author (year)	Treatments	number of patients	Procedure	Efficacy[b] Death during follow-up	Major VTE (DVT + PE)[a]	DVT	PE	Safety[b] Major bleeding	Minor or non-major bleeding
Lassen (2009) [ADVANCE-1] [28]	Enoxaparin	1596	THR	3/1554	20/1216	92/1122	7/1596	22/1588	47/1588
	Apixaban	1599		0/1562	26/1269	89/1142	16/1599	11/1596	35/1596
Lassen (2010a) [ADVANCE-2] [24]	Enoxaparin	1529	TKR	1/1469	26/1199	248/997	0/1529	14/1508	58/1508
	Apixaban	1528		1/1458	13/1195	142/971	4/1528	9/1501	44/1501
Lassen (2010b) [ADVANCE-3] [25]	Enoxaparin	2699	TKR	1/2577	25/2195	68/1911	5/2699	18/2659	120/2659
	Apixaban	2708		2/2598	10/2199	22/1944	3/2708	22/2673	109/2673
Eriksson (2014) [21]	enoxaparin	393	THA	0/393	48/314 (ITT)	6/314	1/314	8/393 (2.0)	20/393 (5.0)
	Darexaban	1529		1/1529	150/1132 (ITT)	9/1132	4/1132	25/1529 (1.6)	61/1529 (4.0)
	15 mg bid	374			42/269 (ITT)	3/269	2/269	5/374	
	30 mg qd	383			39/293 (ITT)	1/293	1/293	4/383	
	30 mg bid	387			33/296 (ITT)	2/296	1/296	9/387	
	60 mg qd	385			36/274 (ITT)	3/274	0/274	7/385	

II. *LMWH vs. direct thrombin inhibitor*

1st author (year)	Treatments	number of patients	Procedure	Efficacy[b] Death during follow-up	Major VTE (DVT + PE)[a]	DVT	PE	Safety[b] Major bleeding	Minor or non-major bleeding
Heit (2001) [10]	Enoxaparin	125	TKR	0/125	23/97	23/97	0/97	1/125	
	Ximelagatran	475	TKR	1/475	77/447	74/447	3/447		
	8 mg	85			17/63	17/63	0/63	0/85	
	12 mg	134			20/202	20/202	0/202	0/134	
	18 mg	126			25/87	23/87	2/87	2/126	
	24 mg	130			15/95	14/95	1/95	0/130	
Eriksson (2003b) [37]	Enoxaparin	957	THR	0/957[c]	45/823			10/942	61/942
	Ximelagatran, 24 mg	966		4/966[c]	14/773			37/915	87/915
	Enoxaparin	432	TKR		29/355			6/445	36/445
	Ximelagatran, 24 mg	433			12/365			9/463	39/463
Colwell (2003) [36]	Enoxaparin	910	THR		36/775	36/775	0/775	8/910	
	Ximelagatran, 24 mg	906			62/782	62/782	0/782	7/906	
Eriksson (2003a) [35]	Enoxaparin	942 (ITT)	THR	0/942[c]	146/801	142/801	4/801	10/942	
	Ximelagatran, 24 mg	914 (ITT)		5/914[c]	99/765	97/765	2/765	37/915	
	Enoxaparin	445 (ITT)	TKR		169/383	167/383	2/383	6/445	
	Ximelagatran, 24 mg	463 (ITT)			132/376	131/376	1/376	9/463	

Table 2 Summary of the efficacy and safety outcomes among the studies (Continued)

1st author (year)	Treatments	number of patients	Procedure	Efficacy[b]				Safety[b]	
				Death during follow-up	Major VTE (DVT + PE)[a]	DVT	PE	Major bleeding	Minor or non-major bleeding
Ginsberg (2009) [RE-MOBILIZE] [26]	Enoxaparin	868	TKR	0	163/868	158/868	5/868	12 (1.4)	
	Dabigatran Etexilate	1728		2	405/1728	399/1728	6/1728		
	220 mg	857		1	187/857		6/857	5 (0.6)	
	150 mg	871		1	218/871		0/871	5 (0.6)	
Eriksson (2007a) [RE-MODEL] [33]	Enoxaparin	694	TKR	1/685 (0.1)			1/685	9/694 (1.3)	69 (9.9)
	Dabigatran Etexilate	1382		2/763			1/1382		
	220 mg	679		1/675 (0.1)			0/675	10/679 (1.5)	60 (8.8)
	150 mg	703		1/696 (0.1)			1/696	9/703 (1.3)	59 (8.4)
Eriksson (2007b) [RE-NOVATE; Europe, Australia, and South Africa] [34]	Enoxaparin	1154	THR	0/1142	36/917	Asymptomatic: 56/894 Symptomatic: 1/1142	3/1142	18	74
	Dabigatran etexilate	2309		6/2293	66/1797	Asymptomatic: 56/894 Symptomatic: 1/1142	6/2293	38	142
	220 mg	1146		3/1137	28/909	Asymptomatic: 40/874 Symptomatic: 6/1137	5/1137	23	70
	150 mg	1163		3/1156	38/888	Asymptomatic: 63/871 Symptomatic: 9/1156	1/1156	15	72
11Eriksson (2011), 220 mg [RE-NOVATE II; North America] [23]	Enoxaparin	1.003	THR	1/951	4/951	67/783	2/992	9/1003	54/1003
	Dabigatran etexilate	1010		0/942	2/942	60/791	1/1001	14/1010	61/1010

Abbreviations: *DVT* deep vein thrombosis, *PE* pulmonary embolism, *THA* total hip arthroplasty, *TKA* total knee arthroplasty, *THR* total hip replacement, *TKR* total knee replacement, *VET* venous thromboembolism;

[a] Major venous thromboembolism was the composite of proximal deep-vein thrombosis and nonfatal pulmonary embolism

[b] Efficacy and safety were summarized as n/N, that n means number of cases and N means number of given treatments

[c] The number of patients dies was the total death in both THR and TKR groups

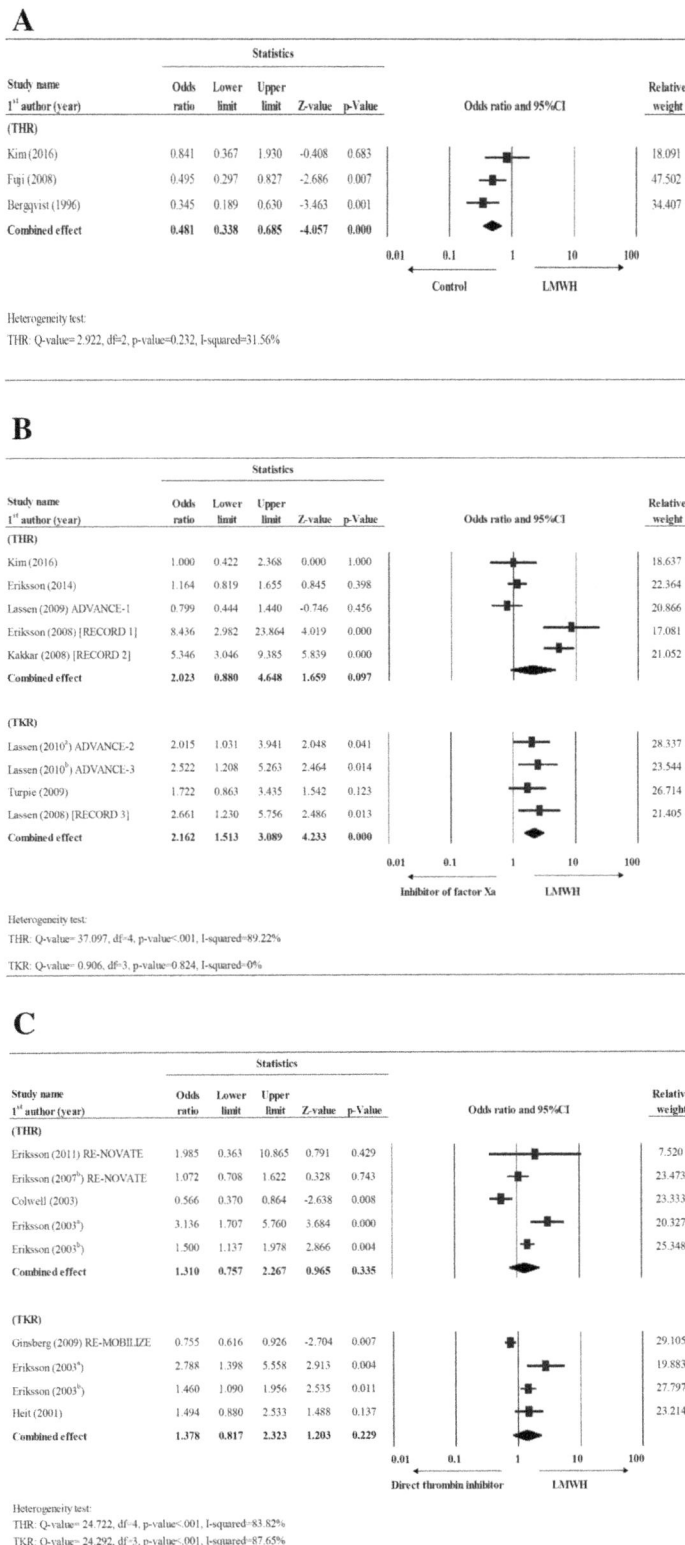

Fig. 2 Forest plot for comparing the total VTE rate between (**a**) LMWH vs. control (placebo), (**b**) LMWH vs. inhibitor of factor Xa, and (**c**) LMWH vs. direct thrombin inhibitor for THR and TKR patients. Abbreviations: CI, confidence interval; Lower limit, lower bound of the 95% CI; Upper limit, upper bound of the 95% CI

A

Study name 1st author (year)	Odds ratio	Lower limit	Upper limit	Z-value	p-Value	Relative weight
(THR)						
Kim (2016)	0.917	0.394	2.134	-0.202	0.840	15.56
Fuji (2008)	0.495	0.297	0.827	-2.686	0.007	42.32
Bergqvist (1996)	0.345	0.189	0.630	-3.463	0.001	30.65
Planes (1996)	0.317	0.119	0.849	-2.286	0.022	11.46
Combined effect	0.464	0.332	0.647	-4.519	0.000	

Odds ratio and 95%CI — Control ↔ LMWH (0.01, 0.1, 1, 10, 100)

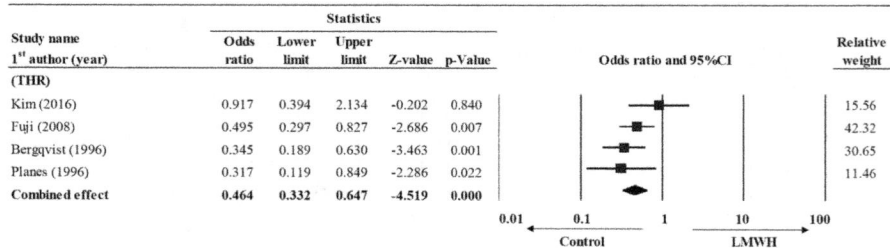

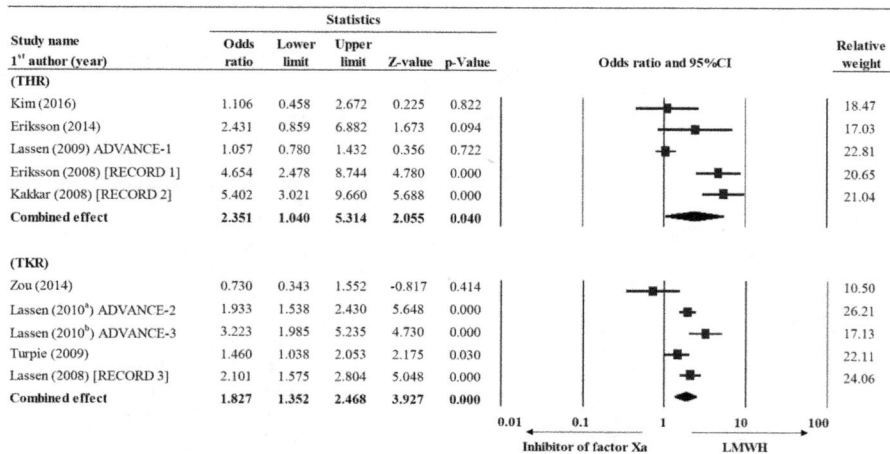

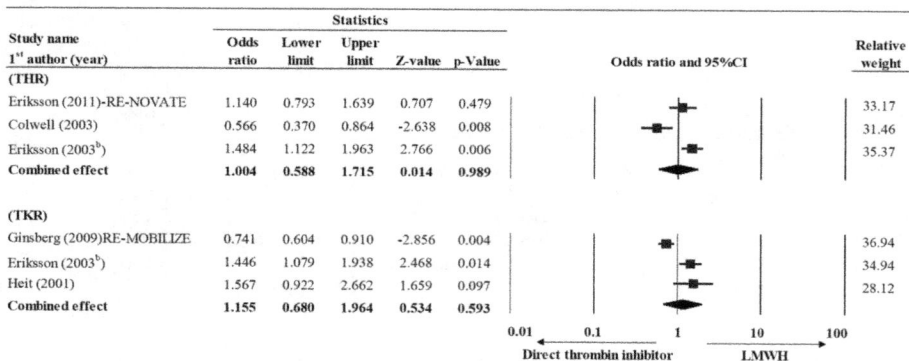

Heterogeneity test:
THR: Q-value= 4.060, df=3, p-value=0.255, I-squared=26.11%

B

Study name 1st author (year)	Odds ratio	Lower limit	Upper limit	Z-value	p-Value	Relative weight
(THR)						
Kim (2016)	1.106	0.458	2.672	0.225	0.822	18.47
Eriksson (2014)	2.431	0.859	6.882	1.673	0.094	17.03
Lassen (2009) ADVANCE-1	1.057	0.780	1.432	0.356	0.722	22.81
Eriksson (2008) [RECORD 1]	4.654	2.478	8.744	4.780	0.000	20.65
Kakkar (2008) [RECORD 2]	5.402	3.021	9.660	5.688	0.000	21.04
Combined effect	2.351	1.040	5.314	2.055	0.040	
(TKR)						
Zou (2014)	0.730	0.343	1.552	-0.817	0.414	10.50
Lassen (2010[a]) ADVANCE-2	1.933	1.538	2.430	5.648	0.000	26.21
Lassen (2010[b]) ADVANCE-3	3.223	1.985	5.235	4.730	0.000	17.13
Turpie (2009)	1.460	1.038	2.053	2.175	0.030	22.11
Lassen (2008) [RECORD 3]	2.101	1.575	2.804	5.048	0.000	24.06
Combined effect	1.827	1.352	2.468	3.927	0.000	

Odds ratio and 95%CI — Inhibitor of factor Xa ↔ LMWH (0.01, 0.1, 1, 10, 100)

Heterogeneity test:
THR: Q-value= 35.701, df=4, p-value<.001, I-squared=88.80%
TKR: Q-value= 13.523, df=4, p-value=0.009, I-squared=70.42%

C

Study name 1st author (year)	Odds ratio	Lower limit	Upper limit	Z-value	p-Value	Relative weight
(THR)						
Eriksson (2011)-RE-NOVATE	1.140	0.793	1.639	0.707	0.479	33.17
Colwell (2003)	0.566	0.370	0.864	-2.638	0.008	31.46
Eriksson (2003[b])	1.484	1.122	1.963	2.766	0.006	35.37
Combined effect	1.004	0.588	1.715	0.014	0.989	
(TKR)						
Ginsberg (2009)RE-MOBILIZE	0.741	0.604	0.910	-2.856	0.004	36.94
Eriksson (2003[b])	1.446	1.079	1.938	2.468	0.014	34.94
Heit (2001)	1.567	0.922	2.662	1.659	0.097	28.12
Combined effect	1.155	0.680	1.964	0.534	0.593	

Odds ratio and 95%CI — Direct thrombin inhibitor ↔ LMWH (0.01, 0.1, 1, 10, 100)

Heterogeneity test:
THR: Q-value= 13.895, df=2, p-value=0.001, I-squared=85.61%
TKR: Q-value= 16.857, df=2, p-value<.001, I-squared=88.14%

Fig. 3 Forest plot for comparing the total DVT rate between (**a**) LMWH vs. control (placebo), (**b**) LMWH vs. inhibitor of factor Xa, and (**c**) LMWH vs. direct thrombin inhibitor for THR and TKR patients. Abbreviations: CI, confidence interval; Lower limit, lower bound of the 95% CI; Upper limit, upper bound of the 95% CI

group in the odds of having a DVT for patients undergoing either THR or TKR (THR: OR = 1.004, 95% CI = 0.588–1.715, p = 0.989; TKR: OR = 1.155, 95% CI = 0.680–1.964, P = 0.593) (Fig. 3c; Additional file 1: Table S1).

Pulmonary embolism

Nine studies in Group II (LMWH vs. inhibitor of factor Xa), five for THR [20, 21, 28, 30, 31] and four for TKR [24, 25, 27, 32] reported complete results for PE . Fixed effect model was used as low heterogeneity was observed among the studies for both THR (Q value = 4.155, df = 4, P = 0.385, I-squared = 3.74%) and TKR (Q value = 4.600, df = 3, P = 0.204, I-squared = 34.78%). The overall effect size showed that LMWH and factor Xa inhibitor group were associated with similar likelihood of developing PE for both THR (OR = 0.554, 95% CI = 0.272–1.127, P = 0.10) and TKR. (OR = 1.680, 95% CI = 0.724–3.896, P = 0.227) (Fig. 4a, Additional file 1: Table S1).

Three studies in Group III (LMWH vs. direct thrombin inhibitor) reported PE data for THR [23, 33, 34] and four had PE data for TKR [10, 26, 33, 34]. Low heterogeneity was observed for both THR and TKR (THR: Q-value = 0.440, df = 2, P value = 0.802, I-squared = 0%; TKR: Q-value = 4.600, df = 3, P value = 0.204, I-squared = 34.78%); hence fixed effect model was used for both. The overall effect size showed that LMWH and direct thrombin inhibitor therapies had similar incidence of PE for either THR (OR = 1.399, 95% CI = 0.524–3.732, P = 0.503) or TKR (OR = 1.588, 95% CI = 0.618–4.080, P = 0.337) (Fig. 4b; Additional file 1: Table S1).

Major bleeding

In Group II (LMWH vs. inhibitor of factor Xa), four studies [21, 28, 30, 31] for THR and four studies [24, 25, 27, 32] for TKR reported the incidence of major bleeding. Fixed effect model was used as low heterogeneity was observed for THR (Q value = 4.236, df = 3, P = 0.237, I-squared = 29.18%) and TKR (Q value = 3.543, df = 3, P = 0.315, I-squared = 15.33%). The overall effect size indicated that the chance of major bleeding was similar between types of treatment both for THR and TKR (THR: OR = 1.370, 95% CI = 0.829–2.265, P = 0.219; TKR: OR = 0.882, 95% CI = 0.577–1.349, P = 0.563) (Fig. 5a; Additional file 1: Table S1).

In Group III (LMWH vs. direct thrombin inhibitor), five studies reported major bleeding data for THR [23, 34–37] and five for TKR [10, 26, 33, 35, 37]. According to the heterogeneity test, random effects and fixed-effect models were applied for both THR and TKR patients, respectively (THR: Q-value = 14.73, df = 4, P = 0.005, I-squared = 72.85%; TKR: Q-value = 5.202, df = 4, P = 0.267, I-squared = 23.11%). The overall effect size showed that LMWH group was associated with a marginal lower rate of major bleeding than direct thrombin

inhibitor for THR subjects (OR = 0.524, 95% CI = 0.277–0.994, P = 0.048) but similar likelihood of major bleeding for TKR subjects (OR = 1.121, 95% CI = 0.716–1.753, p = 0.618) (Fig. 5b; Additional file 1: Table S1).

Safety analyses

a) Major bleeding

Overall incidence of major bleeding events was 1.27% [1.06, 1.48] in this population. In subgroup analysis, Enoxaparin treatment was associated with 1.32% [1.02, 1.63], Dabigatran 1.25% [0.68, 1.81], Rivaroxaban 2.02 [1.00, 3.04], Apixaban [0.70 [0.56, 0.84], and Ximelagatran with 0.93 [– 0.06, 1.91] (Additional file 1: Figure S6).

b) Reoperation rate

Overall reoperation rate was 0.26% [0.21, 0.31] in these patients. Treatment with Enoxaparin treatment was associated with 0.24% [0.17, 0.31], with Dabigatran 0.12% [0.05, 0.19], and with Rivaroxaban 0.28% [0.06, 0.49] reoperation rate (Additional file 1: Figure S7).

c) Mortality

Overall mortality during treatment was 0.13% [0.07, 0.19]. Mortality rate with Enoxaparin was 0.14% [0.04, 0.23], with Dabigatran 0.15% [– 0.01, 0.30], and with Rivaroxaban it was 0.19% [0.08, 0.31] (Additional file 1: Figure S8).

d) Other Adverse events

In this population, 4.31% [2.77, 5.86] patients discontinued treatment due to adverse side effects (4.57% [3.14, 6.00] with Enoxaparin and 5.53% [3.41, 7.66] with Dabigatran) (Additional file 1: Figure S9). Adverse reactions during treatment observed by one or more studies included fever, nausea, vomiting, diarrhea, constipation, urinary tract infections, wound infections, wound complications, wound secretion, wound hematoma, joint dislocation, hypotension, insomnia, edema, anemia, dizziness, headache, urinary problems, hemorrhage, blisters, pyrexia, cardiovascular events, myocardial infarction, and stroke.

Overall incidence of cardiovascular events was 0.36% [0.28, 0.44] (Enoxaparin 0.31% [0.20, 0.43], Dabigatran 1.05% [0.95, 1.15], Rivaroxaban 0.24 [– 0.04, 0.51], and Apixaban 0.15 [0.02, 0.28]) (Additional file 1: Figure S10). Overall incidence of stroke in these patients was 0.08% [0.06, 0.11] (Enoxaparin 0.06% [0.03, 0.10], Rivaroxaban 0.17% [0.09, 0.24], and Apixaban 0.04% [0.01, 0.07]) (Additional file 1: Figure S11).

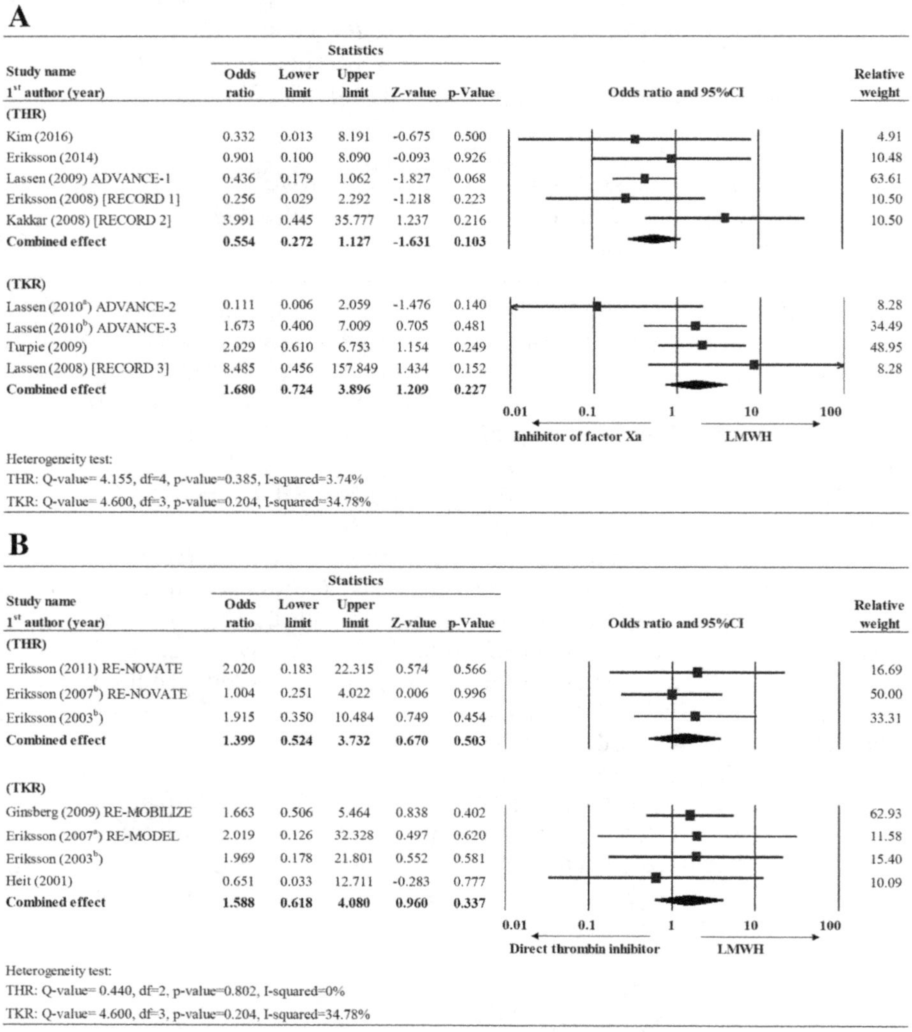

A

Study name 1st author (year)	Odds ratio	Lower limit	Upper limit	Z-value	p-Value	Odds ratio and 95%CI	Relative weight
(THR)							
Kim (2016)	0.332	0.013	8.191	-0.675	0.500		4.91
Eriksson (2014)	0.901	0.100	8.090	-0.093	0.926		10.48
Lassen (2009) ADVANCE-1	0.436	0.179	1.062	-1.827	0.068		63.61
Eriksson (2008) [RECORD 1]	0.256	0.029	2.292	-1.218	0.223		10.50
Kakkar (2008) [RECORD 2]	3.991	0.445	35.777	1.237	0.216		10.50
Combined effect	**0.554**	**0.272**	**1.127**	**-1.631**	**0.103**		
(TKR)							
Lassen (2010ᵃ) ADVANCE-2	0.111	0.006	2.059	-1.476	0.140		8.28
Lassen (2010ᵇ) ADVANCE-3	1.673	0.400	7.009	0.705	0.481		34.49
Turpie (2009)	2.029	0.610	6.753	1.154	0.249		48.95
Lassen (2008) [RECORD 3]	8.485	0.456	157.849	1.434	0.152		8.28
Combined effect	**1.680**	**0.724**	**3.896**	**1.209**	**0.227**		

Inhibitor of factor Xa — LMWH (scale 0.01, 0.1, 1, 10, 100)

Heterogeneity test:
THR: Q-value= 4.155, df=4, p-value=0.385, I-squared=3.74%
TKR: Q-value= 4.600, df=3, p-value=0.204, I-squared=34.78%

B

Study name 1st author (year)	Odds ratio	Lower limit	Upper limit	Z-value	p-Value	Odds ratio and 95%CI	Relative weight
(THR)							
Eriksson (2011) RE-NOVATE	2.020	0.183	22.315	0.574	0.566		16.69
Eriksson (2007ᵇ) RE-NOVATE	1.004	0.251	4.022	0.006	0.996		50.00
Eriksson (2003ᵇ)	1.915	0.350	10.484	0.749	0.454		33.31
Combined effect	**1.399**	**0.524**	**3.732**	**0.670**	**0.503**		
(TKR)							
Ginsberg (2009) RE-MOBILIZE	1.663	0.506	5.464	0.838	0.402		62.93
Eriksson (2007ᵃ) RE-MODEL	2.019	0.126	32.328	0.497	0.620		11.58
Eriksson (2003ᵇ)	1.969	0.178	21.801	0.552	0.581		15.40
Heit (2001)	0.651	0.033	12.711	-0.283	0.777		10.09
Combined effect	**1.588**	**0.618**	**4.080**	**0.960**	**0.337**		

Direct thrombin inhibitor — LMWH (scale 0.01, 0.1, 1, 10, 100)

Heterogeneity test:
THR: Q-value= 0.440, df=2, p-value=0.802, I-squared=0%
TKR: Q-value= 4.600, df=3, p-value=0.204, I-squared=34.78%

Fig. 4 Forest plot for comparing the PE rate between (**a**) LMWH vs. control (placebo), (**b**) LMWH vs. inhibitor of factor Xa, and (**c**) LMWH vs. direct thrombin inhibitor for THR and TKR patients. Abbreviations: CI, confidence interval; Lower limit, lower bound of the 95% CI; Upper limit, upper bound of the 95% CI

Sensitivity analysis

Sensitivity analyses were performed using a leave-one-out approach in which a meta-analysis for total VET (Additional file 1: Figure S1), total DVT (Additional file 1: Figure S2), PE (Additional file 1: Figure S3) and major bleeding (Additional file 1: Figure S4) were performed in which each study for a given analysis was left out in turn. The direction and magnitude of the combined estimates did not markedly differ with the removal of a single study, indicating that the meta-analysis had good reliability and that the data was not overly influenced by any study.

Quality assessment

The results of quality assessment are shown in Additional file 1: Figure S5. In this figure, Panel A shows the potential risk of bias in an individual study, and Panel B shows the summary of bias for included studies. The most potential risk of bias came from attrition bias and selective reporting bias. Also, several studies failed to clearly indicate if they used an intent-to-treat in analysis. Overall, the included studies are of good quality.

Discussion

Anticoagulants are routinely used to prevent deep vein thrombosis following TKR and THR to prevent DVT. However, the relative effectiveness of LMWH and other anticoagulants therapies in patients at risk for DVT has not been comprehensively studied. In the present study, the comparison of LMWH with placebo found that LMWH was associated with lower odds of VTE and DVT compared to placebo in THR subjects, suggesting

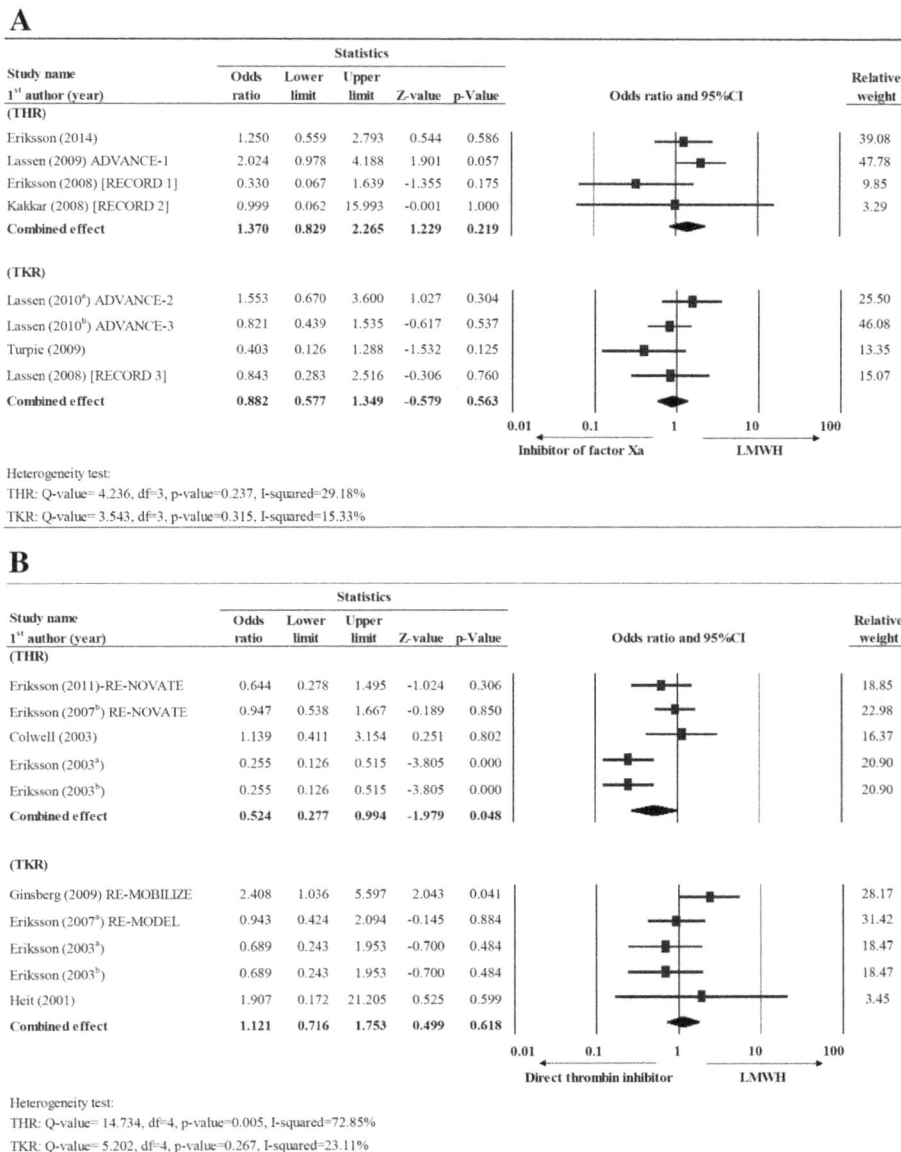

Fig. 5 Forest plot for comparing the major bleeding rate between LMWH vs. (**a**) LMWH vs. inhibitor of factor Xa and (**b**) LMWH vs. direct thrombin inhibitor for THR and TKR patients. Abbreviations: CI, confidence interval; Lower limit, lower bound of the 95% CI; Upper limit, upper bound of the 95% CI

that prophylactic treatment of patients with LMWH could significantly reduce the rate of VTE and DVT but the incidence of PE was similar between the two groups. Compared to factor Xa inhibitors (e.g. rivaroxaban, apixaban, darexaban), LMWH was associated with higher incidence of VTE in TKR subjects, but the odds of VTE was similar between treatment groups in THR subjects. LMWH was associated with higher likelihood of DVT in patients with either THR or TKR, suggesting that factor Xa inhibitors might be superior to LMWH in reducing the rate of VTE and DVT. However, both prophylactic treatments showed a

similar chance of pulmonary embolism and major bleeding in patients with THR and TKR. The odds of VTE, DVT, PE were similar between LMWH and direct thrombin inhibitors (e.g. ximelagatran, dabigatran etexilate); although a marginal benefit in preventing major bleeding was observed for LMWH compared with direct thrombin therapies in patients with THR ($P = 0.048$). These results indicate that LMWH is an effective prophylactic agent for reducing VTE when it was compared with patients without prophylactic treatment. However, LMWH might be less effective than factor Xa inhibitors in reducing the risk of thromboembolic events. In general, LMWH showed effectiveness similar to direct thrombin inhibitors in reducing the risk of thrombo-embolic events as well as major bleeding.

The RCTs for comparing LMWH with placebo in THR or TKR subjects are rare in recent years. A prior systematic review by Hull et al. [40] assessed LMWH in comparison with placebo for the prevention of thrombosis in an out-patient setting in selective hip surgery subjects [40]. They found that compared to placebo, LMWH was associated with decreased episodes of DVT, proximal venous thrombosis, and symptomatic venous thrombosis. These findings support the extended out-of-hospital use of LMWH following hip surgery. A prior meta-analysis by Tasker et al. [41] assessed the in-patient clinical outcomes of LMWH compared to placebo in patients who had THR [41]. They found no difference between LMWH and placebo in affecting the risk of pulmonary embolism, other deaths, all-cause mortality, or major bleeding. They found that compared with placebo, LMWH reduced non-fatal PE at the expense of hematoma formation. Although, our study also assessed in-patient outcomes, it is difficult to compare our findings directly with those of Tasker et al. as we did not evaluate the relative effectiveness of LMWH and placebo with PE or major bleeding due to the limited number of studies reporting these outcomes.

Several systematic reviews and meta-analyses have evaluated the use of different anticoagulant therapies in TKR and THR subjects (see Additional file 1: Table S2) [8, 14, 42–56]. Consistent with the current study, the prior meta-analyses found that the factor Xa inhibitors, rivaroxaban and apixaban, have better anticoagulant effect as compared with the LMWH enoxaparin [42–44]. In contrast to our findings, the prior studies found enoxaparin had a higher incidence of major bleeding compared with some, but not all, of the factor Xa inhibitors. For example, the study of Gomez-Outes et al. [44] found that compared to enoxaparin, the relative risk of clinically relevant bleeding was higher with rivaroxaban, similar with dabigatran, and lower with apixaban. Gomez-Outes et al. concluded that the higher efficacy observed with the factor Xa inhibitors was generally associated with higher bleeding tendency than with LMWH [44]. The meta-analysis of Feng et al. [43] also found that rivaroxaban was associated with a higher bleeding rate [43]. In this meta-analysis, only those RCTs were included which compared the efficacy and safety of any oral direct factor Xa inhibitor with that of enoxaparin for elective THA or TKA. The oral direct factor Xa inhibitor included rivaroxaban, apixaban, darexaban, betrixaban, edoxaban and several developing drugs (e.g. BAY 59–7939, YM150, LY517717). In addition, several trials were open-label and therefore allocation concealment bias may have existed. The author also found that rivaroxaban had a higher bleeding rate, while apixaban and edoxaban did not show significantly higher bleeding risks [43].

Three previous meta-analyses compared the effectiveness of different direct thrombin inhibitors with enoxaparin [14, 45, 46]. In general, our results are similar to those of a few earlier studies which found that dabigatran was similar to enoxaparin with respect to VTE incidence. The same studies also found that the risk of major bleeding was similar between treatments. The meta-analysis of Cohen et al. found that ximelagatran had a significantly lower rate of VTE than with enoxaparin with no difference in bleeding rates [46]. Although, our meta-analysis did not assess individual direct thrombin inhibitors and so the findings are difficult to compare with the prior analyses, we did observe a potentially lower rate of major bleeding associated with LWMH.

The present study has several limitations that should be considered. In addition, the dosing regimens for the different therapies differed across studies. For example, three different regimens of enoxaparin (40 mg once daily or 20 mg or 30 mg bid) were used. A previous meta-analysis compared two different regimens of enoxaparin to oral anticoagulants (apixaban, dabigatran, and rivaroxaban) as thromboprophylaxis in elective TKR or THR [57]. An adjusted indirect comparison showed that bid 40 mg enoxaparin was significantly less effective than 30 mg bid in preventing VTE (relative risk 0.71, $P < 0.001$). The authors concluded that the use of once-daily 40 mg enoxaparin regimen as a control in clinical trials would lead to more favorable estimates of relative efficacy for the new oral anticoagulants than if enoxaparin 30 mg bid had been chosen as a comparator. Our study was able to assess the use of the different drugs in an in-patient setting only. It would be of interest to perform a similar analysis evaluating the long-term use to these therapies in an out-patient setting.

Conclusions

This meta-analysis is the first to our knowledge to evaluate the overall relative effectiveness of LMWH by comparing with placebo control and two major classes of anticoagulants therapy (i.e., factor Xa inhibitors and direct thrombin inhibitor) to treat patient who had TKR or THR surgeries. The findings indicate that prophylactic treatment of patients with LMWH could significantly reduce the rate of VTE and DVT. However, the factor Xa inhibitors might have better anticoagulant effect as compared with the LMWH enoxaparin. Compared to direct thrombin inhibitors, LMWH have similar incidence of VTE, DVT and PE but lower incidence of major bleeding in THR or TKR subjects. In general, LMWH has similar effectiveness to factor Xa inhibitor and direct thrombin inhibitors with respect to clinical outcomes associated with anticoagulation therapy. Factor Xa inhibitors, such as rivaroxaban, is superior to enoxaparin in reducing symptomatic VTE but the trade-offs between thromboprophylaxis versus increased major bleeding should be considered.

Key messages

- In comparison with patients without prophylaxis, low molecular weight heparin (LMWH) effectively reduces venous thromboembolism (VTE) and deep vein thrombosis (DVT) after total hip replacement (TKR).
- Compared to factor Xa inhibitors, LMWH may have higher incidence of VTE and DVT but similar rates of pulmonary embolism and major bleeding in THR or TKR subjects.
- In comparison with direct thrombin inhibitors, LMWH have similar incidence of VTE, DVT and pulmonary embolism but lower incidence of major bleeding in THR or TKR subjects.

Additional file

Additional file 1: Figure S1. Sensitivity analysis using the leave-one-out approach of the influence of each study on the pooled estimate for comparing total VTE rate between LMWH vs. control (A) placebo, (B) inhibitor of factor Xa, and (C) direct thrombin inhibitor for THR and TKR patients. Abbreviations: CI, confidence interval; Lower limit, lower bound of the 95% CI; Upper limit, upper bound of the 95% CI. **Figure S2.** Sensitivity analysis using the leave-one-out approach of the influence of each study on the pooled estimate for comparing total DVT rate between LMWH vs. control (A) placebo, (B) inhibitor of factor Xa, and (C) direct thrombin inhibitor for THR and TKR patients. Abbreviations: CI, confidence interval; Lower limit, lower bound of the 95% CI; Upper limit, upper bound of the 95% CI. **Figure S3.** Sensitivity analysis using the leave-one-out approach of the influence of each study on the pooled estimate for comparing PE rate between LMWH vs. control (A) inhibitor of factor Xa, and (B) direct thrombin inhibitor for THR and TKR patients. Abbreviations: CI, confidence interval; Lower limit, lower bound of the 95% CI; Upper limit, upper bound of the 95% CI. **Figure S4.** Sensitivity analysis using the leave-one-out approach of the influence of each study on the pooled estimate for comparing major bleeding rate (A) inhibitor of factor Xa, and (B) direct thrombin inhibitor for THR and TKR patients. Abbreviations: CI, confidence interval; Lower limit, lower bound of the 95% CI; Upper limit, upper bound of the 95% CI. **Figure S5.** The results of quality assessment for (A) individual studies, and (B) the summary of bias for all included studies. **Figure S6.** Forest graph showing the incidence of major bleeding events. **Figure S7.** Forest graph showing reoperation rate in this population. **Figure S8.** Forest graph showing the immortality rate in this population. **Figure S9.** Forest graph showing the percentage of patients who discontinued treatment due to adverse reaction. **Figure S10.** Forest graph showing the incidence of cardiovascular events. **Figure S11.** Forest graph showing the incidence of stroke. **Table S1.** Summary of meta-analysis results. **Table S2.** Published systematic review and meta-analysis relating to thromboprophylasis after THR and TKR (DOCX 734 kb)

Abbreviations

AAOS: American Association of Orthopedic Surgeons; ACCP: American College of Chest Physicians; DVT: deep vein thrombosis; MWH: low-molecular-weight heparin; RCTs: randomized controlled studies; THR: total hip replacement; TKR: received total knee; VTE: venous thromboembolism

Authors' contributions

We declare that this work was done by the authors named in this article and all liabilities pertaining to claims relating to the content of this article will be borne by the authors. XL and JL designed the study and revised the paper.

XL and JL collected data and carried out the analysis, and JL wrote the paper. Both authors read and approved the final manuscript.

Competing interests

The authors declare that they have no competing interests, and all authors should confirm its accuracy.

References

1. Chapelle C, Rosencher N, Jacques Zufferey P, Mismetti P, Cucherat M, Laporte S. Prevention of venous thromboembolic events with low-molecular-weight heparin in the non-major orthopaedic setting: meta-analysis of randomized controlled trials. Arthroscopy. 2014;30:987–96.
2. Falck-Ytter Y, Francis CW, Johanson NA, Curley C, Dahl OE, Schulman S, et al. Prevention of VTE in orthopedic surgery patients: antithrombotic therapy and prevention of thrombosis, 9th ed: American College of Chest Physicians Evidence-Based Clinical Practice Guidelines. Chest. 2012;141:e278S–325S.
3. Thorlund JB, Juhl CB, Roos EM, Lohmander LS. Arthroscopic surgery for degenerative knee: systematic review and meta-analysis of benefits and harms. BMJ. 2015;350:h2747.
4. Yeo KS, Lim WS, Lee YH. Deep vein thrombosis in arthroscopic surgery and chemoprophylaxis recommendation in an Asian population. Singap Med J. 2016;57:452–5.
5. Sobieraj DM, Coleman CI, Tongbram V, Lee S, Colby J, Chen WT, et al. Venous thromboembolism in orthopedic surgery. Comparative effectiveness review no. 49. AHRQ publication no. 12-EHC020-EF. Rockville: Agency for Healthcare Research and Quality; 2012. www.effectivehealthcare.ahrq.gov/reports/final.cfm. Accessed 19 Sept 2017.
6. Eikelboom JW, Quinlan DJ, O'Donnell M. Major bleeding, mortality, and effi cacy of fondaparinux in venous thromboembolism prevention trials. Circulation. 2009;120:2006–11.
7. Adam SS, McDuffie JR, Lachiewicz PF, Ortel TL, Williams JW Jr. Comparative effectiveness of new oral anticoagulants and standard thromboprophylaxis in patients having total hip or knee replacement: a systematic review. Ann Intern Med. 2013;159:275–84.
8. Kwong LM. Therapeutic potential of rivaroxaban in the prevention of venous thromboembolism following hip and knee replacement surgery: a review of clinical trial data. Vasc Health Risk Manag. 2011;7:461–6.
9. Hirsh J, Levine MN. Low molecular weight heparin: laboratory properties and clinical evaluation. A review Eur J Surg Suppl. 1994:9–22.
10. Heit JA, Colwell CW, Francis CW, Ginsberg JS, Berkowitz SD, Whipple J, et al. Comparison of the oral direct thrombin inhibitor ximelagatran with enoxaparin as prophylaxis against venous thromboembolism after total knee replacement: a phase 2 dose-finding study. Arch Intern Med. 2001;161:2215–21.
11. Wilke T, Muller S. Nonadherence in outpatient thromboprophylaxis after major orthopedic surgery: a systematic review. Expert Rev Pharmacoecon Outcomes Res. 2010;10:691–700.
12. Weitz JI. Low-molecular-weight heparins. N Engl J Med. 1997;337:688–98.
13. Sun Y, Chen D, Xu Z, Shi D, Dai J, Qin J, et al. Deep venous thrombosis after knee arthroscopy: a systematic review and meta-analysis. Arthroscopy. 2014;30:406–12.
14. Huisman MV, Quinlan DJ, Dahl OE, Schulman S. Enoxaparin versus dabigatran or rivaroxaban for thromboprophylaxis after hip or knee arthroplasty: results of separate pooled analyses of phase III multicenter randomized trials. Circ Cardiovasc Qual Outcomes. 2010;3:652–60.
15. Hayden JA, van der Windt DA, Cartwright JL, Cote P, Bombardier C. Assessing bias in studies of prognostic factors. Ann Intern Med. 2013;158:280–6.
16. Higgins JP, Altman DG, Gotzsche PC, Juni P, Moher D, Oxman AD, et al. The Cochrane Collaboration's tool for assessing risk of bias in randomised trials. BMJ. 2011;343:d5928.
17. Hardy RJ, Thompson SG. Detecting and describing heterogeneity in meta-analysis. Stat Med. 1998;17:841–56.
18. Takkouche B, Cadarso-Suarez C, Spiegelman D. Evaluation of old and new tests of heterogeneity in epidemiologic meta-analysis. Am J Epidemiol. 1999;150:206–15.
19. Sterne JA, Sutton AJ, Ioannidis JP, Terrin N, Jones DR, Lau J, et al. Recommendations for examining and interpreting funnel plot asymmetry in meta-analyses of randomised controlled trials. BMJ. 2011;343:d4002.
20. Kim SM, Moon YW, Lim SJ, Kim DW, Park YS. Effect of oral factor Xa inhibitor and low-molecular-weight heparin on surgical complications following total hip arthroplasty. Thromb Haemost. 2016;115:600–7.

21. Eriksson BI, Agnelli G, Gallus AS, Lassen MR, Prins MH, Renfurm RW, et al. Darexaban (YM150) versus enoxaparin for the prevention of venous thromboembolism after total hip arthroplasty: a randomised phase IIb dose confirmation study (ONYX-3). Thromb Haemost. 2014;111:213–25.

22. Zou Y, Tian S, Wang Y, Sun K. Administering aspirin, rivaroxaban and low-molecular-weight heparin to prevent deep venous thrombosis after total knee arthroplasty. Blood Coagul Fibrinolysis. 2014;25:660–4.

23. Eriksson BI, Dahl OE, Huo MH, Kurth AA, Hantel S, Hermansson K, et al. Oral dabigatran versus enoxaparin for thromboprophylaxis after primary total hip arthroplasty (RE-NOVATE II*). A randomised, double-blind, non-inferiority trial. Thromb Haemost. 2011;105:721–9.

24. Lassen MR, Raskob GE, Gallus A, Pineo G, Chen D, Hornick P. Apixaban versus enoxaparin for thromboprophylaxis after knee replacement (ADVANCE-2): a randomised double-blind trial. Lancet. 2010;375:807–15.

25. Lassen MR, Gallus A, Raskob GE, Pineo G, Chen D, Ramirez LM. Apixaban versus enoxaparin for thromboprophylaxis after hip replacement. N Engl J Med. 2010;363:2487–98.

26. Ginsberg JS, Davidson BL, Comp PC, Francis CW, Friedman RJ, Huo MH, et al. Oral thrombin inhibitor dabigatran etexilate vs north American enoxaparin regimen for prevention of venous thromboembolism after knee arthroplasty surgery. J Arthroplast. 2009;24:1–9.

27. Turpie AG, Lassen MR, Davidson BL, Bauer KA, Gent M, Kwong LM, et al. Rivaroxaban versus enoxaparin for thromboprophylaxis after total knee arthroplasty (RECORD4): a randomised trial. Lancet. 2009;373:1673–80.

28. Lassen MR, Raskob GE, Gallus A, Pineo G, Chen D, Portman RJ. Apixaban or enoxaparin for thromboprophylaxis after knee replacement. N Engl J Med. 2009;361:594–604.

29. Fuji T, Ochi T, Niwa S, Fujita S. Prevention of postoperative venous thromboembolism in Japanese patients undergoing total hip or knee arthroplasty: two randomized, double-blind, placebo-controlled studies with three dosage regimens of enoxaparin. J Orthop Sci. 2008;13:442–51.

30. Kakkar AK, Brenner B, Dahl OE, Eriksson BI, Mouret P, Muntz J, et al. Extended duration rivaroxaban versus short-term enoxaparin for the prevention of venous thromboembolism after total hip arthroplasty: a double-blind, randomised controlled trial. Lancet. 2008;372:31–9.

31. Eriksson BI, Borris LC, Friedman RJ, Haas S, Huisman MV, Kakkar AK, et al. Rivaroxaban versus enoxaparin for thromboprophylaxis after hip arthroplasty. N Engl J Med. 2008;358:2765–75.

32. Lassen MR, Ageno W, Borris LC, Lieberman JR, Rosencher N, Bandel TJ, et al. Rivaroxaban versus enoxaparin for thromboprophylaxis after total knee arthroplasty. N Engl J Med. 2008;358:2776–86.

33. Eriksson BI, Dahl OE, Rosencher N, Kurth AA, van Dijk CN, Frostick SP, et al. Oral dabigatran etexilate vs. subcutaneous enoxaparin for the prevention of venous thromboembolism after total knee replacement: the RE-MODEL randomized trial. J Thromb Haemost. 2007;5:2178–85.

34. Eriksson BI, Dahl OE, Rosencher N, Kurth AA, van Dijk CN, Frostick SP, et al. Dabigatran etexilate versus enoxaparin for prevention of venous thromboembolism after total hip replacement: a randomised, double-blind, non-inferiority trial. Lancet. 2007;370:949–56.

35. Eriksson BI, Agnelli G, Cohen AT, Dahl OE, Lassen MR, Mouret P, et al. The direct thrombin inhibitor melagatran followed by oral ximelagatran compared with enoxaparin for the prevention of venous thromboembolism after total hip or knee replacement: the EXPRESS study. J Thromb Haemost. 2003;1:2490–6.

36. Colwell CW Jr, Berkowitz SD, Davidson BL, Lotke PA, Ginsberg JS, Lieberman JR, et al. Comparison of ximelagatran, an oral direct thrombin inhibitor, with enoxaparin for the prevention of venous thromboembolism following total hip replacement. A randomized, double-blind study. J Thromb Haemost. 2003;1:2119–30.

37. Eriksson BI, Agnelli G, Cohen AT, Dahl OE, Mouret P, Rosencher N, et al. Direct thrombin inhibitor melagatran followed by oral ximelagatran in comparison with enoxaparin for prevention of venous thromboembolism after total hip or knee replacement. Thromb Haemost. 2003;89:288–96.

38. Bergqvist D, Benoni G, Bjorgell O, Fredin H, Hedlundh U, Nicolas S, et al. Low-molecular-weight heparin (enoxaparin) as prophylaxis against venous thromboembolism after total hip replacement. N Engl J Med. 1996;335:696–700.

39. Planes A, Vochelle N, Darmon JY, Fagola M, Bellaud M, Huet Y. Risk of deep-venous thrombosis after hospital discharge in patients having undergone total hip replacement: double-blind randomised comparison of enoxaparin versus placebo. Lancet. 1996;348:224–8.

40. Hull RD, Pineo GF, Stein PD, Mah AF, MacIsaac SM, Dahl OE, et al. Extended out-of-hospital low-molecular-weight heparin prophylaxis against deep venous thrombosis in patients after elective hip arthroplasty: a systematic review. Ann Intern Med. 2001;135:858–69.

41. Tasker A, Harbord R, Bannister GC. Meta-analysis of low molecular weight heparin versus placebo in patients undergoing total hip replacement and post-operative morbidity and mortality since their introduction. Hip Int. 2010;20:64–74.

42. Ning GZ, Kan SL, Chen LX, Shangguan L, Feng SQ, Zhou Y. Rivaroxaban for thromboprophylaxis after total hip or knee arthroplasty: a meta-analysis with trial sequential analysis of randomized controlled trials. Sci Rep. 2016;6: 23726.

43. Feng W, Wu K, Liu Z, Kong G, Deng Z, Chen S, et al. Oral direct factor Xa inhibitor versus enoxaparin for thromboprophylaxis after hip or knee arthroplasty: systemic review, traditional meta-analysis, dose-response meta-analysis and network meta-analysis. Thromb Res. 2015;136:1133–44.

44. Gómez-Outes A, Terleira-Fernández AI, Suárez-Gea ML, Vargas-Castrillón E. Dabigatran, rivaroxaban, or apixaban versus enoxaparin for thromboprophylaxis after total hip or knee replacement: systematic review, meta-analysis, and indirect treatment comparisons. BMJ. 2012;344

45. Wolowacz SE, Roskell NS, Plumb JM, Caprini JA, Eriksson BI. Efficacy and safety of dabigatran etexilate for the prevention of venous thromboembolism following total hip or knee arthroplasty. A meta-analysis Thromb Haemost. 2009;101:77–85.

46. Cohen AT, Hirst C, Sherrill B, Holmes P, Fidan D. Meta-analysis of trials comparing ximelagatran with low molecular weight heparin for prevention of venous thromboembolism after major orthopaedic surgery. Br J Surg. 2005;92:1335–44.

47. Ma G, Zhang R, Wu X, Wang D, Ying K. Direct factor Xa inhibitors (rivaroxaban and apixaban) versus enoxaparin for the prevention of venous thromboembolism after total knee replacement: A meta-analysis of 6 randomized clinical trials. Thromb Res. 2015;135:816–22.

48. Neumann I, Rada G, Claro JC, Carrasco-Labra A, Thorlund K, Akl EA, et al. Oral direct Factor Xa inhibitors versus low-molecular-weight heparin to prevent venous thromboembolism in patients undergoing total hip or knee replacement: a systematic review and meta-analysis. Ann Intern Med. 2012;156:710–9.

49. Nieto JA, Espada NG, Merino RG, González TC. Dabigatran, rivaroxaban and apixaban versus enoxaparin for thromboprophylaxis after total knee or hip arthroplasty: pool-analysis of phase III randomized clinical trials. Thromb Res. 2012;130:183–91.

50. Li XM, Sun SG, Zhang WD. Apixaban versus enoxaparin for thromboprophylaxis after total hip or knee arthroplasty: a meta-analysis of randomized controlled trials. Chin Med J. 2012;125:2339–45.

51. Raskob GE, Gallus AS, Pineo GF, Chen D, Ramirez LM, Wright RT, et al. Apixaban versus enoxaparin for thromboprophylaxis after hip or knee replacement: pooled analysis of major venous thromboembolism and bleeding in 8464 patients from the ADVANCE-2 and ADVANCE-3 trials. J Bone Joint Surg Br. 2012;94:257–64.

52. Huang J, Cao Y, Liao C, Wu L, Gao F. Apixaban versus enoxaparin in patients with total knee arthroplasty. A meta-analysis of randomised trials. Thromb Haemost. 2011;105:245–53.

53. Cao YB, Zhang JD, Shen H, Jiang YY. Rivaroxaban versus enoxaparin for thromboprophylaxis after total hip or knee arthroplasty: a meta-analysis of randomized controlled trials. Eur J Clin Pharmacol. 2010;66:1099–108.

54. Melillo SN, Scanlon JV, Exter BP, Steinberg M, Jarvis CI. Rivaroxaban for thromboprophylaxis in patients undergoing major orthopedic surgery. Ann Pharmacother. 2010;44:1061–71.

55. Eriksson BI, Dahl OE, Rosencher N, Clemens A, Hantel S, Feuring M, et al. Oral dabigatran etexilate versus enoxaparin for venous thromboembolism prevention after total hip arthroplasty: pooled analysis of two phase 3 randomized trials. Thromb J. 2015;13:36.

56. Friedman RJ, Dahl OE, Rosencher N, Caprini JA, Kurth AA, Francis CW, et al. Dabigatran versus enoxaparin for prevention of venous thromboembolism after hip or knee arthroplasty: a pooled analysis of three trials. Thromb Res. 2010;126:175–82.

57. Kwok CS, Pradhan S, Yeong JK, Loke YK. Relative effects of two different enoxaparin regimens as comparators against newer oral anticoagulants: meta-analysis and adjusted indirect comparison. Chest. 2013;144:593–600.

9

Validation of the Polish version of the Western Ontario Rotator Cuff Index in patients following arthroscopic rotator cuff repair

Agnieszka Bejer[1,2]* (iD), Mirosław Probachta[1,2], Marek Kulczyk[2], Sharon Griffin[3], Elżbieta Domka-Jopek[1] and Jędrzej Płocki[2,4]

Abstract

Background: The Western Ontario Rotator Cuff Index (WORC) is a joint specific outcome tool that assesses the quality of life in patients with various rotator cuff problems.
Our purpose was to evaluate selected psychometric characteristics (internal consistency, validity, reliability and agreement) of the Polish version of WORC in patients undergoing rotator cuff repair.

Methods: Sixty-nine subjects took part in the study with a mean age 55.5 (range 40–65). All had undergone arthroscopic rotator cuff repair in 2015–2016. Data from 57 patients in whom symptoms in the shoulder joint had not changed within 10–14 days were analyzed in a WORC test-retest using the Intraclass Correlation Coefficient (ICC), Standard Error of Measurement (SEM) and Minimal Detectable Change (MDC). WORC was compared to the short version of the Disabilities of Arm, Shoulder and Hand Questionnaire (QuickDash) and the Short Form-36 v. 2.0 (SF-36).

Results: High internal consistency of 0.94 was found using Cronbach's alpha coefficient. Reliability of the WORC resulted in ICC = 0.99, agreement assessed with SEM and MDC amounted to 1.62 and 4.48 respectively. The validity analysis of WORC showed strong correlations with QuickDash and SF-36 PCS (Physical Component Summary), while moderate with SF-36 MCS (Mental Component Summary). WORC had no floor or ceiling effect.

Conclusions: The Polish version of the WORC is a reliable and valid tool with high internal consistency for assessing the quality of life in patients undergoing arthroscopic rotator cuff repair.

Keywords: WORC, Rotator cuff tear, Quality of life questionnaires, Validity, Reliability

Background

Rotator cuff disorders are one of the most common shoulder problems which can significantly affect a patients' ability to work and other activities of daily life such as dressing, washing hair, driving etc. [1, 2]. Little is known about the incidence of it or associations of its demographic in the general population both in Poland and worldwide. White et al. conducted a large epidemiological study of rotator cuff pathology in the United Kingdom. They observed that the incidence of rotator cuff pathology was 87 per 100,000 person-years. At the same time, it was more common in women (90 cases per 100,000 person-years) than in men (83 cases per 100,000 person-years). They found the highest incidence of 198 per 100,000 person-years in those aged between 55 and 59 years [3]. Mall et al. conducted a systematical review of the literature in 2013 and found that the injury usually causes damage to the tendon of supraspinatus in 84% of tears, infraspinatus in 39% of cases, and the tendon of subscapularis was damaged in 78% of injuries. They also observed that the tear size of the tendon was < 3 cm in 22%, 3 to 5 cm in 36%, and > 5 cm in 42% [4]. In the systematical review Littlewood et al. found the incidence of rotator

* Correspondence: agnbej@wp.pl
[1]Institute of Physiotherapy, Faculty of Medicine, University of Rzeszow, ul. Hoffmanowej 25, 35-016 Rzeszow, Poland
[2]The Holy Family Specialist Hospital, Rudna Mała, Poland
Full list of author information is available at the end of the article

cuff tendinopathy to range from 0.3 to 5.5% and annual prevalence from 0.5 to 7.4%. [5].

A large number of measurement tools for evaluating patients with shoulder problems are available for assessing symptoms, functioning and quality of life, the majority of which were developed in English-speaking countries. Some of those questionnaires available are: the Western Ontario Shoulder Instability Index (WOSI) [6] and the Shoulder Instability Questionnaire (SIQ) [7], the Western Ontario Osteoarthritis of the Shoulder Index (WOOS) [8], the Western Ontario Rotator Cuff Index (WORC) [9] and the Rotator Cuff Quality of Life Index (RC-QOL) [10], the Disabilities of the Arm, Shoulder and Hand Questionnaire (DASH) [11] and its shortened version - QuickDASH [12, 13].

Before being introduced into scientific research and / or clinical practice, outcome tools that were created in a country of a different language or culture need to be adapted. Adaption consists of two phases: a linguistic validation and a psychometric validation and should be conducted according to specific methodology [14–16].

The authors of this paper undertook to adapt and validate the WORC to the Polish version, because up to now there has been no published results of psychometric analysis of the Polish version of questionnaires used to assess the quality of life of patients with rotator cuff disorders. The Western Ontario Rotator Cuff Index is a widely used outcome tool for assessing the quality of life in patients with various problems in the rotator cuff. The analysis of the results of the questionnaire allows for a reliable assessment of the symptoms and functioning (5 domains) of such a patient and verification of the effectiveness of the treatment applied. The questionnaire was originally created in English and published by Kirkley et al. in 2003, who confirmed its high reliability, accuracy and sensitivity [9]. Also, in a systematic review on the patient-reported outcomes used for the evaluation of symptoms and functional limitations in people with rotator cuff problems, St-Pierre et al. concluded that the WORC is one of the most responsive questionnaires and showed good psychometric properties for the targeted population [17].

The WORC questionnaire has been translated into several languages including German [18], Turkish [19], Portuguese for use in Brazil [20], Norwegian [21], Iranian [22], Dutch [23], Japanese [24], Swedish [25] and Chinese [26].

Cultural-linguistic adaptation of the WORC questionnaire to the Polish version was carried out in 2017 by Bejer et al. [27] in accordance with the Mapi Research Institute guidelines [14]. It is proceeded by six stages: preparation of two independent versions of the translation of the WORC questionnaire from English into Polish, reconciliation of the common version, preparation of a back translation into English, comparison of the back translation with the source version of the questionnaire by the original author and

corrections, verification of the received version of the questionnaire by a team of experts, testing the questionnaire in a group of patients diagnosed with rotator cuff injury and making corrections - obtaining the Polish version of WORC-PL [27]. Each stage of linguistic adaptation was completed with a written report sent to the author of the source version.

The purpose of this study was to evaluate selected psychometric properties (internal consistency, reliability and agreement, validity) of the Polish version of the WORC questionnaire.

Methods

Patients were identified from the hospital patient database of the Orthopedic Department in the Specialist Hospital in Rudna Mała, Poland. Patients who had undergone arthroscopic reconstruction of the rotator cuff from 2015 to 2016 by one orthopedic surgeon (supraspinatous, infraspinatous or subscapularis, and additionally after the damage to the tendon of the long head of the biceps brachi), were eligible for the study.

Patients who were ≥ 18 years of age, were native Polish speakers and signed an informed consent participated in the study. Exclusion criteria was: previous surgeries within the shoulder complex and the upper limb, dislocations of the shoulder complex, fractures of the shoulder blade, clavicle or upper limb, and who had co-existing rheumatological or neurological conditions.

Outcome Tools
The Western Ontario Rotator Cuff Index (WORC)
The WORC is a self-reported questionnaire, which contains 21 items grouped into five domains – physical symptoms (six items), sport/recreation (four items), work (four items), lifestyle (four items) and emotions (three items). It also includes instructions for patients on how to complete the questionnaire and in case of problems in fully understanding the questions there are detailed explanations for each. The patients give responses concerning problems and symptoms they have observed over the past week by placing a slash "/" on a 10 cm (100 mm) visual-analogue scale. In order to calculate the result, the distance from the left side of the line is measured and the result calculated out of 100 (with the accuracy of 0.5 mm). The total score for each domain can be calculated (Physical symptoms / 600; Sport and Rrecreation / 400; Work / 400; Lifestyle / 400; Emotions / 300). The best possible result in the whole questionnaire is 0, the worst is 2100. The result presented in a clinically meaningful way is the percentage of the basic result. Since the worst possible result is 2100, the total score is subtracted from 2100, and then divided by 2100 and multiplied by 100, to obtain a percentage. WORC score can therefore vary from 0% - ie the lowest level of

functional status, up to 100%, ie the highest level of functioning [9, 27].

The Short Form-36 v. 2.0 (SF-36 v. 2.0)

The SF-36 v. 2.0 is a generic health related quality of life (HRQOL) questionnaire with 36 questions grouped in eight dimensions: physical functioning, role limitations due to physical health, role limitations due to emotional health, bodily pain, vitality, social functioning, general health and mental health. The score for each domain can range from 0 to 100, the lower the score, the worse the quality of life [28]. From these 8 dimensions, 2 summary scores, 1 for physical health (PCS - Physical Component Summary) and 1 for mental health (MCS - Mental Component Summary), can be computed [29, 30].

The abridged version of the Disabilities of Arm, Shoulder and Hand Questionnaire (QuickDash)

The QuickDash is a self-completed instrument for assessment of disability of the upper limb, viewed as a functional whole. It contains 11 questions: symptoms (3 questions) and the impact of upper limb problems on social activity, limitations at work or everyday activities (8 questions). The response format is a five-point Likert scale, where the lowest value means no restrictions or absence of the symptom, and the highest - lack of possibility to perform the activity or maximum severity of the symptom. The QuickDASH constraint and symptom index is calculated by: summing the circled digits, dividing by the number of responses, subtracting 1 and multiplying by 25. The index takes the form of a number between 0 and 100, where a higher value means a greater limitation in performing activities [12, 13].

Procedure

The subjects were tested two times. The first test consisted of completing the Polish versions of all questionnaires: WORC, QuickDash and the Short Form-36 (SF-36) v. 2.0. The second test was performed 1–2 weeks later. People answered the WORC questionnaire (re-test) and reported whether their symptoms had changed on a 7-point Global Rating of Change Scale (GRC) (1 = much better, 2 = somewhat better, 3 = a little better, 4 = no change, 5 = a little worse, 6 = somewhat worse, 7 = much worse) [31].

The test-retest time interval was used according to the scientific literature, which indicates that an interval of 1–2 weeks is adequate and reasonable in such studies. There is little probability of changes in symptoms during such a period and time is long enough for the respondents to forget their previous answers [32, 33].

Statistical analysis

All analyses were conducted using the Statistica 10.0 software. The level of statistical significance was assumed a priori at $\alpha < 0.05$. Normal distribution of the results of this study was verified using Shapiro-Wilk test. After determining that the data has a non-normal distribution, the non-parametric Wilcoxon test for the basic statistical analysis was used. The dependencies between total and domain scores of the WORC and between total WORC and reference measures (SF-36, QuickDASH) were determined using the non-parametric Spearman's rank correlation coefficient. The sample size was based on the general recommendations of Altman of at least 50 subjects in a methods comparison study [34].

Internal consistency

Internal consistency is a measure of the extent to which items in a questionnaire domain are correlated (homogeneous), thus measuring the same concept. It was calculated by using Cronbach's alpha coefficient and was based on data from a group of 69 patients. The scale shows good internal consistency if value of Cronbach's alpha is between 0.70 and 0.95 [32, 33].

Reliability and agreement

Reliability and agreement concern the degree to which repeated measurements in stable persons (test-retest) provide similar answers. Reliability is the degree to which patients can be distinguished from each other, despite measurement error. Agreement is the absolute measurement error, i.e., how close the scores on repeated measures are. Small measurement error is required for evaluative purposes in which one wants to distinguish clinically important changes from measurement error [33].

The intra class correlation (ICC), with a 95% confidence interval (CI) was used to assess the reliability of the WORC. It was calculated on a group of 57 people who completed the WORC questionnaire two times. According to the guidelines from the literature, we assumed positive rating for reliability when the ICC is ≥ 0.70 [33].

To assess the agreement, we calculated the Standard Error of Measurement (SEM) and the Minimal Detectable Change (MDC) in the group 57 people who completed WORC two times. SEM was calculated using the formula: $SEM = SD \sqrt{(1-R)}$, where SD represents Standard Deviation of the sample and R the reliability parameter (ICC). The MDC is the minimum amount of change in a patient's score that ensures the change is not the result of measurement error. MDC was calculated using the formula. $MDC = SEM \times 1.96 \times \sqrt{2}$, where 1.96 derives from the 0.95% CI of no change, and $\sqrt{2}$ shows two measurements assessing the change [33, 35].

Construct validity

Construct validity refers to the extent to which scores on a particular instrument relate to other measures in a manner that is consistent with theoretically derived hypotheses concerning the concepts that are being measured [33].

To evaluate the construct validity of the Polish version of the WORC, the Spearman's correlation coefficient (SCC) was calculated between total and domain scores of the WORC and a general quality of life questionnaire (SF-36) and the joint-specific questionnaire to assess the functioning of the upper limb (QuickDASH). Correlation coefficients, $r < 0.30$ = low, $0.30 < r < 0.70$ = moderate, $r > 0.70$ = high, were used to assess validity [36]. We hypothesized that correlations between the WORC and the QuickDASH would be stronger than between the WORC and the SF-36. We also expected that the WORC total would be stronger correlated with SF - 36 PCS than MCS, while emotions domain of WORC would be stronger correlated with SF-36 MCS than with PCS and QuickDASH.

Content validity

Floor or ceiling effects are considered to be present if more than 15% of the respondents achieved the lowest or highest possible score, respectively [33]. Floor and ceiling effects were calculated in the group of 69 patients for WORC, SF-36 PCS, SF-36 MCS and QuickDASH.

Results

Participant characteristics

After screening of the database of Specialist Hospital in Rudna Mała we identified 140 patients who were operated on for rotator cuff disorders in 2015–2016 (72 people in 2015 and 68 people in 2016) of which 111 met the inclusion criteria. These patients were contacted by phone, the study explained to them and were asked for their willingness to complete questionnaires. Those that agreed signed an informed consent form and the outcome tools were sent by post according to the measurement protocol. Sixty-nine subjects (62.2%) returned the completed questionnaires. Patient gender, age, operated limb, hand dominance, time from surgery and diagnosis were recorded (Table 1).

In order to assess test-retest reliability and agreement of the scale, the respondents filled in the WORC questionnaire a second time. The median time between administrations was 13 days (range 10–14 days). In the test-retest analyzes, data from 57 people were used; 4 subjects who participated in the first test were excluded due to reporting changes in the functioning of the operated shoulder joint during the assessed period in GRS scale, and 8 people did not return the completed questionnaire for the second time. The absolute values of all scores are given in Table 2.

Internal consistency

Internal consistency was calculated based on the data from test 1. A high degree of internal consistency (α = 0.94) was demonstrated for WORC Total, with an item range of 0.88 to 0.95 and the domain range of 0.92 to 0.95 (Table 3).

Table 1 Patient demographic and clinical characteristics

	N (%)	x̄ (range)
Gender		
Male	49 (71)	
Female	20 (29)	
Age (years)		55.5 (40–65)
Handedness		
Right-handed	58 (84)	
Left-handed	11 (16)	
Time from operation		16.8 mths (6–24)
Diagnosis – Tendon injury in:		
4 muscles:	7 (10.1)	
SST + IST + SScapT+LHBT	7 (100.0)	
3 muscles:	22 (31.9)	
SST + SScapT+LHBT	7 (31.8)	
SST + IST + LHBT	11 (50.0)	
IST + SScapT+LHBT	2 (9.1)	
SST + IST + SScapT	2 (9.1)	
2 muscles:	24 (34.8)	
SST + LHBT	15 (62.5)	
SScapT+LHBT	4 (16.7)	
SST + SScapT	5 (20,8)	
1 muscle:	16 (23.2)	
SST	15 (93.7)	
SScapT	1 (6.3)	

Abbreviations: N number, x̄ Mean, % per cent, SST Supraspinatus Tendon, IST Infraspinatus Tendon, SScapT Subscapularis Tendon, LHBT Long Head Biceps Tendon

Correlations between particular detailed measures and between specific measures and a summary measure were shown using the Spearman's rank correlation coefficient (SCC). All domains are very closely related (from 0.78 to 0.97), as well as very pronounced correlations occur between the domains and WORC Total (from 0.87 to 0.97) (Table 4).

Reliability
Intraclass correlation
The results for the WORC scale were compared in test 1 and test 2 (re-test) for a group of 57 patients. In the domain of Work and Lifestyle there were statistically significant differences between the studies, however in the test 2 the results were slightly higher on average by 0.5 points and 1.2 points respectively. The difference is small in relation to the initial result, which in the domain of Work was 61.5 points, and in the domain of Lifestyle was 73.3 points. The ICC for the WORC Total was 0.99, and the domains ranged between 0.94 and 0.99 suggesting a high consistency of the results of both tests for all WORC domains (Table 5).

Table 2 Absolute values of all scores

Questionnaire	Total group (N = 69)		Group 1 (N = 26)		Group 2 (N = 43)	
	$\overline{x} \pm SD$	Range	$\overline{x} \pm SD$	Range	$\overline{x} \pm SD$	Range
WORC						
Physical symptoms	77.7 ± 20.4	33.5–100.0	56,1 ± 13,7	33,5-81,0	90,8 ± 9,9	62,5-100,0
Sports/recreation	63.8 ± 29.2	7.8–100.0	32,8 ± 15,6	7,8-75,5	82,6 ± 16,6	43,0-100,0
Work	61.5 ± 31.3	0.0–100.0	29,9 ± 15,5	6,5-62,5	80,6 ± 21,3	0,0-100,0
Lifestyle	73.3 ± 26.0	18.8–100.0	46,4 ± 20,0	18,8-100,0	89,5 ± 11,9	62,3-100,0
Emotions	75.8 ± 24.7	18.0–100.0	52,6 ± 21,5	18,0-92,3	89,8 ± 13,3	43,3-100,0
Total	70.9 ± 24.5	24.0–100.0	44,3 ± 13,6	24,0-76,8	86,9 ± 12,7	50,2-100,0
SF-36						
Physical Functioning	77.5 ± 19.5	15.0–100.0	61,5 ± 19,4	15,0-90,0	87,2 ± 11,8	60,0-100,0
Role Physical	58.8 ± 26.3	6.3–100.0	37,0 ± 15,5	6,3-75,0	71,9 ± 22,4	12,5-100,0
Body Pain	64.9 ± 25.2	22.5–100.0	42,0 ± 16,1	22,5-77,5	78,8 ± 18,8	42,5-100,0
General Health	62.0 ± 13.9	25.0–90.0	57,5 ± 13,9	25,0-80,0	64,8 ± 13,4	40,0-90,0
Vitality	63.0 ± 18.2	18.8–100.0	52,4 ± 14,5	18,8-75,0	69,5 ± 17,3	25,0-100,0
Social Functioning	76.3 ± 22.5	25.0–100.0	61,1 ± 21,0	25,0-100,0	85,5 ± 18,1	37,5-100,0
Role Emotional	75.0 ± 24.8	25.0–100.0	57,4 ± 23,4	25,0-100,0	85,7 ± 19,1	41,7-100,0
Mental Health	71.8 ± 17.9	20.0–100.0	61,5 ± 17,9	20,0-85,0	78,0 ± 15,0	40,0-100,0
PCS	63.3 ± 14.7	26.0–85.7	50,5 ± 12,4	26,0-82,4	71,1 ± 9,8	49,5-85,7
MCS	70.6 ± 18.2	21.4–100.0	58,0 ± 16,9	21,4-83,9	78,3 ± 14,5	48,2-100,0
QuickDash	28.6 ± 24.7	0.0–84.1	52,8 ± 19,2	15,9-84,1	14,0 ± 13,6	0,0-50,0

Group 1 - subject evaluated in the period from 6 months to 1 year after the operation, Group 2 - subjects assessed in from over 1 year to 2 years after surgery
Abbreviations: *WORC* Western Ontario Rotator Cuff index, *SF-36 PCS* SF-36 questionnaire Physical Component Summary, *SF-36 MCS* SF-36 questionnaire Mental Component Summary, *QuickDash* an abridged version of the Disabilities of the Arm, Shoulder and Hand questionnaire, *$\overline{x}$* Mean, *SD* Standard Deviation

Agreement
Measurement error and minimal detectable change
The standard error of measurement (SEM) associated with the WORC Total was 1.62 points for measurements of a group of 57 subjects, in two subsequent tests. Minimal detectable change MDC for WORC Total was 4.48 points (95% CI). SEM for the individual domains ranged from 1.62 to 5.65 whereas MDC ranged from 4.48 to 15.66. Based on the above results, it can be concluded that change of state has not occurred in the studied group (Table 5).

Table 3 Cronbach's alpha of WORC calculated for the total score and every domain

WORC	No of items	Cronbach's alpha
Physical symptoms	6	0.931
Sports/recreation	4	0.945
Work	4	0.940
Lifestyle	4	0.915
Emotions	3	0.922
Total	21	0.941

Abbreviations: *WORC* Western Ontario Rotator Cuff index

Validity
Construct validity
Table 6 shows correlations using the Spearman correlation coefficient (SCC), between WORC and reference questionnaires, i.e. SF-36 (results in the domains and in PCS - Physical Component Summary and MCS - Mental Component Summary) and QuickDASH. As expected the WORC Total correlates strongly with SF-36 PCS and moderately with SF-36 MCS. Physical subscales of WORC are more strongly correlated with physical subscales of SF-36. There are strong correlations between WORC domain of Emotions and SF-36 MCS and the correlations with PCS are moderate. However, all correlations between the overall score and the WORC domains and the QuickDash are strong.

Figures 1, 2 and 3 show a scatter plots of WORC Total vs. PCS, WORC Total vs. MCS and WORC Total vs. QuickDash to illustrate the correlation between the scores.

Content validity
The floor effect does not appear in the WORC, SF-36 PCS and SF-36 MCS questionnaire, and the QuickDASH questionnaire is only marked in 5 people (7.2%). The ceiling effect is noted only in 1 person (1.4%) in the WORC questionnaire and SF-36 MCS, and in the other tools it does not occur. These results showed that all the

Table 4 Spearman's correlation coefficient (SCC)

WORC	Physical symptoms	Sports/ recreation	Work	Lifestyle	Emotions	Total
Physical symptoms	1	0.94	0.95	0.90	0.79	0.97
Sports/recreation	0.94	1	0.94	0.87	0.82	0.97
Work	0.95	0.94	1	0.91	0.78	0.97
Lifestyle	0.90	0.87	0.91	1	0.88	0.94
Emotions	0.79	0.82	0.78	0.88	1	0.87
Total	0.97	0.97	0.97	0.94	0.87	1

Spearman correlation coefficients showing the strength of the correlations between individual domains of WORC as well as domains and total score
Abbreviations: WORC Western Ontario Rotator Cuff index
All correlations were significant at $p < 0.001$

outcome tools have similar floor and These results showed that all the outcome tools have similar floor and ceiling effects.

Discussion

All of the hypothesis described in the methodology proved to be true. The WORC had very high test-retest reliability (Total ICC = 0.99, Domains 0.94–0.99). It had a high degree of internal consistency (Cronbach's alpha for Total = 0.94, Domains = 0.92–0.95). Our validity comparisons also proved to be true with the strongest correlation between the Physical domain of the WORC and the SF-36 PCS. All correlations between the Total and the WORC domains and the QuickDash also proved to be strong as expected.

The standard methodology of translation, cultural adaptation and validation of research tools should be taken to ensure that the new language version developed is equivalent to the original version [21]. The use of official language versions of questionnaires or scales is necessary to preserve the comparability of research results carried out between researchers from the developing country as well as from various countries around the world [21, 37].

The WORC questionnaire was adapted to the Polish language due to the good psychometric properties of the original. It includes five domains of health as defined by the World Health Organization and collects information not covered by other research tools. The questionnaire can be used not only in the research setting but also in the clinical setting for monitoring an individual patient's progress and for decision-making about treatment [9]. Bejer et al. [27] found the Polish WORC to be reliable and described the cultural and linguistic adaptation. The internal consistency of the Total WORC was assessed using Cronbach's alpha and was found to be 0.94, with the range for individual items and domains from 0.88 to 0.95. This confirms good internal consistency. Any results lower than 0.70 may indicate a lack of correlation between the items in a scale, while higher might imply redundancy among the questions [33]. Our results are similar to the results of the authors of other the WORC validations. Cronbach's alpha in the overall scale and subscales of the Chinese version of WORC is from 0.872 to 0.954 [26], Japanese version 0.78–0.95 [24], Danish version 0.91–0.97 [23], the Brazilian Portuguese version 0.88–0.97 [20], Swedish 0.89–0.97 [25]. Slightly lower values of the Cronbach's alpha coefficients were obtained in the Turkish version 0.69–0.92 [19].

In our study the ICC for the different domains and for the total WORC ranged from 0.94 and 0.99. According to the literature guidelines, these results are acceptable and suitable for use in both group

Table 5 Reliability of WORC expressed as ICC calculated for WORC total scores and for the individual domains of WORC. Agreement of WORC expressed as Standard Error of Measurement and Minimal Detectable Change of the WORC

WORC	Change test 2 vs. test 1			p	ICC (95% CI)	SEM	MDC
	$\bar{x}$	Me	SD				
Physical symptoms	0.6	0.0	3.2	0.4162	0.9871 (0.9751–0.9934)	2.28	6.32
Sports/recreation	0.4	0.3	2.7	0.1229	0.9960 (0.9923–0.9980)	1.89	5.25
Work	0.5	0.5	4.5	0.0167*	0.9903 (0.9813–0.9950)	3.17	8.78
Lifestyle	1.2	0.3	2.7	0.0209*	0.9935 (0.9855–0.9969)	2.10	5.83
Emotions	−1.4	0.0	8.2	0.4321	0.9491 (0.9041–0.9734)	5.65	15.66
Total	0.4	0.1	2.3	0.1824	0.9955 (0.9913–0.9977)	1.62	4.48

Abbreviations: WORC Western Ontario Rotator Cuff index, $\bar{x}$ mean, *Me* median, *SD* standard deviation, *SEM* Standard Error of Measurement, *MDC* Minimal Detectable Change, *CI* Confidence Interval
All correlations weren't significant, except marked * $p < 0.05$

Table 6 Correlations between WORC (results in domains and overall result) and reference questionnaires

Questionnaire	WORC					
	Physical symptoms	Sports/ recreation	Work	Lifestyle	Emotions	Total
SF-36						
Physical Functioning	0.75***	0.71***	0.74***	0.77***	0.61***	0.76***
Role Physical	0.79***	0.75***	0.78***	0.78***	0.65***	0.80***
Body Pain	0.83***	0.82***	0.79***	0.84***	0.81***	0.85***
General Health	0.22	0.23	0.21	0.19	0.33**	0.24*
Vitality	0.45***	0.51***	0.42***	0.50***	0.61***	0.50***
Social Functioning	0.64***	0.63***	0.62***	0.72***	0.75***	0.68***
Role Emotional	0.53***	0.57***	0.53***	0.65***	0.73***	0.61***
Mental Health	0.47***	0.49***	0.45***	0.52***	0.64***	0.52***
PCS	0.80***	0.76***	0.79***	0.82***	0.63***	0.81***
MCS	0.56***	058***	0.53***	0.63***	0.74***	0.62***
QuickDash	−0.90***	−0.89***	−0.88***	−0.88***	−0.80***	−0.91***

Abbreviations: *WORC* Western Ontario Rotator Cuff index, *SF-36 PCS* SF-36 questionnaire Physical Component Summary, *SF-36 CS* SF-36 questionnaire Mental Component Summary, *QuickDash* an abridged version of the Disabilities of the Arm, Shoulder and Hand questionnaire
Statistically significant correlations * $p < 0.05$, $p < 0,01$**, $p < 0,001$***

comparison studies and for evaluation of change in individuals [38]. Similar results were also obtained by the authors of other adaptations. In research from Norway, the ICC of the total WORC and individual domains ranged between 0,74 and 0.84 [21], in Turkey it ranged between 0.96 and 0.98, in Japan it ranged from 0.72 to 0.84 [19], in Denmark from 0.85–0.94 [23], in Sweden from 0.84 and 0.98 [25], in China from 0.82 and 0.96 [26] and in Brazil from 0.95 and 0.99 [20].

The Standard Error of the Means (SEM) associated with the total WORC was 1.62 points in our study, while Lopes et al. found the Brazilian WORC to be 3.0 points [20]. Our study indicates that clinicians can be confident that the total WORC score falls within 1.62 points (SEM) over a short time interval. We used the Minimal Detectable Change (MDC) to see if true change has occurred in an individual patient's WORC total score. The MDC for the Total WORC was to 4.48 points (95% CI),

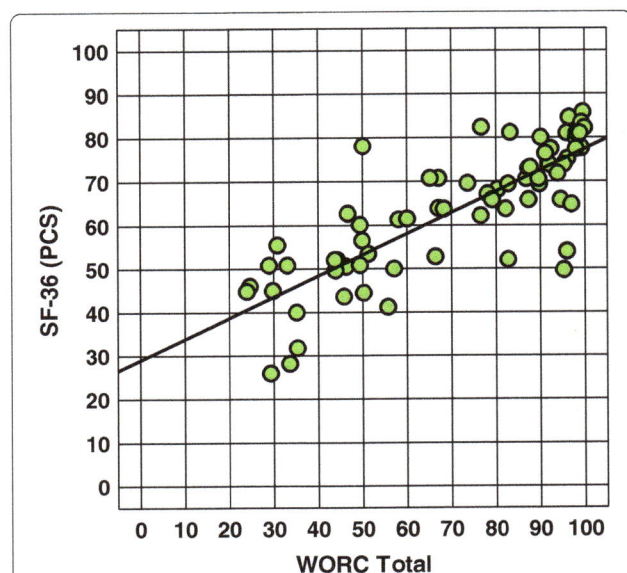

Fig. 1 Scatter plot of WORC total scores vs. SF-36 PCS scores. Spearman's correlation coefficient SCC = 0,81, $p < 0.001$. Abbreviations: *WORC* Western Ontario Rotator Cuff index, *SF-36 (PCS)* SF-36 questionnaire (Physical Component Summary)

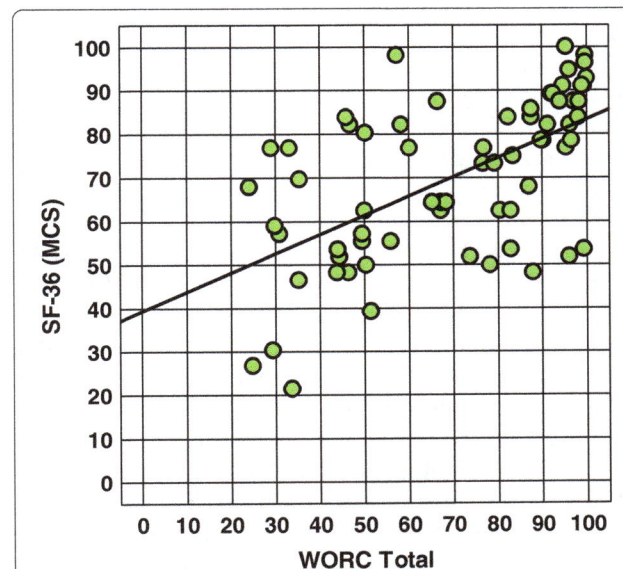

Fig. 2 Scatter plot of WORC total scores vs. SF-36 MCS scores. Spearman's correlation coefficient SCC = 0,62, $p < 0.001$. Abbreviations: *WORC* Western Ontario Rotator Cuff index, *SF-36 (MCS)* SF-36 questionnaire (Mental Component Summary)

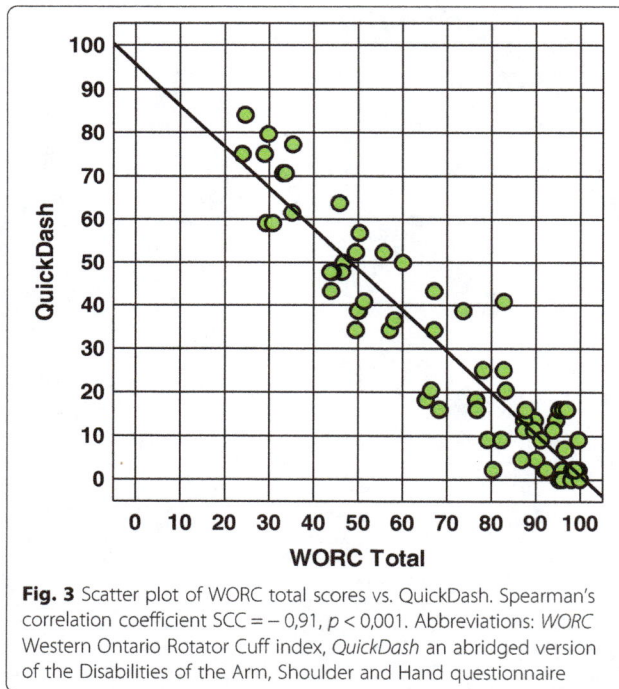

Fig. 3 Scatter plot of WORC total scores vs. QuickDash. Spearman's correlation coefficient SCC = − 0,91, *p* < 0,001. Abbreviations: *WORC* Western Ontario Rotator Cuff index, *QuickDash* an abridged version of the Disabilities of the Arm, Shoulder and Hand questionnaire

while in the Brazilian study by Lopes et al. MDC was 7.1 points (90%CI) [16]. Our research indicates that a real change will occur in a patient if his result changes by more than 4.48 points. In Brazil, this change will occur with a slightly higher result - over 7.1 points [20].

We found that the Polish version of the WORC has good content validity. Floor and ceiling effects are considered to be present if more than 15% of the respondents achieved the lowest or highest possible score [33]. In the WORC questionnaire, there was a small and acceptable ceiling effect (1.4%). The other questionnaires tested (QuickDASH, SF-36 PCS and MCS) also presented a small ceiling and floor effect (max. 7.2%). In a Swedish study, Zhaeentan et al. stated that there were neither floor nor ceiling effects preoperatively but all instruments (WORC, WOOS, OSS and EQ-5D) had some ceiling effect postoperatively of approximately 10%. The EQ-5D had an unacceptably high ceiling effect of 32.3% while the specific health instruments were acceptable [25]. Similarly, Witte et al. found no floor or ceiling effects in the English version of the WORC [39].

Construct validity was assessed by the Spearman correlations coefficient between the WORC and the QuickDASH, a the specific tool to assess disability of the upper limb and the SF-36, a generic tool to assess the quality of life. As expected, correlations with the QuickDASH (0.80–0.91) are stronger than with the SF-36 (0.19–0.84). The WORC Total is moderately correlated with the SF-36 MCS - 0.62 and strongly correlated with the SF-36 PCS - 0.81. Weak correlations or lack of them

only occurs with the SF-36 General Heath domain. Moderate or good correlations (0.47–0.79) were obtained between the physical subscales of the Chinese WORC and the OSS and the physical subscales of SF-36. The emotions subscale of the WORC and the mental subscales of SF-36 (0.52–0.71) correlate similarly [26]. We found similar relations in our study. Kirkley et al. found a moderate correlation between the original English WORC and other shoulder and upper extremity questionnaires: the American Shoulder and Elbow Surgeons Standardized Shoulder Assessment Form (ASES) (*r* = 0.68), the DASH (*r* = 0.63), the Constant Score (*r* = 0.63) and the University of California Los Angeles (UCLA) Shoulder Rating Scale (*r* = 0.48) [9]. The authors of subsequent validations confirm the above relationships. Between the Swedish version of the WORC and the WOOS there are strong correlations (0.97) [25]. The Japanese version of the WORC correlates more strongly with the DASH (*r* = 0.63–0.78) than with the SF-36 (*r* = − 0.24 to − 0.69) [24]. The Brazilian version also has marked strong correlations between the WORC and both the DASH and the UCLA Shoulder Rating Scale (*r* = − 0.86 and *r* = 0.80, respectively). Moderate correlations were found between the WORC and the SF-36 domains. The correlation was stronger with the SF-36 physical health summary score than with the mental health summary score [20].

Limitations and future studies
The current study did not include the assessment of the responsiveness of the WORC and does not contain a control group. Future studies should be undertaken to assess the ability of WORC to detect Minimally Important Changes (MIC) over a period of time longer than 2 weeks and to assess the discriminatory power of the WORC.

Conclusion
The Polish version of the WORC questionnaire can be considered a reliable and valid research tool with high internal consistency used to assess the quality of life in patients with arthroscopic rotator cuff repair. The psychometric properties of the Polish version of the WORC are comparable both with its original version as well as adaptations of WORC published in other countries.

Abbreviations
x̄: (Mean); %: Per cent; ASES: American Shoulder and Elbow Surgeons Standardized Shoulder Assessment Form; CI: Confidence Interval; DASH: Disabilities of the Arm, Shoulder and Hand Questionnaire; GRC: Global Rating of Change Scale; HRQOL: Health Related Quality of Life; ICC: Intraclass Correlation Coefficient; IST: Infraspinatus Tendon; LHBT: Long Head Biceps Tendon; MDC: Minimal Detectable Change; MIC: Minimally Important Changes; N: Number; QuickDash: Disabilities of Arm, Shoulder and Hand Questionnaire (an abridged version); RC-QOL: Rotator Cuff Quality of Life Index; SCC: Spearman's Correlation Coefficient; SEM: Standard Error of Measurement; SF-36 MCS: SF-36 Questionnaire - Mental Component Summary; SF-36 PCS: SF-36 Questionnaire - Physical Component Summary; SF-36 v. 2.0: Short Form-36 Questionnaire - version 2.0; SIQ: Shoulder

Instability Questionnaire; SScapT: Subscapularis Tendon; SST: Supraspinatus Tendon; UCLA: University of California Los Angeles Shoulder Rating Scale; WOOS: Western Ontario Osteoarthritis of the Shoulder Index; WORC: Western Ontario Rotator Cuff Index; WOSI: Western Ontario Shoulder Instability Index

Funding
This study was partly funded by University of Rzeszow. The funding body was not involved in the design, collection, analysis, and interpretation of data, writing the manuscript or decision to publish the manuscript.

Authors' contributions
AB and SG conceived and designed the study. AB, MP, MK, EDJ, JP performed the study, discussed the results. AB, MP, MK, EDJ, JP and SG analyzed the data. AB drafted the manuscript. AB, MP, MK, SG, EDJ and JP revised and approved the final manuscript. SG supervised the study.

Competing interests
The authors declare that they have no competing interests.

Author details
[1]Institute of Physiotherapy, Faculty of Medicine, University of Rzeszow, ul. Hoffmanowej 25, 35-016 Rzeszow, Poland. [2]The Holy Family Specialist Hospital, Rudna Mała, Poland. [3]Fowler Kennedy Sport Medicine Clinic, University of Western Ontario, London, Canada. [4]Faculty of Medicine, University of Information Technology and Management, Rzeszow, Poland.

References
1. Evaluation GDL. Treatment of shoulder pain. Med Clin N Am. 2014;98(3): 487–504.
2. Park K, Bicknell RT. Management of Occupational Shoulder Injuries in primary care Glenn Brown. J Musculoskelet Disord Treat. 2015;1:1.
3. White JJE, Titchener AG, Fakis A, Tambe AA, Hubbard RB, Clark DI. An epidemiological study of rotator cuff pathology using the health improvement network database. Bone Joint J. 2014;96-B:350–3.
4. Mall NA, Lee AS, Chahal J, Sherman SL, Romeo AA, Verma NN, et al. An evidenced-based examination of the epidemiology and outcomes of traumatic rotator cuff tears. Arthroscopy. 2013;29(2):366–76.
5. Littlewood C, May S, Walters S. Epidemiology of rotator cuff tendinopathy: a systematic review. Should Elbow. 2013;5(4):256–65.
6. Kirkley A, Griffin S, McLintock H, Ng L. The development and evaluation of a disease-specific quality of life measurement tool for shoulder instability. The western Ontario shoulder instability index (WOSI). Am J Sports Med. 1998; 26:764–72.
7. Dawson J, Fitzpatrick R, Carr A. The assessment of shoulder instability. The development and validation of a questionnaire. J Bone Joint Surg. 1999;81: 420–6.
8. Lo IK, Griffin S, Kirkley A. The development of a disease-specific quality of life measurement tool for osteoarthritis of the shoulder: the western Ontario osteoarthritis of the shoulder (WOOS) index. Osteoarthr Cartil. 2001;9:771–8.
9. Kirkley A, Alvarez C, Griffin S. The development and evaluation of a disease-specific quality-of-life questionnaire for disorders of the rotator cuff: The Western Ontario Rotator Cuff Index. Clin J Sport Med. 2003;13(2):84–92.
10. Hollinshead RM, Mohtadi NG, Vande Guchte RA, Wadey VM. Two 6-year follow-up studies of large and massive rotator cuff tears: comparison of outcome measures. J Shoulder Elb Surg. 2000;9:373–81.
11. Hudak P, Amadio PC, Bombardier C. The upper extremity collaborative group. Development of an upper extremity outcome measure: the DASH (disabilities of the arm, shoulder, and hand). Am J Ind Med. 1996;29:602–8.
12. Beaton DE, Wright JG, Katz JN. The upper extremity collaborative group. Development of the QuickDASH: comparison of three item-reduction approaches. J Bone Joint Surg Am. 2005;87(5):1038–46.
13. Golicki D, Krzysiak M, Strzelczyk P. Translation and cultural adaptation of the polish version of the disabilities of the arm, shoulder and hand (DASH) and QuickDASH questionnaires. Ortop Traumatol Rehabil. 2014;16(4):387–95.
14. Acquadro C, Conway K, Giroudet C, Mear I. Linguistic validation manual for patient-reported outcomes (PRO) instruments. Lyon: Mapi research institute; 2004.
15. Beaton DE, Bombardier C, Guillemin F, Bosi FM. Guidelines for the process of cross-cultural adaptation of self-report measures. Spine. 2000;25(24):3186–91.
16. Wild D, Grove A, Martin M, Eremenco S, McElroy S, Verjee-Lorenz A, et al. Principals of good practice for translation and cultural adaptation process for patient-reported outcomes (PRO) measures: report of the ISPOR task force translation and cultural adaptation. Value Health. 2005;8(2):94–104.
17. St-Pierre C, Roy J, Dionne F, Frémont P, MacDermid JC, Roy JS. Patient-reported outcomes for the evaluation of symptoms and functional limitation in individuals with rotator cuff disorders: a systematic review. Disabil Rehabil. 2016;38(2):103–22.
18. Huber W, Hofstaetter JG, Hanslik-Schnabel B, Posch M, Wurnig C. Translation and psychometric testing of the Western Ontario Rotator cuff index (WORC) for use in Germany. Z Orthop Ihre Grenzgeb. 2005;143(4):435–60.
19. El O, Bircan C, Gulbahar S, Demiral Y, Sahin E, Baydar M, et al. The reliability and validity of the Turkish version of the Western Ontario rotator cuff index. Rheumatol Int. 2006;26(12):1101–8.
20. Lopes AD, Ciconelli RM, Carrera EF, Griffin S, Faloppa F, Dos Reis FB. Validity and reliability of the Western Ontario Rotator Cuff Index (WORC) for use in Brazil. Clin J Sport Med. 2008;18(3):266–72.
21. Ekeberg OM, Bautz-Holter E, Tveita EK, Keller A, Juel NG, Brox JI. Agreement, reliability and validity in 3 shoulder questionnaires in patients with rotator cuff disease. BMC Musculoselet Disord. 2008;9:68.
22. Mousavi SJ, Hadian MR, Abedi M, Montazeri A. Translation and validation study of the Persian version of the Western Ontario Rotator Cuff Index. Clin Rheumatol. 2009;28(3):293–9.
23. Wessel RN, Lim TE, Mameren H, Bie RA. Validation of the Western Ontario Rotator Cuff Index in patients with arthroscopic rotator cuff repair: A study protocol. BMC Musculoskelet Disord. 2011;12:64.
24. Kawabata M, Miyata T, Nakai D, Sato M, Tatsuki H, Kashiwazaki Y, et al. Reproducibility and validity of the Japanese version of the western Ontario rotator cuff index. J Orthop Sci. 2013;18(5):705–11.
25. Zhaeentan S, Legeby M, Ahlström S, Stark A, Salomonsson BA. A validation of the Swedish version of the WORC index in the assessment of patients treated by surgery for subacromial disease including rotator cuff syndrome. BMC Musculoskelet Disord. 2016;17:165.
26. Wang W, Xie Q, Jia Z, Cui L, Liu D, Wang C, et al. Cross-cultural translation of the western Ontario cuff index in Chinese and its validation in patients with rotator cuff disorders. BMC Musculoskel Disord. 2017;18:178.
27. Bejer A, Probachta M, Kulczyk M, Griffin S. The western Ontario rotator cuff index (WORC) – the polish language version. The polish language version of the WORC. Issue Rehabil. Orthop. Neurophysiol. Sport Promot. 2017;20:20–9.
28. Hays RD, Morale LS. The RAND-36 measure of health-related quality of life. Ann Med. 2001;33:350–7.
29. Ware JE. SF-36 health survey update. Spine. 2000;25(24):3130–9.
30. Tylka J, Piotrowicz R. SF-36 life quality assessment questionnaire – polish version. Pol Heart J. 2009;67:1166–9. Polish
31. Fischer D, Stewart AL, Bloch DA, Lorig K, Laurent D, Holman H. Capturing the patient's view of change as a clinical outcome measure. JAMA. 1999; 282(12):1157–62.
32. Tsang S, Royse CF, Terkawi AS. Guidelines for developing, translating, and validating a questionnaire in perioperative and pain medicine. Saudi J Anaesth. 2017;11(Suppl 1):80–9.
33. Terwee CB, Bot SD, de Boer MR, van der Windt DA, Knol DL, Dekker J, et al. Quality criteria were proposed for measurement properties of health status questionnaires. J Clin Epidemiol. 2007;60(1):34–42.
34. Altman DG. Practical statistics for medical research. Boca Raton: Chapman & Hall/CRC; 1999.
35. Paradowski PT, Witoński D, Klęska R, Roos E. Cross-cultural translation and measurement properties of the polish version of the knee injury and osteoarthritis outcome score (KOOS) following anterior cruciate ligament reconstruction. Health Qual Life Outcomes. 2013;11:107.
36. Portney LG, Watkins MP. Foundations of clinical research: applications to practice. 3rd ed. Upper Saddle River: New Jersey Pearson Prentice Hall Health; 2009.
37. Ćwirlej-Sozańska A, Wilmowska-Pietruszyńska A, Sozański B. Validation of the Polish version of theWorld Health Organization Disability Assessment Schedule (WHODAS 2.0) in an elderly population (60–70 years old). Int J Occup Saf Ergon (JOSE). 2017; https://doi.org/10.1080/10803548.2017.1316596
38. Streiner DL, Norman GR. Health measurement scales: a practical guide to their development and use. 3rd ed. Oxford: Oxford University Press; 2003.

10

Diagnostic strategy for elderly patients with isolated greater trochanter fractures on plain radiographs

Nam Hoon Moon[1], Won Chul Shin[2]* (iD), Min Uk Do[2], Seung Hun Woo[2], Seung Min Son[2] and Kuen Tak Suh[2]

Abstract

Background: Isolated greater trochanter (GT) fractures are relatively rare and few studies have assessed the appropriate diagnostic and therapeutic strategies for these fractures. When initial plain radiographs show an isolated GT fracture, underestimation of occult intertrochanteric extension may result in displacement of a previously non-displaced fracture. This study examined the clinical results and value of different diagnostic strategies in elderly patients with isolated GT fractures on plain radiographs.

Methods: Between January 2010 and January 2015, 30 patients with initial plain radiographs showing isolated GT fractures were examined using MRI, bone scanning and/or CT for suspected occult intertrochanteric extension. We assessed the sensitivity, specificity, and positive and negative predictive value of each test. In addition, we noted the location of the fracture or soft-tissue injury on MRI in addition to treatment results.

Results: All 30 patients had osteoporosis and fractures caused by minor trauma. MRI revealed isolated GT fractures in nine patients and occult intertrochanteric fractures in 21 patients. Using the MRI-based diagnosis as a reference, the results showed that plain radiographs, bone scans, and CT scans can be used for supplementary examination but they are not appropriate as confirmatory tests for these fractures. However, in patients with both isolated GT fractures seen on plain radiographs and increased uptake in only the GT area on bone scans, MRI revealed isolated GT fractures. The fractures were treated surgically in 20 patients and conservatively in 10 patients with satisfactory clinical results.

Conclusions: We confirmed that MRI-based examination is useful in all symptomatic elderly patients whose plain radiographic findings reveal isolated GT fractures. However, we suggest that there is a need to establish a diagnostic strategy through increased understanding of the available diagnostic methods. We believe that surgical treatment should be considered in patients with occult intertrochanteric fractures that are detected on MRI.

Keywords: Greater trochanter fracture, Occult intertrochanteric fracture, Diagnosis, Radiographs

Background

Proximal femoral or "hip" fractures are a serious medical problem in orthopedic practice due to the increasing elderly population [1]. The approximate incidence of proximal femoral fractures is > 28,000 per year in the Korean population [2] and growing rapidly. Correct early diagnosis is very important for appropriate treatment and recovery in elderly patients because of a high first-year mortality rate (14–36%) and poor outcomes [3–5]. In 2–10% of patients presenting with symptomatic hip fractures, initial plain radiographs do not show the fracture line and are thus termed "occult fractures" [4]. Many epidemiological studies have reported that proximal femoral fractures are commonly related to osteoporosis that develops with age [2, 6]. Although isolated greater trochanter (GT) fractures are relatively rare [7, 8], the intertrochanteric extension of fractures has been demonstrated when plain radiographs show only an isolated GT fracture [8–10]. The diagnosis of occult

* Correspondence: dreami3e5t@pusan.ac.kr
[2]Department of Orthopedic Surgery, Research Institute for Convergence of Biomedical Science and Technology, Pusan National University Yangsan Hospital, Pusan National University School of Medicine, 20 Geumo-ro, Mulgeum-eup, Yangsan, Gyeongsangnam-do 626-770, Republic of Korea
Full list of author information is available at the end of the article

intertrochanteric fractures of the femur on plain radiographs can be challenging, especially in elderly individuals with osteoporosis because of their poor bone quality [10, 11].

In most clinical institutes, the diagnosis of proximal femoral fractures is based on clinical history and physical examination, whereas confirmation is achieved by initial plain radiographs. However, when the initial plain radiograph shows an isolated GT fracture, underestimating the extent of the fractures may result in displacement of a previously non-displaced fracture, which will alter the treatment plan and necessitate more complicated surgery [3, 12]. Therefore, when an occult intertrochanteric fracture is clinically suspected, especially in elderly patients with osteoporosis, additional diagnostic examinations are necessary.

According to some recent reports, magnetic resonance imaging (MRI), which is becoming increasingly accepted and available, can more accurately define the anatomical extent of occult fractures and is routinely recommended for further evaluation in these situations [12, 13]. In addition, MRI is useful for the detection of soft-tissue injuries, especially in patients with clinical suspicion of occult intertrochanteric fractures [14]. However, the routine use of MRI for the detection of occult fractures is costly and requires a trained radiologist to review the images. Bone scans generally play a supplementary role in the detection of occult fractures but may produce false positive or negative results [15]. In addition, bone scans cannot show the precise extent of the fracture, often necessitating further imaging. Computed tomography (CT) scans are another alternative imaging option, and are more readily available and less expensive to perform. However, CT can lead to the misdiagnosis of occult hip fractures due to the resolution of the trabecular structure of severe osteoporotic bone compared with MRI [4, 16]. CT may also underestimate the full extent of injury in identified occult hip fractures [17, 18].

No protocol has yet been developed for the second-line investigation of isolated GT fractures identified on plain radiographs in elderly patients. The present study was designed retrospectively to examine the diagnostic strategy and clinical results in elderly patients with isolated GT fractures identified on plain radiographs. Therefore, we proposed the following questions: (1) what are the sensitivity, specificity, and positive and negative predictive value of each test and (2) what are the locations of the fracture or soft-tissue injury on MRI and results of treatment in these fractures.

Methods

Between January 2010 and January 2015, we treated 455 consecutive patients with proximal femoral fractures affecting the femoral head, neck, GT, intertrochanteric, or subtrochanteric areas at our university hospital. Thirty patients with initial plain radiographs (anteroposterior, lateral, and Lorenz view) showing isolated GT fractures were examined by bone scans, CT, and MRI for suspicion of occult intertrochanteric extension. Patients with a definite intertrochanteric extension of the fracture line on plain radiographs were excluded. The patients were 65–91 years old (average 77 years) and 17 women (Table 1). Bone mineral density was measured in all cases preoperatively at an unaffected trochanteric region using dual-energy X-ray absorptiometry. Patient information was reviewed by the university human subjects committee, and Institutional Review Board approval was obtained prior to commencing the study.

MRI was performed at a mean of 5.3 days (range, 1–21 days) after trauma and was conducted on a 3.0-T magnet (MAGNETOM Verio, Siemens Healthineers) device using a commercially available pelvic phase array surface coil as a receiver. Sequence protocols included T1-weighted spin-echo in the coronal plane (slice thickness 3 mm with a gap of 0.5–1 mm, matrix 384×269) and axial plane (slice thickness 4 mm with a gap of 0.5–1 mm, matrix 384×176), and T2-weighted Turbo Inversion Recovery Magnitude in the coronal plane (slice thickness 3 mm with a gap of 0.5–1 mm, matrix 320×224), axial plane (slice thickness 4 mm with a gap of 0.5–1 mm, matrix 320×224), and sagittal plane (slice thickness 4 mm with a gap 0.5–1 mm, matrix 320×146). All MRI images were evaluated for the presence and extension of bone or soft-tissue injury. We determined the presence of a fracture when linear low signal intensity focus was surrounded by an intermediate signal on T1-weighted images and surrounded by high signal on T2-weighted images [19]. T2-weighted images facilitated the identification of soft tissue injuries and bone marrow edema [14, 20] (Fig. 1). The bone scan protocol consisted of both whole-body and hip pin-hole images. The bone scan was performed at a mean of 5.5 days (range, 2–21 days) after trauma. CT scans were performed using multidetector CT scanners (SOMATOM Definition Flash, Siemens Healthineers) with 128 detector rows. CT scanning from 2 cm cranial to the acetabulum and including the lesser trochanter distally was performed at a 2.0-mm slice thickness, and reconstructive images of the bone, soft, coronal, and sagittal views were obtained with high-spatial-resolution bone algorithms. CT scans were not performed in four patients because MRI was performed at the time of admission to the emergency room without additional CT scans. All MRI, CT, bone scans and plain radiographic images were reviewed by three observers (two authors and an experienced musculoskeletal radiologist).

We noted the location of the fracture or soft-tissue injury on MRI. Clinical instability was defined when a

Table 1 Demographic data of the patients

Number	Sex	Type of trauma	BMD (T-score)	Presence of pain	Presence of ecchymosis	Time from trauma to admission (days)
1	F	Slip in bathroom	−2.5	+	−	< 1
2	M	Slip in hospital	− 3.4	+	−	2
3	F	Slip in bathroom	−2.7	+	+	10
4	F	Slip in bathroom	−2.5	+	−	< 1
5	F	Slip in home	−4.0	+	−	< 1
6	F	Slip in home	−3.5	+	−	3
7	F	Slip in home	−3.9	+	−	< 1
8	F	Slip in home	−3.1	+	−	1
9	F	Slip in bathroom	−4.2	+	−	5
10	F	Slip in home	−2.8	+	−	< 1
11	F	Slip in home	− 2.6	+	+	< 1
12	M	Slip in hospital	−2.9	+	−	2
13	F	Slip in hospital	−2.5	+	−	13
14	F	Slip in home	−2.8	+	+	2
15	M	Slip in home	−4.0	+	−	7
16	F	Slip in home	−2.7	+	−	1
17	M	Slip in home	−2.5	+	+	0
18	F	Slip in home	−4.0	+	+	15
19	M	Bicycle accident	−3.0	+	−	16
20	M	Bicycle accident	−3.2	+	−	0
21	F	Slip in home	−3.1	+	−	4
22	M	Slip in home	−3.2	+	−	1
23	M	Slip in home	−3.5	+	−	1
24	M	Slip in home	−3.2	+	−	1
25	F	Slip in home	−3.5	+	−	19
26	M	Bicycle accident	−3.5	+	−	1
27	M	Slip in home	−3.5	+	−	2
28	F	Slip in hospital	−3.3	+	−	2
29	M	Pedestrian accident	−3.5	+	+	2
30	M	Slip in home	−3.5	+	−	< 1

BMD bone mineral density, *M* male, *F* female

fracture line extended through more than 50% of the longitudinal axis on coronal images, and surgical treatment was conducted [10].

All data were collected in a structured database using SPSS software (version 20.0; IBM Corp.) Using MRI findings as the reference, the overall accuracy, sensitivity, specificity, and positive and negative predictive values (PPV, NPV) of each test were calculated. Categorical data were statistically analyzed by Fisher's exact test. We performed receiver operating characteristic analysis to analyze and compare diagnostic performance between each test for occult intertrochanteric extension. In all tests, P-values < 0.05 were considered statistically significant. Data were reported with 95% confidence intervals.

Results

Twenty-six of 30 (87%) fractures were caused by minor trauma that occurred indoors, such as through slipping. Only eight patients were admitted within 24 h after trauma; seven patients were admitted 7 days after trauma. All patients were elderly, > 65 years old, and had osteoporosis preoperatively (average T-score: − 3.2, range − 2.5 to − 4.2) (Table 1). Clinically, all patients presented with hip or proximal thigh pain. However, ecchymosis was evident in only six (20%) patients.

Initial plain radiographs of all 30 patients were interpreted as depicting minimally or non-displaced GT fracture. The types of fractures were finally identified by MRI (Table 2). Isolated GT fractures were present in

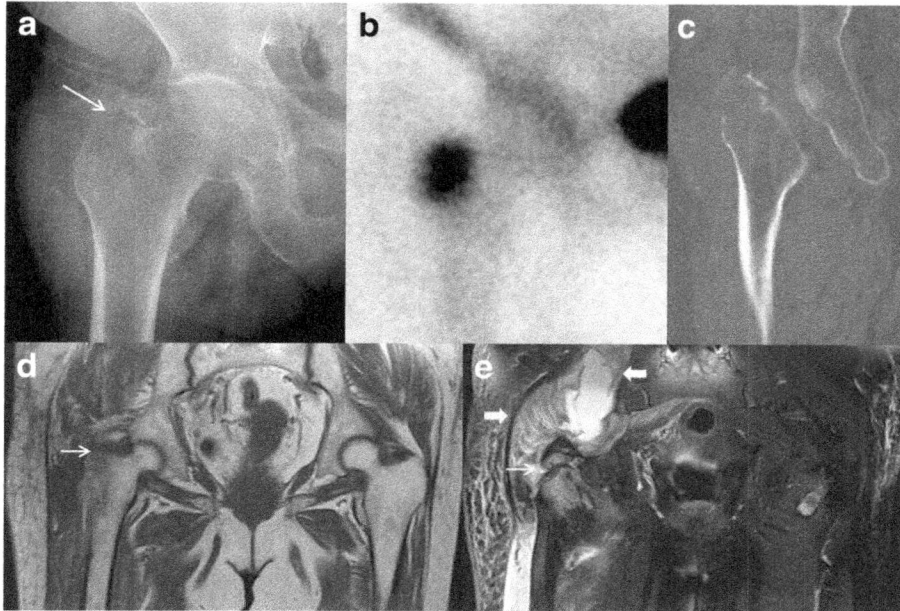

Fig. 1 Case of a 72-year-old who presented at the outpatient department with right hip pain after slipping at home. **a** A plain radiograph of the right hip shows only an isolated greater trochanter fracture (*arrow*). **b** A bone scan obtained 3 days after the trauma shows radionuclide predominantly concentrated in the greater trochanter. **c** A computed tomography scan shows no occult intertrochanteric fracture. **d** A T1-weighted coronal image shows a linear low-signal intensity focus (*arrow*) indicating a fracture. **e** A T2-weighted coronal image shows a fracture surrounded by high signal intensity (*arrow*) and abnormal signal in the muscles around the hip. These findings are compatible with interstitial hemorrhage and hematoma (*bold arrows*)

only nine patients (30%) and occult intertrochanteric fractures in 21 patients (70%). In our overall data, the incidence of isolated GT fracture and occult intertrochanteric fracture was 2.0 and 4.6%, respectively, among 455 hip fractures in the same period. Seven patients' bone scans showed increased uptake only in the GT region, 19 patients had extension into the intertrochanteric region, and four patients had normal findings. In 26 of 30 patients (87%), the MRI and bone scan results agreed. However, none of the bone scans definitively showed fracture propagation. On CT, 13 of 26 patients had isolated GT fractures, two had normal findings, and 11 had an occult intertrochanteric extension. In 20 of 26 patients (77%), the MRI and CT scan results agreed. Only 7 of 30 patients (23%) had isolated GT fractures on all imaging modalities (plain radiograph, bone scan, CT scan, and MRI) (Fig. 1).

The diagnostic characteristics of the imaging modalities are shown in Table 3. Bone scans demonstrated the highest nominal sensitivity but low specificity for occult intertrochanteric fractures. The sensitivity of plain radiographs and CT scans was below 80%. The specificity was 77.8–100% and did not show significant differences across the three modalities ($p = 0.157$). The PPV was acceptable ($\geq 80\%$) for most modalities, as was NPV for

bone scans. In contrast, NPV was 69.2% for CT scans and only 30% for plain radiographs. MRI was the most accurate methodology, followed by bone scans, CT scans, and plain radiographs for occult intertrochanteric fractures. However, in patients with isolated GT fractures seen on both plain radiographs and bone scans, MRI also revealed isolated GT fractures.

On MRI images, soft tissue injuries such as hematoma or muscle injury were visible in all 30 cases (100%) with fracture (Fig. 2). Muscle edema, hemorrhage, and partial tears represented accounted for most muscle injuries of the obturator externus and the other external rotators, which include the gluteus maximus, piriformis, obturator internus, gemelli, and quadratus femoris. Nine patients with isolated GT fractures were treated conservatively and had satisfactory results, achieving bone union without any complications on follow-up radiographs. These patients commenced gradual weight bearing while ambulating with crutches or a walker after pain relief. Surgical treatment was conducted in 20 of 21 patients with occult intertrochanteric fractures using a proximal femoral nail (Fig. 3). All operations were performed by a single surgeon in the same technique using a Proximal Femoral Nail Antirotation (Synthes, Solothrun, Switzerland) system with the patient lying supine on a fracture table. No complications related to implant fixation were observed in the follow-up

Table 2 Radiologic findings and managements in the study group

Number	Plain radiograph	Uptake site on bone scan	CT	MRI	Presence of soft tissue injury	Type of management
1	Isolated GT fx.	No uptake	No data	IT fx.	+	Surgical
2	Isolated GT fx.	IT	No fx.	IT fx.	+	Surgical
3	Isolated GT fx.	No uptake	No data	IT fx.	+	Surgical
4	Isolated GT fx.	IT	No data	IT fx.	+	Surgical
5	Isolated GT fx.	IT	No data	IT fx.	+	Surgical
6	Isolated GT fx.	Isolated GT	Isolated GT fx.	Isolated GT fx.	+	Conservative
7	Isolated GT fx.	IT	No fx.	IT fx.	+	Surgical
8	Isolated GT fx.	IT	IT fx.	IT fx.	+	Surgical
9	Isolated GT fx.	IT	IT fx.	IT fx.	+	Surgical
10	Isolated GT fx.	IT	IT fx.	IT fx.	+	Surgical
11	Isolated GT fx.	IT	IT fx.	IT fx.	+	Surgical
12	Isolated GT fx.	IT	IT fx.	IT fx.	+	Surgical
13	Isolated GT fx.	Isolated GT	Isolated GT fx.	Isolated GT fx.	+	Conservative
14	Isolated GT fx.	IT	IT fx.	IT fx.	+	Surgical
15	Isolated GT fx.	IT	IT fx.	IT fx.	+	Surgical
16	Isolated GT fx.	IT	IT fx.	IT fx.	+	Surgical
17	Isolated GT fx.	No uptake	Isolated GT fx.	Isolated GT fx.	+	Conservative
18	Isolated GT fx.	IT	Isolated GT fx.	IT fx.	+	Conservative
19	Isolated GT fx.	Isolated GT	Isolated GT fx.	Isolated GT fx.	+	Conservative
20	Isolated GT fx.	IT	IT fx.	IT fx.	+	Surgical
21	Isolated GT fx.	IT	Isolated GT fx.	IT fx.	+	Surgical
22	Isolated GT fx.	IT	IT fx.	IT fx.	+	Surgical
23	Isolated GT fx.	IT	IT fx.	IT fx.	+	Surgical
24	Isolated GT fx.	Isolated GT	Isolated GT fx.	Isolated GT fx.	+	Conservative
25	Isolated GT fx.	No uptake	Isolated GT fx.	Isolated GT fx.	+	Conservative
26	Isolated GT fx.	Isolated GT	Isolated GT fx.	Isolated GT fx.	+	Conservative
27	Isolated GT fx.	IT	Isolated GT fx.	IT fx.	+	Surgical
28	Isolated GT fx.	Isolated GT	Isolated GT fx.	Isolated GT fx.	+	Conservative
29	Isolated GT fx.	IT	Isolated GT fx.	IT fx.	+	Surgical
30	Isolated GT fx.	Isolated GT	Isolated GT fx.	Isolated GT fx.	+	Conservative

GT greater trochanteric, *Fx.* Fracture, *IT* intertrochanteric

Table 3 Diagnostic characteristics of the imaging modalities of occult intertrochanteric fracture of the femur (reported with 95% confidence interval)

	Plain radiograph (n = 30)	Bone scan (n = 30)	CT (n = 26)	P-value
Sensitivity	0.0 (0.0–22.8)	100.0 (77.2–100.0)	76.5 (50.1–93.2)	0.045
Specificity	100.0 (55.5–100.0)	77.8 (40.0–97.2)	100.0 (55.5–100.0)	0.157
Accuracy	30.0 (14.7–49.4)	93.3 (77.9–99.2)	84.6 (65.1–95.6)	0.046
PPV	NaN	91.3 (72.0–98.9)	100.0 (66.1–100.0)	
NPV	30.0 (14.7–49.4)	100.0 (47.3–100.0)	69.2 (38.6–90.9)	

PPV positive predictive value, *NPV* negative predictive value

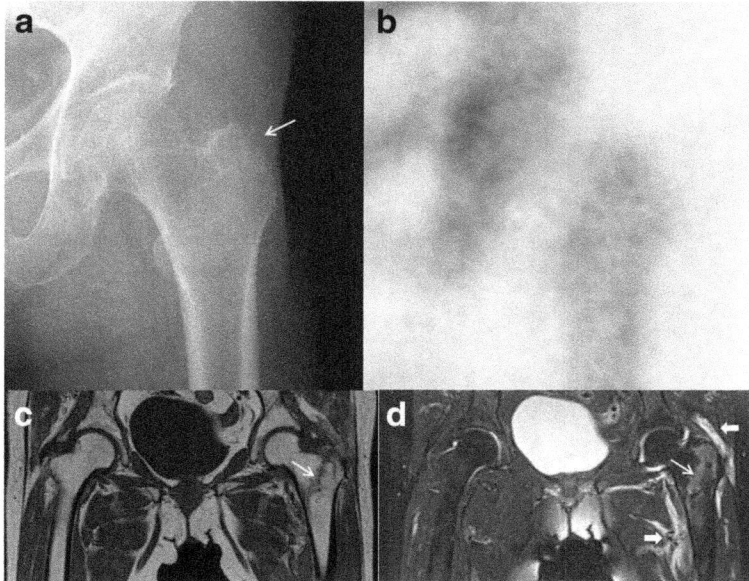

Fig. 2 Case of an 84-year-old woman who presented at the emergency department with left hip pain after slipping in the bathroom. **a** A plain radiograph of the left hip only shows an isolated greater trochanter fracture (*arrow*). **b** A bone scan obtained 2 days after the trauma was unremarkable. **c** The T1-weighted coronal image shows an intertrochanteric fracture (*arrow*) that extends to the medial cortex. **d** The T2-weighted coronal image shows a fracture at the same level (*arrow*) and abnormal signal in the muscles around the hip (*bold arrows*)

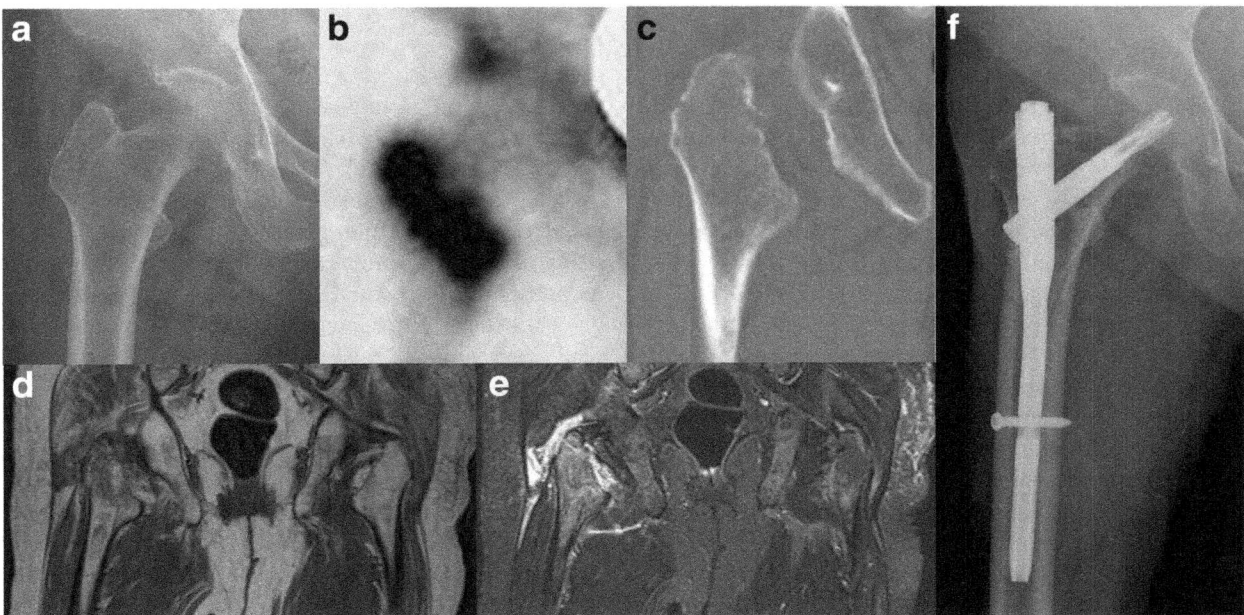

Fig. 3 Case of a 73-year-old woman presented at the emergency department with right hip pain after slipping in a convalescent hospital. **a** A plain radiograph of the right hip shows an isolated greater trochanter fracture. **b** A bone scan performed 6 days after the trauma reveals that the fracture extended into the intertrochanteric region. **c** A computed tomography scan shows an isolated greater trochanteric fracture without intertrochanteric extent. **d, e** Magnetic resonance imaging shows an intertrochanteric fracture that crosses the midline to the medial cortex. **f** Internal fixation was performed using proximal femoral nail antirotation

Table 4 Clinical results in the study group

	Preoperative	Recovery
Charnley hip pain score[a]		4.9
Walking ability		
Independent community ambulator	16	14
Community ambulator with cane	8	9
Community ambulator with walker	2	1
Independent household ambulator	2	3
Household ambulator with cane	1	1
Household ambulator with walker	0	1
Nonfunctional ambulator	1	1
Death within 1 year		0

[a]Best possible score = 6 and worst possible score = 1

period. One patient was treated conservatively because she had high risks for surgical and anesthesia-related complications because of terminal lung cancer. All patients were instructed to walk with partial weight-bearing with the aid of crutches or a walker on the second day, with full weight-bearing as tolerated. Follow-up was possible in all 30 patients. The mean follow-up was 2.9 years (range, 1–5.5 years). The clinical results were good, as subjectively rated by both the patients and clinician. In this study, the first-year mortality rate of occult intertrochanteric fracture in elderly patients was 0% (Table 4).

Discussion

In the current study, we reviewed 30 patients with isolated GT fractures initially evaluated by plain radiographs and then further evaluated by either bone scanning, CT, or MRI. This retrospective, observational study describes 6 years of our experience with these fractures in elderly patients. We presented an efficient diagnostic strategy using the second-line investigations and integrated these data with a selection of established treatment methods.

The incidence of proximal femoral or "hip" fractures increases with age. Such fractures are associated with increased mortality [1, 3–5, 21]. Elderly patients are generally fragile and can experience hip fractures without major trauma. In addition, osteoporosis is strongly associated with increased risks for hip fracture [22]. Therefore, identifying osteoporosis as a potential risk factor for mortality after hip fracture is important because this can help to identify patients at high risk for mortality. Furthermore, hip fractures in elderly people with osteoporosis may present with occult or equivocal features due to poor bone quality [3, 6, 22]. For these reasons, correct early diagnosis is very important for the appropriate treatment and recovery of elderly patients with osteoporosis.

The demographic results of this patient series were consistent with those in other published studies [10, 12, 16]. The incidences of occult intertrochanteric femur fracture and isolated GT fracture among hip fractures were 4.6 and 2.0%, respectively. Only 9 of 30 patients (30%) had true isolated GT fractures on MRI. All fractures occurred in elderly individuals and all patients had osteoporosis preoperatively. Most fractures were caused by minor trauma that occurred indoors, such as that resulting from slipping. From these results, it is reasonable to assume that GT fractures with occult intertrochanteric extension are commonly related to osteoporosis because of clinical features, including increased incidence with age and associated minor trauma.

Most proximal femoral fractures are diagnosed based on clinical examination and a routine plain radiograph in the emergency department. However, in cases of occult intertrochanteric fracture of the femur, initial plain radiographs may show only GT fractures, especially in patients with osteoporosis [6, 9, 10]. To avoid the misdiagnosis of these fractures, second-line investigations such as bone scan, CT, or MRI are required. Bone scans have some advantages, including a short half-life, good availability, cost effectiveness, and relatively high detection rate (sensitivity 93%, specificity 95% [15]). As described by Matin [11], bone scans in elderly patients with closed fractures may appear normal if performed within 24 h of the injury. The interval from the injury to bone scan in this retrospective study was 2–21 days; therefore, our results have the advantage of excluding this problem. In patients with both isolated GT fractures seen on plain radiograph and increased uptake only in the GT area on a bone scan, MRI also revealed isolated GT fractures. Although our sample size was too small to determine the efficacy of bone scans, the technique is deemed to have diagnostic value due to the lack of false positive results in the present study. However, bone scans usually play only a supplementary role in the detection of occult fractures because they cannot show the precise extent of the fracture [12, 15]. In addition, bone scans may produce false negative results. In this study, four bone scans showed normal findings that represented false negatives. CT scanning is another alternative imaging option. Although CT excludes or verifies a fracture in most cases with inconclusive radiographs, CT is more likely than MRI to lead to the misdiagnosis of occult hip fractures. The evidence supporting the use of newly developed CT scanners with much better resolution than older scanners for the diagnosis of occult fractures is limited [4, 23, 24]. Lubovsky et al. [4] reported that CT led to misdiagnosis in 66% of patients with occult hip fractures, and noted that using CT before MRI caused a delay in diagnosis. Cabarrus et al. [24] reported that occult fractures were detected by

3D-CT in only 34 of 64 (53%) hips. Our results show that CT led to misdiagnosis in 6 of 26 (23%) patients despite using multidetector CT scanners with 128 detector rows. Failure to promptly diagnose the exact extension of fractures can result in the displacement of a previously non-displaced fracture, which can complicate the clinical situation.

Although MRI, an increasingly accepted and available method, is more expensive than other diagnostic imaging tools and susceptible to over-interpretation, it is recommended for the further evaluation and confirmation of occult hip fractures [4, 12–14, 19, 20, 25]. MRI has been considered as the "gold standard" in diagnosing occult and suspected proximal femoral fractures, with a reported sensitivity of 100%. It provides anatomical information as well as the identification of soft-tissue injuries [4, 16, 26, 27]. Using MRI diagnosis as a reference in this study, neither plain radiographs, bone scans, nor CT scans could be used as a single confirmatory test for the detection of occult intertrochanteric extension in elderly patients with osteoporosis. Of the 35 patients with fractures on MRI studied by Oka and Monu [14], 24 (69%) had muscle injuries such as edema, hemorrhage, muscle tears, or hematoma. Unlike their report, all patients in our series with isolated GT or occult intertrochanteric femoral fractures had accompanying soft tissue injuries. However, ecchymosis was evident in only six (20%) patients.

There are no standard treatment guidelines for occult intertrochanteric fractures of the femur. It is undisputed that isolated GT fractures in elderly patients are most often treated conservatively when they occur in isolation. The nine patients with isolated GT fractures in this study were treated conservatively and the results were clinically and radiographically satisfactory. Omura et al. [9] reported that seven patients with occult intertrochanteric fractures were treated conservatively with 1–3 weeks of bed rest followed by progressive walker-assisted ambulation. In a similar study, five patients with normal plain radiographs who had occult intertrochanteric fractures on MRI were managed conservatively [28]. The authors recommended that these patients with occult intertrochanteric fractures should be considered for conservative treatment. In contrast, in another study involving 10 patients with more complex injuries than apparently isolated GT fractures, six underwent surgery because of extension into the intertrochanteric region [29]. Schultz et al. [10] emphasized that incomplete intertrochanteric fractures that crossed the midline in the MRI coronal plane were treated surgically. Surgery was also carried out for all patients with no medical contraindications, regardless of the fracture pattern [12]. The authors determined that surgery for these patients focused on their underlying medical conditions

and patient consent. Twenty of 21 patients with no medical contraindications underwent surgery because MRI showed extension into the intertrochanteric region through > 50% of the longitudinal axis on coronal images. In general, weight-bearing ambulation can cause incomplete intertrochanteric fractures to progress to complete fractures [28], which may lead to more complicated surgery, longer hospitalization, and delayed rehabilitation [3]. For these reasons, the authors prefer surgical internal fixation if possible. In the group of patients with occult intertrochanteric extension that received conservative treatment, one had a poor medical condition and refused surgery. The clinical results were subjectively good in all cases, and the first-year mortality rate of occult intertrochanteric fracture with osteoporosis was 0%.

This study had some limitations that should be discussed. First, the main limitation of this study is that it was retrospective in design. Second, the study population of 30 cases was too small to allow the general incidence of occult intertrochanteric femoral fracture and definitive criteria for treatment options to be established. Third, all images should be reviewed by different blinded radiologists with different experiences, and repeated measures should be obtained, in order to strengthen the research design. The investigation was, however, performed by an experienced senior experienced radiologist and the evaluation was performed together with two orthopaedic surgeons, limiting bias and the risk of false negative results. Finally, there was no control group to compare results between surgical and conservative treatment in patients with occult intertrochanteric fractures. The identification of more specific criteria for performing surgery or conservative management will require a larger prospective, case-control series and further analysis of the influence of fracture features on treatment options. As in Western countries, the number of Korean osteoporosis patients with proximal femoral fractures is increasing rapidly as the population ages. As a result, this study is thought to represent a valuable contribution to the literature despite the limitations described above.

Conclusion

This study confirmed that MRI examination is useful in all symptomatic elderly patients when plain film radiographs show isolated GT fractures because of the inability of the film to reveal the geographic extent of the lesion, leading to questions regarding safe treatment. However, we suggest that there is a need to establish a diagnostic strategy through understanding the respective test methods. We also believe that surgical treatment and early ambulation in elderly patients is possible following the early detection of occult intertrochanteric fractures using proper diagnostic approaches.

Abbreviations
CT: Computed tomography; GT: Greater trochanter; MRI: Magnetic resonance imaging; NPV: Negative predictive value; PPV: Positive predictive value

Acknowledgements
This study was supported by the Research Institute for Convergence of Biomedical Science and Technology (30-2016-010), Pusan National University Yangsan Hospital.

Funding
No funding was obtained for this study.

Authors' contributions
NHM and WCS were responsible for the study design and writing the manuscript. MUD, SHW, and SMS contributed to the data collection and literature reviwe. NHM and KTS analyzed the data. SWC revised the manuscript and organized the surgeries. All authors read and approved the final manuscript.

Competing interests
The authors declare that they have no competing interests.

Author details
[1]Department of Orthopedic Surgery, Pusan National University Hospital, Pusan National University School of Medicine, Busan, Republic of Korea. [2]Department of Orthopedic Surgery, Research Institute for Convergence of Biomedical Science and Technology, Pusan National University Yangsan Hospital, Pusan National University School of Medicine, 20 Geumo-ro, Mulgeum-eup, Yangsan, Gyeongsangnam-do 626-770, Republic of Korea.

References
1. Rudman N, McIlmail D. Emergency department evaluation and treatment of hip and thigh injuries. Emerg Med Clin North Am. 2000;18:29–66.
2. Yoon BH, Lee YK, Kim SC, Kim SH, Ha YC, Koo KH. Epidemiology of proximal femoral fractures in South Korea. Arch Osteoporos. 2013;8:157–61.
3. Koval KJ, Zuckerman JD. Current concept review: functional recovery after fracture of the hip. J Bone Joint Surg Am. 1994;76:751–8.
4. Lubovsky O, Liebergall M, Mattan Y, Weil Y, Mosheiff R. Early diagnosis of occult hip fractures MRI versus CT scan. Injury. 2005;36:788–92.
5. Diamantopoulos AP, Hoff M, Skoie IM, Hochberg M, Haugeberg G. Short- and long-term mortality in males and females with fragility hip fracture in Norway. Apopulation-based study. Clin Interv Aging. 2013;8:817–23.
6. Cummings SR, Melton LJ. Epidemiology and outcomes of osteoporotic fractures. Lancet. 2002;359:1761–7.
7. Lee KH, Kim HM, Kim YS, Jeong C, Moon CW, Lee SU, et al. Isolated fractures of the greater trochanter with occult intertrochanteric extension. Arch Orthop Trauma Surg. 2010;130:1275–80.
8. Kim SJ, Ahn J, Kim HK, Kim JH. Is magnetic resonance imaging necessary in isolated greater trochanter fracture? A systemic review and pooled analysis. BMC Musculoskelet Disord. 2015;16:395–400.
9. Omura T, Takahashi M, Koide Y, Ohishi T, Tamanashi A, Kushida K, et al. Evaluation of isolated fractures of the greater trochanter with magnetic resonance imaging. Arch Surg. 2000;120:195–7.
10. Schultz E, Miller T, Boruchov S, Schmell EB, Toledano B. Incomplete intertrochanteric fractures: imaging features and clinical management. Radiology. 1999;211:237–40.
11. Matin P. The appearance of bone scans following fractures, including immediate and long-term studies. J Nucl Med. 1979;20:1227–31.
12. Feldman F, Staron RB. MRI of seemingly isolated greater trochanteric fractures. AJR Am J Roentgenol. 2004;183:323–9.
13. Feldman F, Staron R, Zwass A, Rubin S, Haramati N. MRI: its role in detecting occult fractures. Skelet Radiol. 1994;23:439–44.
14. Oka M, Monu JU. Prevalence and pattern of occult hip fractures and mimic revealed by MRI. AJR Am J Roentgenol. 2004;182:283–8.
15. Holder LE, Schwarz C, Wernicke PG, Michael RH. Radionuclide bone imaging in the elderly detection of fractures of the proximal femur (hip): multifactorial analysis. Radiology. 1990;174:509–15.
16. Cannon J, Silvestri S, Munro M. Imaging choices in occult hip fractures. J Emerg Med. 2009;37:144–52.
17. Haubro M, Stougaard C, Torfing T, Overgaard S. Sensitivity and specificity of CT- and MRI-scanning in evaluation of occult fracture of the proximal femur. Injury. 2015;48:1557–61.
18. Collin D, Geijer M, Göthlin JH. Computed tomography compared to magnetic resonance imaging in occult or suspected hip fracture. A retrospective study in 44 patients. Eur Radiol. 2016;26:3932–8.
19. Quinn SF, McCarthy JL. Prospective evaluation of patients with suspected hip fracture and indeterminate radiographs: use of T1-weighted MR images. Radiology. 1993;187:469–71.
20. Bogost GA, Lizerbram EK, Cruse JV 3rd. MR imaging in evaluation of suspected hip fracture: frequency of unsuspected bone and soft-tissue injury. Radiology. 1995;197:263–7.
21. Abrahamsen B, van Staa T, Ariely R, Olson M, Cooper C. Excess mortality following hip fracture: a systematic epidemiological review. Osteoporos Int. 2009;20:1633–50.
22. Browner WS, Pressman AR, Nevitt MC, Cummings SR. Mortality following fractures in older women. The study of osteoporotic fractures. Arch Intern Med. 1996;156:1521–5.
23. Gill SK, Smith J, Fox R, Chesser TJ. Investigation of occult hip fractures: the use of CT and MRI. Sci World J. 2013;830319.
24. Cabarrus MC, Ambekar A, Lu Y, Link TM. MRI and CT of insufficiency fractures of the pelvis and the proximal femur. AJR Am J Roentgenol. 2008;191:995–1001.
25. Verbeeten KM, Hermann KL, Hasselqvist M, Lausten GS, Joergensen P, Jensen CM, et al. The advantages of MRI in the detection of occult hip fractures. Eur Radiol. 2005;15:165–9.
26. National Clinical Guideline Centre (UK). The Management of Hip Fracture in Adults. London: Royal College of Physicians (UK); 2011.
27. Iwata T, Nozawa S, Dohjima T, Yamamoto T, Ishimaru D, Tsugita M, et al. The value of T1-weighted coronal MRI scans in diagnosing occult fracture of the hip. J Bone Joint Surg (Br). 2012;94:969–73.
28. Alam A, Willett K, Ostlere S. The MRI diagnosis and management of incomplete intertrochanteric fractures of the femur. J Bone Joint Surg (Br). 2005;87:1253–5.
29. Craig JG, Moed BR, Eyler WR, van Holsbeeck M. Fractures of the greater trochanter: intertrochanteric extension shown by MR imaging. Skelet Radiol. 2000;29:572–6.

11

Incidence of deep vein thrombosis before and after total knee arthroplasty without pharmacologic prophylaxis: a 128-row multidetector CT indirect venography study

Moon Jong Chang, Min Kyu Song, Min Gyu Kyung, Jae Hoon Shin, Chong Bum Chang and Seung-Baik Kang[*]ⓘ

Abstract

Background: We sought to document the incidences of deep vein thrombosis (DVT) before and after total knee arthroplasty (TKA). In addition, we aimed to explor whether routine preoperative DVT evaluation was useful to establish DVT treatment strategies after TKA. Finally, we wanted to evaluate whether the incidences of DVT differed between patients undergoing unilateral and staged bilateral TKA within the same hospitalization period.

Methods: The retrospective study included 153 consecutive patients (253 knees) with osteoarthritis who underwent primary TKA. After surgery, mechanical compression devices (only) were used for DVT prophylaxis. DVT status before and after TKA was determined via 128-row, multidetector, computed tomography/indirect venography.

Results: Overall, the preoperative DVT incidence was 2.6% per patient and 1.6% per knee. All preoperative DVTs were distal in nature and asymptomatic. After TKA, newly developed thrombi were evident in various calf veins, without propagation of any pre-existing thrombi. Postoperatively, the overall incidences of DVT were 69.9% per patient and 58.5% per knee. The DVT incidences were 66% per patient and 69.8% per knee in the unilateral TKA group. In contrast, the incidences were 72% per patient and 55.5% per knee in the staged bilateral TKA group. There was one case of symptomatic distal (unilateral TKA; 0.65% per patient and 0.4% per knee) and proximal DVT (bilateral TKA; 0.65% per patient and 0.4% per knee), respectively.

Conclusions: The incidence of symptomatic DVT was low in Asian patients treated with mechanical compression devices alone, although substantial portion of patients had DVT after surgery. Routine preoperative DVT evaluation is probably not necessary; preoperative DVT was rare and of limited clinical relevance. Furthermore, staged bilateral TKA during a single period of hospitalization does not increase the incidence of DVT.

Keywords: Venous thromboembolism, Deep vein thrombosis, Total knee arthroplasty, Mechanical compression device, Indirect venography

Background

Deep vein thrombosis (DVT) is a frequent and significant complication after total knee arthroplasty (TKA) [1, 2]. However, the incidence, diagnosis, prevention, and treatment of DVT remain controversial [1, 3–9]. Differences in the DVT incidence between Asian and Western populations may have aggravated the controversies [10–14].

Most recent studies have recorded lower incidences of DVT in Asian patients; routine pharmacological prophylaxis is not recommended [1, 2, 6]. Indeed, studies on the use of mechanical compression devices (alone) to prevent DVT have become more common [1, 2, 6, 15]. However, theoretically, the use of such devices alone, thus without pharmacological treatment, would be less effective than the combination.

It was important to calculate the incidences of DVT before and after surgery in patients undergoing TKA to establish appropriate treatment strategies. A previous

* Correspondence: ossbkang@gmail.com
Department of Orthopedic Surgery, Seoul National University College of Medicine, SMG-SNU Boramae Medical Center, 5 Gil 20, Boramae-road, Dongjak-gu, Seoul 07061, South Korea

study found preoperative, asymptomatic vascular disease in 4.6% of patients scheduled for TKA [16]. Furthermore, 8% of patients had DVT before TKA [17]. Therefore, the incidence of preoperative DVT must be calculated to allow accurate estimation of the incidence after surgery. In addition, a prior history of venous thromboembolism (VTE) is a well-known risk factor for DVT development after surgery [18]. Furthermore, if a preexisting DVT can propagate after surgery, additional prophylactic treatment may be required.

The incidence and characteristics of DVT may differ between patients undergoing unilateral and staged bilateral TKA. Patients who undergo the bilateral procedure during a single hospitalization period may have to endure prolonged immobilization and a longer hospital stay than the former patients. Furthermore, in contrast to those who undergo bilateral TKA in a single operation, patients undergoing the staged procedure are subjected to repeat surgery with additional anesthesia. Several studies have compared the incidences of DVT between patients undergoing unilateral and simultaneous bilateral TKA [19, 20]. However, it is not clear whether staged bilateral TKA during a single period of hospitalization increases the incidence of DVT compared to that after unilateral TKA.

Therefore, we documented the incidence of DVT before and after TKA. In addition, we explored whether routine preoperative DVT evaluation was useful when establishing treatment strategies for DVT developing after TKA. Finally, we examined whether the incidence of DVT differed between patients undergoing unilateral or staged bilateral TKA during a single hospitalization period. We hypothesized that a considerable proportion of patients undergoing TKA would exhibit DVT both before and after surgery, and that routine preoperative DVT evaluation would thus be valuable. We also hypothesized that patients undergoing staged bilateral TKA would develop postoperative DVT more often than patients undergoing unilateral TKA.

Methods

This retrospective study included 153 consecutive patients (253 knees) with osteoarthritis who underwent primary TKA. From April 2016 to November 2016, 198 patients underwent primary TKA, due to osteoarthritis, at our institution. Of these, 45 were excluded because of previous surgery on the same knee joint (8); the use of anticoagulants (including aspirin) for thromboprophylaxis due to the presence of cardiovascular and/or cerebrovascular disease (30); contraindications for CT angiographic evaluation (2); and refusal to participate in the study (5). Ultimately, 153 patients (253 knees) were included. There were 130 females (85%) and 23 (15%) males of mean age 71.4 years (standard deviation [SD], 6.4 years; range, 53–84 years). Fifty-three patients (34.6%) underwent unilateral TKA and 100 (65.4%) staged bilateral TKA. The mean preoperative height and weight were 153.5 cm (SD, 7.4; range; 132.3–177 cm) and 63.9 kg (SD, 11.0; range, 43–95.2 kg). The mean body mass index was 27.1 kg/m^2 (SD, 3.8; range, 18.6–44.8 kg/m^2). No demographic difference including number of comorbidities was apparent between patients undergoing unilateral and staged bilateral TKA (Table 1). The study protocol was approved by our institutional review board.

All surgeries were performed by a single surgeon using a standard medial parapatellar approach with inflation of a pneumatic tourniquet, and all patients underwent identical postoperative rehabilitation. The tourniquet pressure was set to 300 mmHg and the tourniquet was inflated until skin closure was attained. Intramedullary guides were used during surgery on both the femora and tibiae. All TKAs featured placement of a fixed-bearing posterior stabilized prosthesis. All components were fixed with cement. A closed suction drain was inserted into the subcutaneous space, and tranexamic acid was not used. Periarticular injections and intravenous patient-controlled analgesia (PCA) were used to control postoperative pain. Active ankle flexion and extension

Table 1 Demographic data on patients in the unilateral and staged bilateral TKA groups

Variable	Unilateral TKA group (n = 53)	Bilateral TKA group (n = 100)	P value
Age (years)	71.3(range, 55–84; SD, 6.3)	71.5 (range, 53–84; SD, 6.4)	0.891
Proportion of female patients	45 (84.9)*	85 (85)*	0.988
BMI (kg/m^2)	26.9 (range, 20.9–44.8; SD, 4.1)	27.2 (range, 18.6–36; SD, 3.7)	0.684
Proportion undergoing general anesthesia	45 (84.9)*	95 (95)*	0.063
Operation time (min)	95.4 (range, 66–175; SD, 19)	91.2 (range, 43–140; SD, 16.2)	0.159
Length of hospital stay (days)	13.9 (range, 8–23; SD 2.7)	20.7 (range, 11–32; SD 3.9)	< 0.001
Number of comorbidities[a]	1.4 (range, 0–5; SD, 1.0)	1.3 (range, 0–4; SD, 1.1)	0.331

Data are presented as means or numbers of patients. Ranges, standard deviations, and proportions* are shown in parentheses. *Abbreviations = TKA* Total knee arthroplasty, *BMI* Body mass index, *SD* standard deviation
[a]Comorbidities include previous venous thromboembolism, varicose vein and previous operation on the leg, which are the major risk factors for deep vein thrombosis

exercises, and quadriceps strengthening exercises, were encouraged immediately after surgery. On the second postoperative day, after removal of the drain, all patients began walking with a walker, and commenced both active and passive range-of-motion (ROM) exercises. The second operation for those undergoing staged bilateral TKA was performed 1 week later, during the same hospitalization period.

Mechanical compression devices were applied to both lower legs of all patients after surgery. The Kendall SCD™ 700 Sequential Compression System (Kendall, Mansfield, MA, USA) was used, commencing on the day of surgery and continuing for 2 weeks thereafter. The device was discontinued at the time of discharge. For patients who underwent staged bilateral TKA, the device was placed on the day of the first operation, and continued to be used for 2 weeks after the second operation. The device has a sleeve for the leg, surrounded by three air chambers, and covers the lower limb from the ankle to the thigh. The device allows bilateral, sequential, circumferential, and gradient leg compression. All patients were fully compliant with treatment delivered by the device during their hospitalization periods.

We screened for DVT in both legs before and after TKA using 128-row, multidetector computed tomography-indirect venography (MDCT-indirect venography) (Philips Healthcare, Cleveland, OH, USA). The preoperative evaluation was performed in the outpatient clinic within 2 weeks prior to surgery, and the postoperative evaluation was performed on day 4 after surgery for patients undergoing unilateral TKA and on day 4 after the second operation for patients undergoing staged bilateral TKA [5]. All scans were obtained with the patient supine after injection of 2 mL/kg of the Optiray® 350 contrast agent (741 mg/mL) at 4–5 mL/s. Scanning was performed in a craniocaudal direction, from the diaphragm to the foot, 3 min after contrast injection. The slice thickness was 2 mm, the window level 50, and the window width 350.

A single radiologist blinded to the study protocol interpreted all venographs. The interpreter was a professor and a board-certified radiologist who had undergone fellowship training. Radiographic evaluation was performed with the aid of a picture archiving and communication system (PACS) (Maroview™, Marotech, Seoul, Korea). On MDCT-indirect venography, a DVT was defined as a low-attenuating partial or complete filling defect in the lumen of a vein, surrounded by a highly attenuating enhanced ring, evident on at least two consecutive images (Fig. 1) [18, 21]. A proximal DVT was defined as a DVT at the level of the popliteal vein or proximal to that vein, and a distal DVT as a DVT involving a calf vein. In principle, we intended to delay surgery if a symptomatic VTE was detected during preoperative evaluation. During the study period, we did not prescribe pharmacological treatment even if an asymptomatic preoperative DVT was evident, based on the recommendation of a previous study on Asian patients [20]. However, if DVT was evident on routine MDCT-indirect venography performed after surgery, we prescribed an anticoagulant regardless of symptoms.

Clinical symptoms and signs of DVT or a PE were recorded by the orthopedic residents in charge. Symptomatic DVT was considered present when DVT was apparent on MDCT-indirect venography, and the patient fulfilled at least one of the following criteria (suggested in a previous study): 1) swelling of all lower extremities; 2) abnormal lower leg swelling; 3) pitting edema; or, 4) a positive Homans' sign [6]. Imaging to detect PE was performed as described in a previous study; the relevant symptoms were: 1) tachycardia (heart rate > 100 beats/ min); 2) dyspnea or tachypnea; 3) sudden chest pain; or,

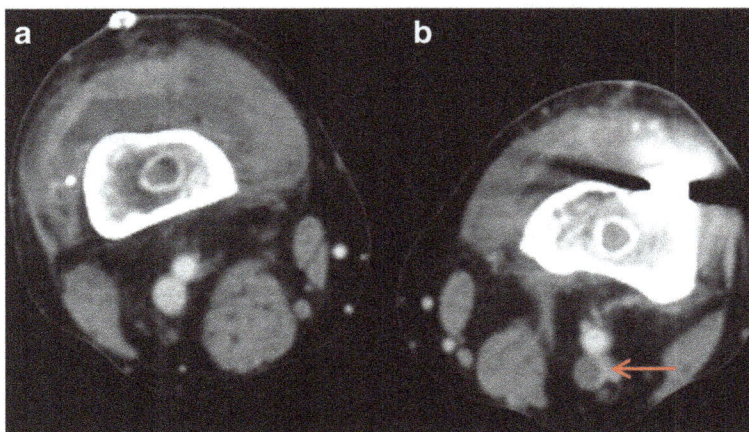

Fig. 1 Deep vein thrombosis (DVT) in the left popliteal vein. The image shows that the DVT exhibited a filling defect in the lumen of the vein, surrounded by a highly attenuating enhanced ring

4) decreased oxygen saturation [6]. Routine clinical follow-up was performed at six weeks, three months, six months, and annually thereafter.

All statistical analyses were performed using SPSS for Windows (version 18.0; SPSS Inc., Chicago, IL, USA) and a p-value < 0.05 was considered statistically significant. Demographic data were summarized and compared between the unilateral and staged bilateral TKA groups. Statistical significance was explored using the t-test for two independent samples, and the chi-squared test (or Fisher's exact test if necessary). The incidences of DVT before and after TKA were described as numbers with percentages. The statistical significance of any difference in the incidence or location (proximal or distal) of DVT between the unilateral and staged bilateral TKA groups was explored using the chi-squared test (or Fisher's exact test if necessary). The tests obtained more than 80% power within the proper sample size and significance level, α value, of 0.05.

Results

The overall preoperative incidences of DVT were 2.6% (four patients) per patient and 1.6% (four knees) per knee. All cases of preoperative DVT were distal and asymptomatic. Only one patient had concomitant varicose veins in the index limb prior to surgery. After TKA, they developed new thrombi in different calf veins (three of them also developed new thrombi in the opposite leg) without any propagation to proximal DVT of the preexisting thrombi (Table 2).

Postoperatively, the overall incidences of DVT were 69.9% (107 patients) per patient and 58.5% (148 knees) per knee, respectively. There was one case of symptomatic distal (unilateral TKA; 0.65% per patient and 0.4% per knee) and proximal DVT (bilateral TKA; 0.65% per patient and 0.4% per knee), respectively. The incidences of proximal DVT were 9.8% (fifteen patients) per patient and 7.1% (eighteen knees) per knee, respectively. Only one symptomatic PE with proximal DVT in a unilateral TKA was noted.

The incidence of DVT after TKA did not increase in the staged bilateral TKA group than the unilateral TKA

group. The incidences of DVT were 66% (35 of 53) per patient and 69.8% (37 of 53) per knee in the unilateral TKA group. In contrast, the incidences were 72% (72 of 100) per patient and 55.5% (111 of 200) per knee in the staged bilateral TKA group (per patient, $p = 0.444$; per knee, $p = 0.021$). In the unilateral TKA group, 88.6% (31/35) of DVT cases were diagnosed in the operated limb, and 5.7% of DVT cases were (2/35) bilateral DVT. In contrast, bilateral DVT was evident in 54.2% of patients (39/72) in the staged bilateral TKA group. In the bilateral TKA group, the incidence of DVT did not differ between the first and second TKA (55% vs. 56%; $p = 0.887$). In contrast, patients with DVT in the first-operated limb developed DVT more frequently in the second-operated limb (37 of 54 patients) compared with those with no DVT in the first-operated limb (17 of 46 patients) ($p = 0.001$).

Discussion

The guidelines of the American Academy of Orthopedic Surgeons (AAOS) state that "Patients undergoing elective hip and knee arthroplasty are already at high risk for venous thromboembolism." [22] Nonetheless, no consensus exists in terms of any of the incidence, diagnosis, prevention, or treatment of DVT, especially in Asian patients [10, 11, 23]. In the present study, we sought to accurately determine the incidences of DVT pre- and post-TKA using 128-row MDCT-indirect venography. In addition, we explored whether routine preoperative DVT evaluation was useful when planning postoperative treatment strategies. Finally, we examined whether the incidence and characteristics of DVT differed between those undergoing unilateral and staged bilateral TKA. Our principal findings were: 1) the incidence of preoperative DVT was low (2.6%) and of limited clinical significance; all affected patients also developed postoperative DVT at different sites; 2) although a considerable proportion of patients developed postoperative DVT, most was distal and asymptomatic; we found one example of symptomatic PE; and, 3) staged bilateral TKA during a single period of hospitalization does not increase the incidence of DVT.

Our findings did not support the hypotheses that a considerable proportion of patients undergoing TKA would have preoperative DVT, or that routine preoperative DVT evaluation would be useful. A previous study found that the preoperative incidence of DVT, diagnosed via Doppler ultrasound, in patients scheduled for TKA was 4.5% [11]. Another study using a 16-row MDCT reported an overall incidence of 8% [17]. As a 128-row MDCT is more accurate than the devices used in earlier studies, we initially hypothesized that the preoperative incidence would be higher than reported previously [23, 24]. However, the incidence of preoperative DVT in our current study was only 2.6%; such DVT was

Table 2 Details of the four patients with preoperative DVT

Case	Index knee	Preoperative DVT	Postoperative DVT
Case 1	Right	Right calf muscle vein	Right peroneal and calf muscle veins
Case 2	Left	Right calf muscle vein	Left below knee veins
Case 3	Right	Left calf muscle vein	Right peroneal, posterior tibial and calf muscle vein, Left calf muscle vein
Case 4	Right	Left calf muscle vein	Right tibioperoneal and calf muscle vein

Abbreviations = DVT Deep vein thrombosis

asymptomatic and did not propagate after surgery. In addition, only one patient with preoperative DVT had concomitant varicose veins, which are known to be a risk factor for postoperative VTE [18]. Thus, routine preoperative DVT evaluation did not yield useful information. Furthermore, the preoperative incidence of DVT did not affect the postoperative incidence; the four patients with preoperative DVT exhibited newly developed DVT after surgery. Therefore, preoperative DVT evaluation is of limited clinical utility.

The incidence of DVT in the current study was higher than the incidence previously reported in Asian patients. In a recent meta-analysis, the overall incidence of DVT in Asians was lower than in Westerners [10]. The incidence of postoperative DVT attained 80% in Western patients [25]. In contrast, in a meta-analysis of data on Asian populations, the incidences of overall, proximal, and symptomatic DVT were only 40.4, 5.8, and 1.9%, respectively [10]. A possible explanation for the higher incidence of DVT in the present study is that we used an intramedullary guide during both femoral and tibial resection. Many surgeons use such guides during femoral resection only even if no consensus on the use of guides during tibial resection has yet emerged [26]. Theoretically, an intramedullary guide may be more invasive than an extramedullary guide [27]. However, no study has yet explored whether the incidence of DVT increases after TKA using an intramedullary guide. Furthermore, previous studies on the incidence of DVT do not mention whether intramedullary or extramedullary guides were used during surgery on femora and/or tibiae. Therefore, the issue requires further evaluation.

We found no increase of DVT incidence in the staged bilateral TKA than in the unilateral TKA. In contrast to the hypothesis, unilateral TKA group showed higher DVT incidence per knee. It remains unclear whether simultaneous bilateral TKA is a risk factor for DVT development. When selected patients with DVT symptoms were examined, DVT was more common in those undergoing simultaneous bilateral TKA (12.4% vs. 25.9%) [19]. In contrast, when venography was used to perform routine DVT examinations, no difference in DVT incidence was evident between the unilateral and simultaneous bilateral TKA groups (41.4% of unilateral TKAs vs. 41.8% of simultaneous bilateral TKAs) [20]. In our present study, staged bilateral TKA during a single period of hospitalization does not increase the incidence of DVT. However, patients with DVT in the first-operated limb tended to exhibit DVT in the second-operated limb. This was probably because prior VTE is a risk factor for DVT development [22]. Furthermore, the fact that we found no difference in the incidence of postoperative DVT between the first- and second-operated limbs indirectly suggests that surgery

per se is the most significant risk factor for DVT, not prolonged immobilization or hospitalization.

Our study had several limitations. First, our sample size was relatively small and we did not have a control group undergoing pharmacological treatment. However, all patients underwent pre- and post-operative MDCT-indirect venography, which detects DVT more accurately than the methods used in previous studies [18]. Second, we prescribed anticoagulant therapy when DVT was evident on MDCT-indirect venography after surgery. This may have prevented late systematic complications associated with DVT. However, we believe that our findings are still valuable, because we did not prescribe any pharmacological treatment prior to DVT evaluation. In addition, withholding of anticoagulant therapy would have been unethical. Third, since the CT indirect venography was performed on the day 4 after surgery, we were not able to provide the incidence of late onset DVT using this study. Finally, all subjects were Asian, and females predominated. It is well-known that the incidence of overall DVT, those of symptomatic DVT and PE differ between Asians and Westerners. Thus, caution is appropriate when seeking to apply our findings to populations differing in ethnicity and/or sex ratio.

Conclusion

The incidence of symptomatic DVT was low in Asian TKA patients treated with a mechanical compression device alone, although a considerable proportion of patients exhibited DVT after surgery. Routine preoperative DVT evaluation is probably not required; preoperative DVT was rare and of limited clinical relevance. Furthermore, staged bilateral TKA during a single period of hospitalization did not increase the incidence of DVT.

Abbreviations
DVT: Deep vein thrombosis; MDCT: Multidetector computed tomography; PACS: Picture archiving and communication system; PCA: Patient controlled analgesia; PE: Pulmonary embolism; ROM: Range of motion; SD: Standard deviation; TKA: Total knee arthroplasty; VTE: Venous thromboembolism

Funding
This research was supported by the Bio & Medical Technology Development Program of the National Research Foundation (NRF) funded by the Ministry of Science & ICT (2017M3A9D8063538) in writing the manuscript.

Authors' contributions
MJC: design of the study, analysis and interpretation of data, drafting the article, revising the manuscript for important intellectual content; MKS: acquisition of data, analysis and interpretation of data, drafting the article; MGK: acquisition of data, analysis and interpretation of data; JHS: analysis and interpretation of data; CBC: design of the study, revising the manuscript for important intellectual content; SBK: design of the study, revising the manuscript for important intellectual content. All authors have read and approved the manuscript.

92

Musculoskeletal Disorders: Diagnosis, Prevention and Treatment

Competing interests

The authors declare that they have no competing interests.

References

1. Kim YH, Kulkarni SS, Park JW, Kim JS. Prevalence of deep vein thrombosis and pulmonary embolism treated with mechanical compression device after Total knee arthroplasty in Asian patients. J Arthroplast. 2015;30:1633–7.

2. Park SH, Ahn JH, Park YB, Lee SG, Yim SJ. Incidences of deep vein thrombosis and pulmonary embolism after Total knee arthroplasty using a mechanical compression device with and without low-molecular-weight heparin. Knee Surg Relat Res. 2016;28:213–8.

3. Wilson DG, Poole WE, Chauhan SK, Rogers BA. Systematic review of aspirin for thromboprophylaxis in modern elective total hip and knee arthroplasty. Bone Joint J. 2016;98-b:1056–61.

4. Tay K, Bin Abd Razak HR, Tan AH. Obesity and venous thromboembolism in Total knee arthroplasty patients in an Asian population. J Arthroplast. 2016;31:2880–3.

5. Song K, Xu Z, Rong Z, Yang X, Yao Y, Shen Y, et al. The incidence of venous thromboembolism following total knee arthroplasty: a prospective study by using computed tomographic pulmonary angiography in combination with bilateral lower limb venography. Blood Coagul Fibrinolysis. 2016;27:266–9.

6. Park YG, Ha CW, Lee SS, Shaikh AA, Park YB. Incidence and fate of "symptomatic" venous thromboembolism after knee arthroplasty without pharmacologic prophylaxis in an Asian population. J Arthroplast. 2016;31:1072–7.

7. Mori N, Kimura S, Onodera T, Iwasaki N, Nakagawa I, Masuda T. Use of a pneumatic tourniquet in total knee arthroplasty increases the risk of distal deep vein thrombosis: a prospective, randomized study. Knee. 2016;23:887–9.

8. Hamilton WG, Reeves JD, Fricka KB, Goyal N, Engh GA, Parks NL. Mechanical thromboembolic prophylaxis with risk stratification in total knee arthroplasty. J Arthroplast. 2015;30:43–5.

9. Charters MA, Frisch NB, Wessell NM, Dobson C, Les CM, Silverton CD. Rivaroxaban versus enoxaparin for venous thromboembolism prophylaxis after hip and knee arthroplasty. J Arthroplast. 2015;30:1277–80.

10. Lee WS, Kim KI, Lee HJ, Kyung HS, Seo SS. The incidence of pulmonary embolism and deep vein thrombosis after knee arthroplasty in Asians remains low: a meta-analysis. Clin Orthop Relat Res. 2013;471:1523–32.

11. Kim KI, Cho KY, Jin W, Khurana SS, Bae DK. Recent Korean perspective of deep vein thrombosis after total knee arthroplasty. J Arthroplast. 2011;26:1112–6.

12. Kanchanabat B, Stapanavatr W, Meknavin S, Soorapanth C, Sumanasrethakul C, Kanchanasuttirak P. Systematic review and meta-analysis on the rate of postoperative venous thromboembolism in orthopaedic surgery in Asian patients without thromboprophylaxis. Br J Surg. 2011;98:1356–64.

13. Brookenthal KR, Freedman KB, Lotke PA, Fitzgerald RH, Lonner JH. A meta-analysis of thromboembolic prophylaxis in total knee arthroplasty. J Arthroplast. 2001;16:293–300.

14. Westrich GH, Haas SB, Mosca P, Peterson M. Meta-analysis of thromboembolic prophylaxis after total knee arthroplasty. J Bone Joint Surg Br. 2000;82:795–800.

15. Bin Abd Razak HR, Tan HC. The use of pneumatic tourniquets is safe in Asians undergoing total knee arthroplasty without anticoagulation. Knee. 2014;21:176–9.

16. Park IH, Lee SC, Park IS, Nam CH, Ahn HS, Park HY, et al. Asymptomatic peripheral vascular disease in total knee arthroplasty: preoperative prevalence and risk factors. J Orthop Traumatol. 2015;16:23–6.

17. Watanabe H, Sekiya H, Kariya Y, Hoshino Y, Sugimoto H, Hayasaka S. The incidence of venous thromboembolism before and after total knee arthroplasty using 16-row multidetector computed tomography. J Arthroplast. 2011;26:1488–93.

18. Shin WC, Woo SH, Lee SJ, Lee JS, Kim C, Suh KT. Preoperative prevalence of and risk factors for venous thromboembolism in patients with a hip fracture: an indirect multidetector CT venography study. J Bone Joint Surg Am. 2016;98:2089–95.

19. Chung LH, Chen WM, Chen CF, Chen TH, Liu CL. Deep vein thrombosis after total knee arthroplasty in asian patients without prophylactic anticoagulation. Orthopedics. 2011;34:15.

20. Kim YH, Kim JS. Incidence and natural history of deep-vein thrombosis after total knee arthroplasty. A prospective, randomised study J Bone Joint Surg Br. 2002;84:566–70.

21. Cham MD, Yankelevitz DF, Shaham D, Shah AA, Sherman L, Lewis A, et al. Deep venous thrombosis: detection by using indirect CT venography. The pulmonary angiography-indirect CT venography cooperative group. Radiology. 2000;216:744–51.

22. Jacobs JJ, Mont MA, Bozic KJ, Della Valle CJ, Goodman SB, Lewis CG, et al. American Academy of Orthopaedic surgeons clinical practice guideline on: preventing venous thromboembolic disease in patients undergoing elective hip and knee arthroplasty. J Bone Joint Surg Am. 2012;94:746–7.

23. Park KH, Cheon SH, Lee JH, Kyung HS. Incidence of venous thromboembolism using 64 channel multidetector row computed tomography-indirect venography and anti-coagulation therapy after total knee arthroplasty in Korea. Knee Surg Relat Res. 2012;24:19–24.

24. Duarte R, Fernandez G, Castellon D, Costa JC. Prospective coronary CT angiography 128-MDCT versus retrospective 64-MDCT: improved image quality and reduced radiation dose. Heart Lung Circ. 2011;20:119–25.

25. Wang CJ, Huang CC, Yu PC, Chen HH. Diagnosis of deep venous thrombosis after total knee arthroplasty: a comparison of ultrasound and venography studies. Chang Gung Med J. 2004;27:16–21.

26. Han HS, Kang SB, Jo CH, Kim SH, Lee JH. The accuracy of intramedullary tibial guide of sagittal alignment of PCL-substituting total knee arthroplasty. Knee Surg Sports Traumatol Arthrosc. 2010;18:1334–8.

27. Zhou F, Ji J, Song Q, Peng Z, Zhang G, Wang Y. Pulmonary fat embolism and related effects during femoral intramedullary surgery: an experimental study in dogs. Exp Ther Med. 2013;6:469–74.

12

Cyclic bisphosphonate therapy reduces pain and improves physical functioning in children with osteogenesis imperfecta

Melissa D. Garganta[1], Sarah S. Jaser[2], Margot A. Lazow[3], Jonathan G. Schoenecker[2], Erin Cobry[2], Stephen R. Hays[2] and Jill H. Simmons[2,4*] (iD)

Abstract

Background: Children with osteogenesis imperfecta (OI) experience pain and impaired physical functioning. The longitudinal effect of cyclic bisphosphonate treatment on these symptoms has not been described. We serially evaluated pain and functioning in pediatric patients with OI treated with intravenous bisphosphonate therapy.

Methods: Pain and physical functioning were assessed at multiple time-points over two infusion cycles in 22 OI patients (median age 10 years [range 2–21 years]; 8 girls) receiving cyclic intravenous bisphosphonate therapy. Pain was assessed using the FACES® visual analogue scale; physical functioning, including self-care, was assessed using the PedsQL™ Generic Core inventory.

Results: Pain scores decreased significantly immediately following infusion and remained reduced at 4 weeks post-infusion, increasing before and decreasing again after subsequent infusion ($F = 25.00$, $p < 0.001$). Physical functioning scaled scores improved 4 weeks after infusion and declined before subsequent infusion across patients ($F = 10.87$, $p = 0.007$). Exploratory analyses indicated significantly different effects between mild and moderate-severe OI types for pain, but not for physical functioning. No fractures occurred during the study.

Conclusion: In children with OI, cyclic intravenous bisphosphonate therapy transiently reduces pain and improves functional abilities. Pain relief occurs immediately following infusion with functional improvements observed 4 weeks later. Both pain and physical functioning return to pretreatment levels by the subsequent infusion.

Keywords: Osteogenesis imperfecta, Bisphosphonate, Pamidronate, Zoledronic acid, Pain, Faces®, Quality of life, PedsQL™, Pediatrics

Background

Osteogenesis imperfecta (OI) is a genetic disorder that affects type 1 collagen and has variable manifestations including low bone mineral density, skeletal deformities, recurrent bone fractures, scoliosis, and chronic pain [1–3]. The majority of patients with OI have a mutation in the *COL1A1* or *COL1A2* gene encoding the alpha 1 and alpha 2 chains of type 1 collagen, producing either defective type 1 collagen or a deficient quantity of normal type 1 collagen; more than 200 mutations in multiple genes have been identified [4, 5]. The widely accepted Sillence classification distinguishes the four most common phenotypic presentations (Types I-IV) (Table 1), although up to 17 types have been described based upon either unique phenotype or molecular etiology [6–8]. Regardless of type, many patients with OI report pain on a chronic basis, even during periods without fractures [4, 9]. The specific etiology of the pain that occurs in patients with OI in the absence of an acute fracture is not entirely clear; however, it has been hypothesized that inflammatory cytokines, such as prostaglandins or thromboxanes, may contribute to bone turnover and therefore result in pain symptoms [10]. Chronic pain may result in delayed motor development, missed school days and significant psychosocial stress for patients and their families [11, 12]. Furthermore, children

* Correspondence: jill.h.simmons@vanderbilt.edu
[2]Vanderbilt University Medical Center, Nashville, TN, USA
[4]Division of Pediatric Endocrinology and Diabetes, Village at Vanderbilt, 1500 21st Avenue South, Suite 1514, Nashville, TN 37212-3157, USA
Full list of author information is available at the end of the article

Table 1 Sillence classification system for osteogenesis imperfecta

OI Type	Features
Type I	Mildest form. Limited bone deformity and fragility.
Type II	Lethal in perinatal period.
Type III	Most severe form in patients who survive the newborn period.
Type IV	Moderate severity. Spectrum of severity between types I and III.
Additional OI types	Range in severity. Etiology is typically due to mutations in genes involved with collagen formation other than *COL1A1* or *COL1A2*.

with OI experience reduced physical functioning, such as poor mobility and inability to perform routine activities of daily living [2, 13].

The current mainstay of pharmacologic treatment for OI is nitrogen-containing bisphosphonate therapy, which has been shown to decrease bone turnover, improve bone mineral density and reduce fracture rates [14, 15]. Bisphosphonate therapy is typically initiated when children with OI have two fragility fractures per year. Although dosing schedules vary between institutions, pamidronate is typically given every 2 months until age 2 years, every 3 months in the third year of life, and every 4 months thereafter; zoledronic acid is generally given every 6 months. The choice of bisphosphonate administered is typically dependent upon provider and patient comfort [16]. It has previously been reported that bisphosphonate therapy relieves bone pain acutely following infusion in children with OI, but a sustained long-term effect, if any, is unclear [2, 3, 14, 17–19]. A recent study reported decreased pain at 1 week post-infusion with zoledronate compared to pre-infusion [20]. Previous studies have demonstrated that cyclic bisphosphonate treatment with pamidronate may improve mobility and muscle force in children with moderate to severe types of OI and may reduce the number of days per week with pain [8], but the effect on severity of pain between infusion cycles has not been well- assessed. Some studies have reported improvement in mobility and independence of activities following bisphosphonate treatment, whereas others have not demonstrated any beneficial effects on physical functioning [2, 3, 13, 21]. Therefore, we assessed the effect of cyclic intravenous bisphosphonate treatment on patient-reported pain levels and parent-assessed physical functioning over time and compared effects between children with mild and moderate-to-severe forms of OI.

Methods
Patient population and study design
The sample in this prospective longitudinal cohort study consisted of 22 children with a diagnosis of OI receiving intravenous bisphosphonate therapy at the Monroe Carell Jr. Children's Hospital at Vanderbilt between November

2014 and February 2016. Patients that had experienced at least 2 fragility fractures within the 12 months prior to starting therapy were included and patients naïve to bisphosphonate treatment were excluded. All patients approached agreed to be enrolled.

OI Type (Type I, Type III or Type IV) was defined clinically, and one patient had genetic testing consistent with OI Type VIII. Patients were followed under real-world conditions through two cycles of bisphosphonate treatment with pain assessed by patient report immediately before and after each infusion and 4 weeks following the initial infusion. Physical functioning was assessed immediately before each infusion and 4 weeks after the first infusion by a parent-completed survey. This study was approved by the Institutional Review Board at Vanderbilt University Medical Center. The authors have no conflicts of interest to disclose.

Treatments
Patients received either pamidronate or zoledronic acid per their chronic regimen. Pamidronate was administered in a single-day infusion dosed in a weight- and age-dependent manner. Children ages 2–3 years received 1.1 mg/kg every 3 months and those > 3 years received 1.5 mg/kg/dose every 4 months (maximum dose ≤45 mg/ infusion and 4.5 mg/kg/year). Zoledronic acid was administered in a single-day infusion of 0.05 mg/kg every 6 months for all ages. The treatment regimen was selected prior to study participation by patients and families after discussion about long-term knowledge of the effects of pamidronate compared with ease of administration of zoledronic acid.

Assessments
Pain was evaluated using the FACES® visual analogue scale, a validated tool for assessing patient-perceived pain on a scale of 0–10 with 0 indicating no pain and 10 indicating worst possible pain [22]. The specific location of pain was not recorded. Physical functioning was assessed using the Pediatric Quality of Life Inventory 4.0 Generic Core Scales for Physical Functioning (PedsQL™) Parent Reports for Young Children ages 5–7, Children ages 8–12 and Teens ages 13–17 years. The PedsQL™ is a health-related quality of life measure that has demonstrated validity and reliability in a wide variety of general populations and in several disease-specific pediatric populations [23–25]. The Physical Functioning Core Scale consists of eight items related to daily activities specific to age group (e.g., walking, running, bathing, lifting items, energy level). Physical Functioning Core Scale score is calculated as a scaled score ranging from 0 to 100, with 100 indicating the highest level of health-related quality of life and physical functioning [25].

Statistical analyses

Descriptive analyses were conducted to determine the means and standard deviations of the measures at each time point. To assess changes in pain and physical functioning over time (within subjects), we conducted repeated measures analysis of variance. The repeated measures design provides greater statistical power to detect effects with a smaller number of patients by controlling for individual differences. We also conducted exploratory analyses to determine whether there were differences in changes in pain across OI types (Type I vs. Types III and IV). Analyses were performed using IBM SPSS software, version 23 (SPSS, Chicago, IL).

Results

Clinical characteristics of the 22 children analyzed in this study are presented in Table 2. Patients were 2–21 years old (median age 10 years); 36% had mild OI (Type I, $N = 8$) while 64% had moderate-severe OI (Type III, $N = 7$; Type IV, $N = 6$; Type VIII, $N = 1$), as defined by clinical characteristics (Sillence classification (Table 1)), except for the patient with Type VIII, who was classified based upon genetic testing (moderate-severe). Not all patients were able to complete all study visits, though this was never due to patient/parent refusal. As these patients were not seen under specific study conditions, but rather were followed at their regularly scheduled appointments, some patients missed study windows due to cancellations, rescheduling or no-shows to their appointments, or research staff being unavailable during their appointment times. The median time

Table 2 Clinical characteristics of the study population

Characteristic	$N = 22$
Age (years) [a]	10 (2–21)
Male/Female	14/8 (64%/36%)
White	14 (64%)
Black	4 (18%)
Asian	2 (9%)
Latino	1 (5%)
Multiracial	1 (5%)
OI Type I	8 (36%)
OI Type III	7 (32%)
OI Type IV	6 (27%)
OI Type VIII	1 (5%)
Height z-score [a]	− 2.96 (− 12.43–4.16)
Weight z-score [a]	− 1.64 (− 11.89–3.29)
BMI z-score [a]	0.81 (− 0.95–2.51)
Able to ambulate without assistance	14/21 (67%)
Receiving pamidronate	16 (73%)
Receiving zoledronic acid	6 (27%)

[a] Median (range)

between Visit 1 (initial infusion during study) and Visit 2 (per protocol, 4 weeks post infusion) was 30.5 days. The median time between Visit 1 (initial infusion during study) and Visit 3 (2nd infusion) was 206 days (6.9 months). Overall, 73% ($N = 16$) of patients were treated with pamidronate, while 27% ($N = 6$) were treated with zoledronic acid. There were no significant differences between patients treated with pamidronate and zolendronic with respect to child age, sex, or OI Type. No fractures occurred during the study.

Pain

Eighteen patients completed the pre- and immediately post- infusion pain assessments, 12 patients completed the 4-week post-infusion assessment, and eight patients completed the subsequent pre-infusion pain assessment. One patient sustained acute trauma by falling from a chair during his infusion and his pain scores were excluded.

For patients who had data for all time points ($n = 6$), there was a significant change in self-reported pain scores over time associated with bisphosphonate infusion ($F = 10.19$, $P < 0.001$) (Fig. 1). Pain scores decreased from 2.00 ± 2.00 immediately pre-infusion to 0.50 ± 0.84 immediately post-infusion. Pain scores remained decreased from baseline at 4 weeks post-infusion, with a mean score of 0.67 ± 0.82. A diminished analgesia was observed with pain scores returning to pre-infusion levels (2.50 ± 2.43) immediately prior to subsequent infusion, approximately 6 months later. Significant analgesia was again noted immediately following subsequent infusion (pain scores 1.00 ± 1.27). For the 12 patients who had pain assessments only at the first pre- and post- infusion and 4-week follow-up visit, there was a significant change in self-reported pain scores from the first infusion to the follow-up visit, about 4 weeks later ($F = 25.00$, $P < .001$). Pain scores decreased from 2.17 ± 1.53 prior to infusion to 0.42 ± 0.79 post-infusion and remained decreased from baseline at 4 weeks post-infusion, with a mean score of 0.50 ± 0.67. It is notable that there was a significant difference between pre-infusion pain scores at the first visit and follow-up visit ($t = -.2.65$, $P = 0.033$).

Exploratory subgroup analysis indicated that the effect of bisphosphonate infusion on pain scores differed according to type of OI (Fig. 1). We identified a significant Time x OI Type interaction effect for pain ($F = 3.82$, $P = 0.023$): children with more severe forms of OI (Types III/IV, $n = 3$) reported significantly higher levels of pain at baseline, and a greater decrease in pain following bisphosphonate infusion, than children with milder OI (Type I, $n = 3$). In patients with Types III/ IV OI, mean pain scores decreased from 3.33 ± 2.08 pre-infusion to 1.00 ± 1.00 post-infusion, and remained decreased at 1.33 ± 0.58 4 weeks post-infusion. In patients with Type I OI, mean pain scores decreased from 0.67 ± 0.58 pre-infusion to 0.00 ± 0.00 post-infusion, and remained decreased at 0.00 ± 0.00 4 weeks post- infusion. A similar pattern was seen with the second infusion cycle.

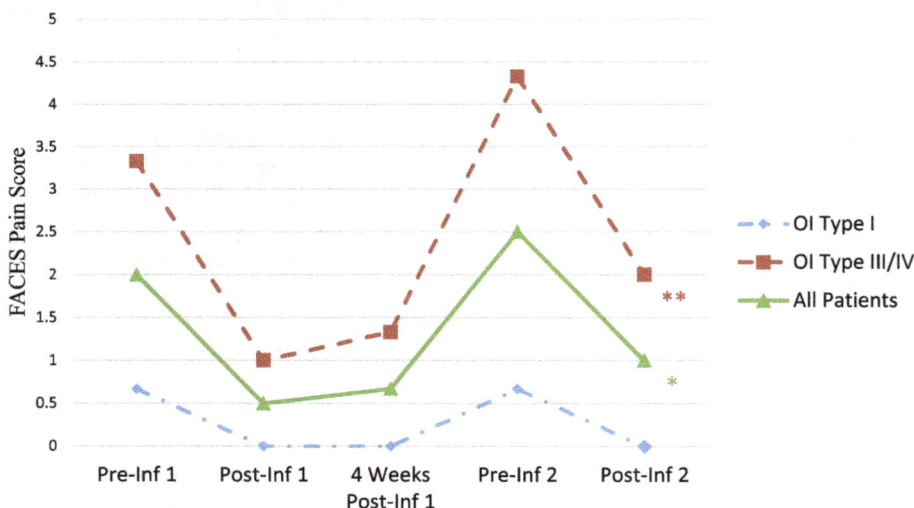

Fig. 1 Mean pain scores over time by osteogenesis imperfecta (OI) type, assessed by FACES® visual analogue scale immediately pre- / immediately post-infusion, 4 weeks post-infusion, and immediately pre- / immediately post subsequent infusion. Scale reduced (maximum pain score 5) for visual effect. * $P < 0.001$ for effect over time in all patients. ** $P = 0.023$ for difference in pain over time between patients with milder (Type I) and more severe (Types III/IV) OI

Children with more severe OI (Types III/IV) reported mean pain scores of 4.33 ± 2.08 prior to infusion, decreasing to 2.00 ± 1.00 immediately after the second infusion; children with milder OI (Type I) reported mean pain scores of 0.67 ± 0.58 pre-infusion, decreasing to 0.00 ± 0.00 immediately after infusion. These results must be interpreted with caution and are therefore considered exploratory; given the observed effect size and our sample of six participants measured across five time points, we had power of .24 to detect a significant effect. A sample size of 16 (8 per group) was needed to have sufficient power to detect significant effects.

Physical functioning

Parents of all 22 patients completed the pre-infusion physical functioning assessment, 12 parents completed the 4-week post-infusion assessment, and seven parents completed the subsequent pre-infusion physical functioning assessment.

For the patients who had data for only the first two visits ($n = 12$, Fig. 2a), we observed significant change from the first visit to the post-visit assessment in parent-reported physical functioning scaled scores associated with bisphosphonate infusion ($F = 10.87$, $P = .007$). Mean scaled score for physical functioning was 49.48 ± 25.49 before infusion, and increased to 57.03 ± 25.29 4 weeks after infusion.

For the patients who had data from all time points ($n = 5$, Fig. 2b), we observed a significant change in parent-reported physical functioning scaled scores. This effect was quadratic ($F = 24.61$, $P = .008$), such that physical functioning improved after the first infusion, and diminished to pre-infusion levels by Visit 3. Specifically, mean scaled score for physical functioning was 46.25 ± 31.59 before infusion,

increased to 53.75 ± 29.60 4weeks after infusion, and returned to 46.88 ± 28.13 by the second infusion cycle. We were not able to evaluate differences in physical function between OI types due to small sample size.

Discussion

We demonstrate that treatment with cyclic bisphosphonate infusions in a real-world setting reduces pain and improves reported physical functioning in children with both mild and moderate-severe OI. Patients experience pain relief immediately following infusion, with sustained analgesia for several weeks. This effect eventually wanes over time, with pain returning at least to pre-infusion baseline prior to the next infusion. The children in the current study also experience a similar improvement in parental reports of physical functioning, including the ability to participate in exercise, play, household chores and self-care activities, such as bathing, following infusions, but these gains appeared to decrease back to baseline prior to the next cycle.

Our findings are consistent with the results of previous studies investigating the short-term effect of bisphosphonate infusions on pain relief in children with OI, in which consecutive three-day infusions reduced the number of days with pain per week in the weeks following the infusion, with recurrence of pain preceding the next treatment cycle [14, 17]. A recent study which evaluated pain in patients who were administered zoledronic acid in the hospital setting similarly showed reduction in both pain scores and number of pain quality descriptors measured following infusions, but neither were statistically significant [20]. Similar to our findings, these aforementioned studies also demonstrated improvements in physical functioning,

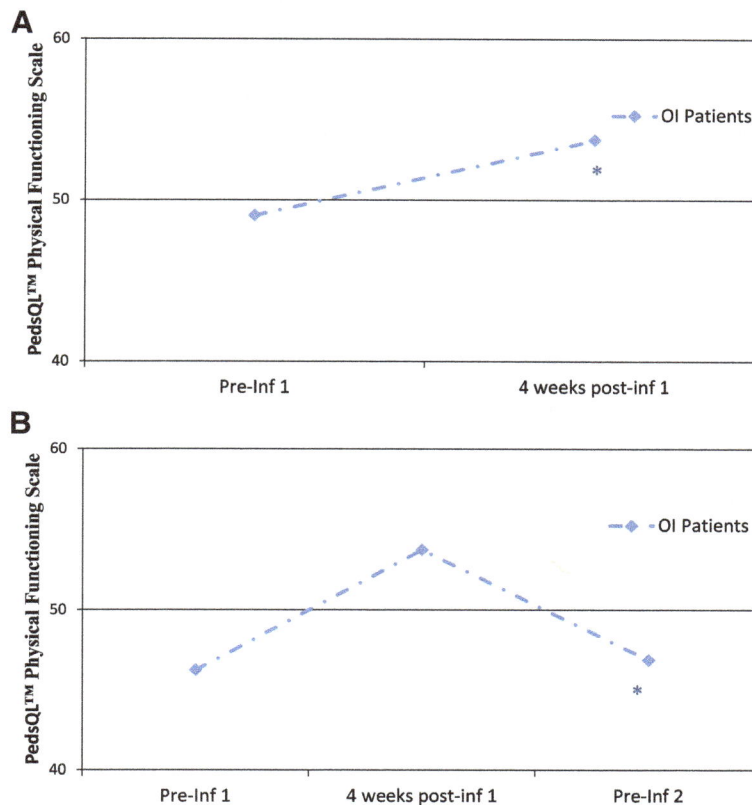

Fig. 2 a Mean physical functioning scaled scores over time, assessed using the PedsQL™ Generic Core Scale for Physical Functioning pre-infusion and 4 weeks post-infusion ($n = 12$). * $P = 0.007$. **b** Mean physical functioning scaled scores over time, assessed using the PedsQL™ Generic Core Scale for Physical Functioning pre-infusion, 4 weeks post-infusion, and pre-subsequent infusion ($n = 5$). * $P = 0.008$. Scale reduced (minimum scaled score 40) for visual effect

notably mobility and ambulation, following bisphosphonate infusions, with decline in functioning prior at the time of the subsequent infusion [14, 17, 20]. However, these studies were not performed in patients receiving outpatient single-day infusions of bisphosphonate therapy [26]. Our results indicate that reduced pain and improved physical functioning can be achieved using single-day outpatient treatment, which is less cumbersome for patients and families than the traditional consecutive three-day infusion cycle. Other potential areas of investigation include determining if these effects on pain and functioning can be achieved with oral bisphosphonate therapy.

The results of the current study contribute to growing evidence supporting temporary gains in pain relief and physical functioning following bisphosphonate infusions, but it remains unclear if and how these improvements after bisphosphonate use can be sustained long-term. Prior studies did not demonstrate significant long-term improvements in pain, mobility, or functioning at time points of 12 months or more following administration of bisphosphonates [2, 3, 18, 19], though two of these trials utilized different bisphosphonate types (risedronate and alendronate) than the ones administered in this study. Further research investigating the optimal bisphosphonate cycle duration and type as well as supplementary therapies to ensure sustained pain and functional improvements is therefore needed.

As expected, children with more severe forms of OI have more pain at baseline than children with milder forms of OI. While exploratory, our findings suggest that more severely affected OI patients have greater improvement in pain scores after infusions, while patients with milder OI experience less dramatic pain relief. Why patients with more severe forms of OI should obtain greater pain relief following bisphosphonate infusion than patients with milder OI is unclear. Additionally, the mechanism through which bisphosphonate treatment provides pain relief is unclear. Previous studies have suggested that decreased rates of fracture and bone turnover may provide relief from pain, but this does not explain the significant analgesia reported immediately following a single-day infusion as demonstrated in this study. Reduction of inflammatory cytokines such as serum prostaglandins or thromboxanes may play a role, as suggested by previous studies [10]. Future studies should include objective laboratory data such as measurement of the inflammatory cytokine prostaglandin E2, which has been implicated as a potent contributor to bone remodeling [10, 27], correlated with subjective measures of pain and functioning.

In the current cohort, patients with mild OI had experienced fractures prior to initiation of treatment with bisphosphonate therapy, as fragility fractures are typically considered a requirement for treatment. Further studies are needed to examine the effect of bisphosphonate therapy on pain, physical functioning and quality of life in patients with mild forms of OI who do not have fragility fractures.

Limitations of this study include small sample size and lack of either a placebo-controlled or non-treatment control group. The small sample size provided insufficient statistical power to evaluate for racial or gender differences in pain and functioning, or to determine differences between the two bisphosphonates used in this cohort. Patients were on chronic bisphosphonate therapy, so we were unable to evaluate the effect of first bisphosphonate infusion, as patients undergoing their first bisphosphonate infusion were excluded due to the flu-like reaction that often occurs in this setting. It would be appropriate in other investigations to evaluate effects on pain and physical functioning of first bisphosphonate infusion after this flu-like reaction has resolved. Additionally, the patient sample size was too small to determine whether there is a cumulative effect of bisphosphonate therapy on pain and physical functioning. The time between infusions was a mean of 6 months, making it difficult to determine exactly when the pain began to increase again following the initial infusion. In addition, while the timing between infusions varies depending on the type of bisphosphonate administered (zoledronate vs pamidronate), the current study did not have a large enough population to evaluate whether there was a significant difference in pain relief or improved functioning between these two groups. However, understanding both the exact time at which pain starts to worsen as well as whether analgesia is impacted by bisphosphonate type could be important in determining the duration and type of therapy which maximally reduces pain and improves physical functioning in these patients. Additionally, the exact locations of pain were not assessed, but would be useful to identify in future studies, in order to more specifically evaluate the impact of bisphosphonates. Physical functioning was not assessed by medical provider evaluation, but by parental survey. The PedsQL™ is an inventory not approved specifically for OI, but has been used in other chronic pediatric disease-specific populations [28, 29]. The FACES® scale used to evaluate pain is not specific for a population with OI; unfortunately, there is no pain assessment available specifically for children and adolescents with OI [30].

Conclusions

Our data indicate that chronic cyclic treatment with single-day bisphosphonate infusions acutely reduces pain and improves parental reports of daily functioning, including ability to participate in self-care, in children with OI regardless of type. Effects on pain appear to differ according to type of OI. Pain relief occurs immediately following infusion with functional improvements observed 4 weeks later. Both pain and physical functioning return to pretreatment levels by the subsequent infusion.

Abbreviations
OI: osteogenesis imperfecta; PedsQL™: Pediatric Quality of Life Inventory 4.0 Generic Core Scales for Physical Functioning

Funding
The project was supported by CTSA award # UL1TR000445 from the National Center for Advancing Translational Sciences. Funding for this study was used for urine sample analysis (data not shown in this manuscript).

Authors' contributions
This manuscript has seven authors. MDG made substantial contributions to study design, acquisition of data, analysis and interpretation of data, and drafted the manuscript. SSJ contributed substantially to analysis of interpretation of the data. MAL and EC contributed substantially through data acquisition. SRH and JGS contributed substantially to study design. JHS contributed substantially to study design, data acquisition and interpretation of the data as well as mentorship of MDG. All authors critically revised the manuscript for important intellectual content and approved the final version of the manuscript.

Competing interests
The authors declare that they have no competing interests.

Author details
Medical University of South Carolina, Greenville, SC, USA. ²Vanderbilt University Medical Center, Nashville, TN, USA. ³Cincinnati Children's Hospital Medical Center, Cincinnati, OH, USA. ⁴Division of Pediatric Endocrinology and Diabetes, Village at Vanderbilt, 1500 21st Avenue South, Suite 1514, Nashville, TN 37212-3157, USA.

References
1. Ben Amor M, Rauch F, Monti E, Antoniazzi F. Osteogenesis imperfecta. Pediatr Endocrinol Rev. 2013;10(Suppl 2):397–405.
2. Land C, Rauch F, Montpetit K, Ruck-Gibis J, Glorieux FH. Effect of intravenous pamidronate therapy on functional abilities and level of ambulation in children with osteogenesis imperfecta. J Pediatr. 2006;148(4):456–60.
3. Letocha AD, Cintas HL, Troendle JF, Reynolds JC, Cann CE, Chernoff EJ, et al. Controlled trial of pamidronate in children with types III and IV osteogenesis imperfecta confirms vertebral gains but not short-term functional improvement. J Bone Miner Res. 2005;20(6):977–86.
4. Ben Amor IM, Glorieux FH, Rauch F. Genotype-phenotype correlations in autosomal dominant osteogenesis imperfecta. J Osteoporos. 2011;2011:540178.
5. Rauch F, Glorieux FH. Osteogenesis imperfecta. Lancet. 2004;363(9418):1377–85.
6. Van Dijk FS, Silence DO. Osteogenesis imperfecta: clinical diagnosis, nomenclature and severity assessment. Am J Med Genet A. 2014; 164a(6):1470–81.
7. Symoens S, Malfait F. D'hondt S, Callewaert B, Dheedene a, Steyaert W, et al. deficiency for the ER-stress transducer OASIS causes severe recessive osteogenesis imperfecta in humans. Orphanet J Rare Dis. 2013;8(1):1–6.
8. Mendoza-Londono R, Fahiminiya S, Majewski J, Tétreault M, Nadaf J, Kannu P, et al. Recessive osteogenesis imperfecta caused by missense mutations in SPARC. Am J Hum Genet. 2015;96(6):979–85.

9. Zack P, Franck L, Devile C, Clark C. Fracture and non-fracture pain in children with osteogenesis imperfecta. Acta Paediatr. 2005;94(9):1238–42.

10. D'Eufemia P, Finocchiaro R, Celli M, Zambrano A, Tetti M, Villani C, et al. High levels of serum prostaglandin E2 in children with osteogenesis imperfecta are reduced by neridronate treatment. Pediatr Res. 2008; 63(2):203–6.

11. Cole DE. Psychosocial aspects of osteogenesis imperfecta: an update. Am J Med Genet. 1993;45(2):207–11.

12. Huguet A, Miro J. The severity of chronic pediatric pain: an epidemiological study. J Pain. 2008;9(3):226–36.

13. Sousa T, Bompadre V, White KK. Musculoskeletal functional outcomes in children with osteogenesis imperfecta: associations with disease severity and pamidronate therapy. J Pediatr Orthop. 2014;34(1):118–22.

14. Forin V, Arabi A, Guigonis V, Filipe G, Bensman A, Roux C. Benefits of pamidronate in children with osteogenesis imperfecta: an open prospective study. Joint Bone Spine. 2005;72(4):313–8.

15. Devogelaer JP, Coppin C. Osteogenesis imperfecta : current treatment options and future prospects. Treat Endocrinol. 2006;5(4):229–42.

16. Palomo T, Fassier F, Ouellet J, Sato A, Montpetit K, Glorieux FH, et al. Intravenous bisphosphonate therapy of young children with osteogenesis imperfecta: skeletal findings during follow up throughout the growing years. J Bone Miner Res. 2015;30(12):2150–7.

17. Glorieux FH, Bishop NJ, Plotkin H, Chabot G, Lanoue G, Travers R. Cyclic administration of pamidronate in children with severe osteogenesis imperfecta. N Engl J Med. 1998;339(14):947–52.

18. Ward LM, Rauch F, Whyte MP, D'Astous J, Gates PE, Grogan D, et al. Alendronate for the treatment of pediatric osteogenesis imperfecta: a randomized placebo-controlled study. J Clin Endocrinol Metab. 2011; 96(2):355–64.

19. Rauch F, Munns CF, Land C, Cheung M, Glorieux FH. Risedronate in the treatment of mild pediatric osteogenesis imperfecta: a randomized placebo-controlled study. J Bone Miner Res. 2009;24(7):1282–9.

20. Tsimicalis A, Boitor M, Ferland CE, Rauch F, Le May S, Carrier JI, et al. Pain and quality of life of children and adolescents with osteogenesis imperfecta over a bisphosphonate treatment cycle. Eur J Pediatr. 2018; 177(6):891–902.

21. Sakkers R, Kok D, Engelbert R, van Dongen A, Jansen M, Pruijs H, et al. Skeletal effects and functional outcome with olpadronate in children with osteogenesis imperfecta: a 2-year randomised placebo-controlled study. Lancet. 2004;363(9419):1427–31.

22. Tomlinson D, von Baeyer CL, Stinson JN, Sung L. A systematic review of faces scales for the self-report of pain intensity in children. Pediatrics. 2010; 126(5):e1168–98.

23. Varni JW, Seid M, Kurtin PS. PedsQL 4.0: reliability and validity of the pediatric quality of life inventory version 4.0 generic core scales in healthy and patient populations. Med Care. 2001;39(8):800–12.

24. Varni JW, Burwinkle TM, Seid M, Skarr D. The PedsQL 4.0 as a pediatric population health measure: feasibility, reliability, and validity. Ambul Pediatr. 2003;3(6):329–41.

25. Varni JW, Seid M, Rode CA. The PedsQL: measurement model for the pediatric quality of life inventory. Med Care. 1999;37(2):126–39.

26. Steelman J, Zeitler P. Treatment of symptomatic pediatric osteoporosis with cyclic single-day intravenous pamidronate infusions. J Pediatr. 2003;142(4):417–23.

27. Liu XH, Kirschenbaum A, Yao S, Levine AC. Cross-talk between the interleukin-6 and prostaglandin E(2) signaling systems results in enhancement of osteoclastogenesis through effects on the osteoprotegerin/receptor activator of nuclear factor-{kappa}B (RANK) ligand/RANK system. Endocrinology. 2005; 146(4):1991–8.

28. Engsberg JR, Ross SA, Collins DR. Increasing ankle strength to improve gait and function in children with cerebral palsy: a pilot study. Pediatr Phys Ther. 2006;18(4):266–75.

29. Bayle-Iniguez X, Audouin-Pajot C, Sales de Gauzy J, Munzer C, Murgier J, Accadbled F. Complex regional pain syndrome type I in children. Clinical description and quality of life. Orthop Traumatol Surg Res. 2015;101(6):745–8.

30. Nghiem T, Louli J, Treherne SC, Anderson CE, Tsimicalis A, Lalloo C, et al. Pain experiences of children and adolescents with osteogenesis imperfecta: an integrative review. Clin J Pain. 2017;33(3):271–80.

13

Somatosensation in OA: exploring the relationships of pain sensitization, vibratory perception and spontaneous pain

Anisha B. Dua[1][*] iD, Tuhina Neogi[2,1], Rachel A. Mikolaitis[3], Joel A. Block[4] and Najia Shakoor[4]

Abstract

Background: Pain in osteoarthritis (OA) remains poorly understood. Different types of somatosensory alterations exist in OA including hyperesthesia and increased sensitivity to painful stimuli as well as those of decreased sensitivity to cutaneous stimuli including vibratory perception threshold. The relationship between these different somatosensory measures has not been previously evaluated in OA. In this observational study, we evaluated relationships between vibratory perception (VPT), pressure pain detection thresholds (PPT), allodynia and subjective pain in knee OA.

Methods: Forty-two persons with moderate to severe knee OA and 12 controls without OA were evaluated. VPT was measured using a biothesiometer. Allodynia was measured by application of a 60 g Von Frey monofilament repeatedly to predetermined sites. PPTs were measured using a pressure algometer.

Results: Increased vibratory acuity was associated with lower PPTs and presence of allodynia. Allodynia was more common in OA than controls (54.8% vs 16.6%, $p = 0.024$ in the ipsilateral knee, and 42.9% vs 0%, $p = 0.005$ in the contralateral knee). OA participants with allodynia had lower PPTs than those without allodynia. In those with OA, spontaneous knee pain was associated with lower PPTs and with allodynia.

Conclusion: This study confirms the presence of somatosensory alterations in OA. Sensory alterations (vibratory perception) were shown to be related to nociceptive alterations (sensitization) in OA, showing a general increased sensitivity to cutaneous mechanical stimulation. Understanding these relationships is an important step in delineating the complicated pathophysiology of pain processing in OA.

Keywords: Osteoarthritis, Pain, Somatosensory measures, Allodynia

Background

Osteoarthritis (OA) is the most common chronic arthropathy worldwide, and pain is the most disabling symptom [1]. Mechanisms of pain in OA are poorly understood, and there is only a weak association between pain and radiographic knee OA [2]. A better understanding of somatosensory pathways and their roles in OA and OA-related pain may help improve our understanding of OA pathogenesis and our management of OA.

"Somatosensory" has a broad application when referring to alterations of the nervous system that have been shown to be present in clinical OA. First, "somatosensory alterations" could refer to those of specific pain processing pathways. Studies have suggested that abnormal excitability in the pain pathways of the peripheral and central nervous system play an important role in OA pain [3–5]. Continuous nociceptive input in OA could affect neuropeptide release from nerve endings, neuroplasticity, increases in synaptic strength and lowered firing thresholds of the dorsal horns. This could lead to changes in pain thresholds, and spreading of pain to uninjured sites [6]. The continuous input in chronic painful states such as OA can lead to heightened responsiveness, or "sensitization", of peripheral nociceptors (i.e., peripheral sensitization) and nociceptors in the central nervous system resulting in hypersensitivity to stimuli, responsiveness to non-noxious stimuli, and increased pain response evoked by stimuli outside the area of injury (i.e., central

* Correspondence: adua@uchicago.edu
[1]Section of Rheumatology, University of Chicago, 5841 S Maryland Ave, MC0930, Chicago, IL 60637, USA
Full list of author information is available at the end of the article

sensitization) [7–9]. Sensitization may be expressed clinically as allodynia (painful response resulting from a normally innocuous stimulus) and hyperalgesia (enhanced pain response to a noxious stimulus). Previous studies of symptomatic knee OA have demonstrated findings suggestive of sensitization or heightened pain sensitivity, including lower pressure pain thresholds (PPT) and the presence of mechanical allodynia [8, 10–12].

In addition to the nociceptive sensory alterations in OA, there is extensive literature of other types of "somatosensory" alterations that exist in OA, including deficits in such functions as vibratory perception and proprioception [13, 14]. We have previously shown that subjects with knee OA and hip OA have generalized vibratory sense deficits with impaired vibratory perception threshold (VPT) at both the upper and lower extremities compared to age-matched control subjects [14, 15].

Interestingly, the paradox between the different types of somatosensory alterations in OA is the existence of both "increased sensitivity" to some cutaneous stimuli (pressure and pain) while there is "decreased" sensory function in other measures such as sensation of vibration and proprioceptive acuity. Some studies in neuropathic pain have previously demonstrated the coexistence of somatosensory "profiles" with both loss and gain of sensation or sensitivity [16]. The relationships between pain sensitization and vibratory sense alterations in OA are not clear and have not been previously evaluated. Although vibratory sense may have a mechanical role similar to the hypothesized role of proprioceptive deficits in OA, alterations in vibratory sense may also play a role in pain processing in OA.

Here we explore the relationship between nociceptive alterations and other somatosensory alterations, specifically, vibratory sense in OA. We evaluate vibration sense, allodynia, pressure pain and subjective pain in knee OA participants and in healthy, pain-free controls. Our primary hypothesis is that vibratory acuity will be inversely associated with other somatosensory measures that may be reflective of sensitization. Specifically, we hypothesized that those with greater vibratory deficits will also have lower PPTs and evidence of allodynia. Our secondary hypothesis is that sensitization as well as worse vibratory acuity, indicative of chronic pain and severe OA [17–19], respectively, will be associated with higher subjective pain measures in knee OA.

Methods

Study sample

This study was approved through the institution's review board for studies involving human subjects and written informed consent was obtained from all subjects. Study subjects were recruited from a single large urban academic medical center in the United States between 2011 and 2013. Subjects were recruited through referral from the Rheumatology clinic and the department's clinical studies center. None of the subjects declined participation in the study. Study subjects were those with *symptomatic* OA of the knee, which was defined by the American College of Rheumatology's Clinical Criteria for Classification and Reporting of OA of the knee [20] and by the presence of at least 20 mm of pain (on a 100 mm scale) while walking (corresponding to question 1 of the visual analog format of the knee-directed Western Ontario and McMaster Universities Arthritis Index (WOMAC)) [21]). In subjects with bilateral knee OA, the most symptomatic side was considered the "affected" side. Radiographic OA of the index knee was documented by anterior-posterior standing radiographs of the knees in full extension, of grade greater than or equal to 2 as defined by the Kellgren-Lawrence (KL) grading scale [22, 23]. All KL evaluations and assessments were performed by a single trained investigator (NS). Knee OA participants were excluded if they demonstrated greater than 20 mm (of 100 mm) pain while walking (corresponding to question 1 of the VAS format of the site-directed WOMAC) at any other joint besides the knees. Other exclusion criteria included the presence of an inflammatory arthropathy or neuropathy, history of any lower extremity joint replacement or diabetes mellitus.

Controls were recruited from Rheumatology clinic as well as personal referrals from clinic staff age-matched control participants were included in the study if they had pain less than 20 mm (of 100 mm) at the knee, hip and ankle while walking (corresponding to question 1 of the VAS format of the site-specific WOMAC) and did not have radiographic knee OA, documented by KL grade of 0 or 1 on knee radiograph. The index knee in the control group was the right knee and the contralateral knee was the left knee. They had the same exclusion criteria as the OA participants.

Mechanical allodynia to repetitive stimulation

Allodynia was assessed using a 60 g Von Frey monofilament, which is an innocuous mechanical stimulus in healthy individuals. The sites evaluated were the tibial tuberosities and the right radial styloid. The Von Frey monofilament was applied perpendicularly to the skin with enough pressure to make it bend. The monofilament was then applied repeatedly to the same site at a rate of 1 Hz for 30 s. Subjects provided a numerical pain rating at the end of this train of stimulations. Allodynia was considered to be present when participants answered "yes" to the question "do you consider this painful?" Participants provided a numerical pain rating at the end of this train of stimulations, rating the extent of their pain on a scale of 0 to10 after each trial ("0" representing no pain). The procedure was repeated twice at each site and the mean of the pain rating values was used for analysis. The intraclass correlation coefficient (ICC) for this method at our center was 0.49–0.66 between initial and repeat testing on separate days.

Pressure pain detection thresholds

Pressure pain detection thresholds (PPT) were defined by applying a pressure algometer (FPIX, Wagner Instruments, Greenwich, CT; 1cm² hard rubber tip) on each anatomic site at a rate of 0.5 kg/second as the point at which the subject reported the pressure first changed to pain [24]. The sites tested were the medial joint line and tibial tuberosity of each knee and both radial styloids. The PPT in kilograms of force (kg/force) was obtained three times at each site. The mean value of the three trials was used in analysis. The ICC for PPT evaluation at our center was 0.70–0.96 between initial and repeat testing on separate days.

Subjective pain assessments

All participants completed questionnaires regarding knee pain and function, including the question "Do you feel spontaneous pain in your knee?" Subjects completed the WOMAC visual analog scale for evaluation of pain at both knees, both ankles and both hips. The WOMAC is a standardized and validated questionnaire for assessment of pain and function in lower extremity OA [21, 25, 26] and site-specific adaptation of the WOMAC has proven useful and feasible [27, 28].

Vibration perception

VPT was measured using a biothesiometer (Bio-Medical Instrument Co., Newberry, Ohio) operating at a frequency of 120 Hz according to previously published methods [14]. The following anatomic sites were tested: the first metatarsophalangeal joint, medial malleolus, lateral malleolus, medial femoral condyle, tibial tuberosity, and lateral femoral condyle bilaterally. The bilateral radial styloids were used as control sites. The applicator tip of the machine was placed at the predetermined anatomic site. The biothesiometer voltage was set at "0" volts and the voltage output was increased by 1 V/second until subjects verbally reported their first sensation of vibration. Each site was tested twice and the mean value was recorded and used for analysis. Higher voltage represented worse vibratory sense acuity. The ICC was high, 0.96–0.99, between initial and repeat testing on separate days.

All qualitative sensory testing (QST) assessments were performed by one of two trained investigator (AD, RM), and subjects were given standardized instructions prior to testing.

Statistical analyses

Power calculations were based upon the difference in means in previous studies available in 2011 at initiation of the study that had evaluated allodynia and PPT's in OA subjects [10, 12]. Using conservative estimates, we based our power calculation on a mean PPT (kg/cm²) in the control group of 5 and the OA group of 3.8 with a combined standard deviation of 1.3. Inclusion of 37 participants with OA and 10 age-matched healthy controls was estimated to provide 80% power to detect differences between the groups (α = 0.05 and sampling ratio of approximately 3:1 OA to control participants). There are no prior studies evaluating the correlations between VPT, PPTs, and allodynia in OA participants. Therefore, estimating a small to moderate effect size (0.15), power of 0.80 and α = 0.05, 40 participants with OA would be needed to examine these relationships.

Independent samples t-test and Chi-square tests were used to compare the OA with the control group. Pearson and Spearman correlations were used to evaluate bivariate associations within the OA group. $P < 0.05$ was considered to be statistically significant. All values are reported as mean ± standard deviation.

Results

Forty-two OA participants (mean age 54 ± 8 years, 13 males/29 females) and twelve controls (mean age 53 ± 11 years, 3 males/9 females) were studied. A majority of the participants had bilateral knee OA. The KL grade at the index knee included 26 KL 2 and 16 KL 3 knees and at the contralateral knee, 2 KL 1, 28 KL 2, and 12 KL 3. Mean WOMAC pain score at the index knee (0 to 100 mm ± SD) was 183 ± 110 mm and at the contralateral knee was 129 ± 111 mm. WOMAC pain at the ankles and hips was less than 60 mm out of 500 mm in the OA group. The control participants had no knee pain on full WOMAC evaluation (mean < 1 mm out of 500 mm at both knees).

Significantly more OA participants demonstrated mechanical allodynia (responded yes to the question "do you consider this painful?" after completion of the Von Frey filament stimulus, (n = 23) compared with controls at the ipsilateral knee (54.8% vs 16.6%, p = 0.024) and contralateral knee (42.9% vs 0%, p = 0.005). Pressure pain thresholds (PPT) were lower in the OA group but did not reach statistical significance (affected tibial tuberosity 3.81 ± 1.63 vs 4.62 ± 1.37 kg/force, p = 0.09 and affected medial joint line 2.73 ± 1.55 vs 3.65 ± 1.57 kg/force, p = 0.09).

VPT and PPT were directly correlated at several anatomic sites (Table 1), in that those with increased sensitivity to vibration also had lower pressure pain thresholds. Similarly, VPT was lower at the first metatarsophalangeal joint (MTP) in those who had allodynia at the ipsilateral

Table 1 Correlation between VPT at Multiple Sites with PPT at the Ispilateral Tibial Tuberosity and Medial Joint Line in OA participants*

	PPT Ipsilateral tibial tuberosity Spearman's rho (p value)	PPT Ipsilateral medial joint line Spearman's rho (p value)
VPT Ipsilateral MTP	0.272 (0.081)	0.310 (0.046)
VPT Ipsilateral medial ankle	0.416 (0.006)	0.476 (0.001)
VPT Ipsilateral lateral ankle	0.210 (0.182)	0.193 (0.221)
VPT Ipsilateral medial knee	0.338(0.030)	0.389 (0.010)
VPT Ipsilateral lateral knee	0.432 (0.004)	0.405 (0.008)
VPT Ipsilateral tibial tuberosity	0.350 (0.023)	0.268 (0.086)

*Association between increased sensitivity to vibration and lower pressure detection thresholds

tibial tuberosity compared with those that did not (8.2 ± 3.3 vs 12.1 ± 4.8 V, p = 0.005).

OA participants with allodynia at the ipsilateral tibial tuberosity (n = 23) had higher WOMAC pain scores at the affected knee compared to OA participants without allodynia (217 ± 111 vs 142 ± 97 mm, p = 0.025). This relationship was not seen at the other anatomic sites.

Bivariate correlations showed no relationship between WOMAC pain score at the ipsilateral knee in OA participants and PPT (rho = − 0.115 to − 0.139, p > 0.05) or VPT (rho = − 0.051 to − 0.219, p > 0.05) at any of the several sites tested.

Further exploratory analyses were performed. OA participants with allodynia at the ipsilateral tibial tuberosity had significantly lower PPTs at multiple sites compared with those without allodynia (Table 2). Information regarding spontaneous pain was also evaluated and was available in 35 of the 42 OA participants due to the questionnaire being added later in the study. It was available on all control participants. The experience of spontaneous pain in the knee was only observed in OA participants (74.3% in OA vs 0% in controls, p = 0.001). In the OA group, participants with spontaneous knee pain had significantly lower PPTs than those without spontaneous knee pain at all ipsilateral and contralateral

sites (Table 3). Spontaneous knee pain was also associated with presence of allodynia as well as the pain rating post-stimulation at the ipsilateral and contralateral tibial tuberosities (Table 3). An association between VPT with spontaneous pain was not observed.

Discussion

Understanding relationships between various somatosensory measures as well as subjective pain in knee OA can provide insights into pain processing in OA [10]. Central and peripheral sensitization, which are due to alterations in central and peripheral pain processing resulting in allodynia and hyperalgesia [6], have been increasingly recognized as a potential contributor to the experience of pain in those with knee OA.

We hypothesized that in OA participants, poor vibratory sense would be associated with higher pain sensitivity (lower pain threshold) and allodynia. Instead, our study demonstrated that *increased* vibratory acuity, or increased sensitivity to vibration, was associated with increased pain sensitivity (lower pain detection thresholds) as well as the presence of allodynia to repetitive stimulation.

Poor VPT [14], lower PPT and hyperalgesia have been reported in OA [10–12]. The association between these different somatosensory measures is likely complicated as has been suggested by previous studies in chronic neuropathies in which combinations of heightened responses to one somatosensory measure coexisted with dampened responses to a different measure [16]. This is initially what we hypothesized to be the case in OA. However, in this study, the direction of alterations appeared to parallel one another, such that when vibration was felt more easily (higher acuity), so was pain (lower PPTs) as well as the experience of pain with a usually non-noxious stimulus (allodynia). This suggests that the OA participants may have had widespread sensitization to a variety of types of mechanical stimulation. This was a surprising observation in light of our previous findings that subjects with painful symptomatic knee OA have decreased sensitivity to vibration compared with age-matched controls [14]. Thus far, vibratory deficits in

Table 2 Relationship between Allodynia and Pain Pressure Threshold in OA participants

Pressure Pain Threshold (kilograms of force), (Mean ± SD)	Presence of Allodynia at Ipsilateral tibial tuberosity		P-value
	Yes (n = 23)	No (n = 19)	
Ispilateral radial styloid	2.56 ± 1.19	3.71 ± 1.53	0.01
Contralateral radial styloid	2.51 ± 1.26	3.75 ± 1.50	0.007
Ispilateral tibial tuberosity	3.16 ± 1.56	4.59 ± 1.39	0.003
Contralateral tibial tuberosity	3.57 ± 1.61	4.48 ± 1.32	0.052
Ispilateral medial joint line	2.16 ± 1.23	3.44 ± 1.64	0.008
Contralateral medial joint Line	2.54 ± 1.46	3.77 ± 11.81	0.02

*significant relationship between allodynia at the ipsilateral tibial tuberosity and lower PPT at tested site

Table 3 Relationship Between Spontaneous pain and Pressure Pain Thresholds and Allodynia in OA participants

	Spontaneous Pain		P value
	Yes (n = 26)	No (n = 9)	
Pressure Pain Threshold, Radial Styloid (kgf)*, (Mean ± SD)	2.42 ± 1.07	4.39 ± .1.25	0.001
Pressure Pain Threshold, Medial Joint Line (kgf), (Mean ± SD)	2.05 ± 1.08	3.98 ± 1.61	0.001
Pressure Pain Threshold Tibial Tuberosity (kgf), (Mean ± SD)	3.52 ± 1.44	5.01 ± 1.11	0.005
Presence of Allodynia, Ipsilateral Tibial Tuberosity	69.20%	30.70%	0.012
Pain Rating, Ipsilateral Tibial Tuberosity Scale after Repeated Mechanical Stimulus (Mean ± SD)	4.3 ± 2.6	1.6 ± 1.7	0.003
Presence of Allodynia, Contralateral Tibial Tuberosity	65.40%	11.10%	0.007
Pain Rating, Contalateral Tibial Tuberosity Scale after Repeated Mechanical Stimulus (Mean ± SD)	3.7 ± 2.3	1.4 ± 1.3	0.001

*kgf kilogram force

OA have been hypothesized to play a mechanical role in OA with suggestion that alterations in sensory input would lead to aberrant mechanics and possible OA progression [18]. However, vibratory acuity may have a different nociceptive role or association in OA and may be involved in or be affected by central pain processing in OA, as suggested by this study's results. In larger groups, it would be important to examine whether these relationships between vibration and other somatosensory or sensitization measures vary depending on the severity or stage of OA. Notably, the OA participants in this study had primary knee OA without much pain at other lower extremity joints. Populations with multi-articular lower extremity OA or chronic widespread pain may differ on these associations.

In our cohort, OA participants with allodynia at the ipsilateral knee had significantly lower pressure pain thresholds at all ipsilateral and contralateral sites, suggesting that there is a relationship between these different measures of sensitization/pain sensitivity. Further, those with OA and spontaneous pain had significantly lower pressure pain thresholds at ipsilateral and contralateral sites, greater likelihood of allodynia and higher pain ratings with repeated mechanical stimulation than those without spontaneous pain. These relationships suggest that the presence of spontaneous pain in knee OA correlates with measures thought to reflect sensitization. With repeated nocicecptive stimulation, high threshold polymodal C fibers may undergo changes that result in enhanced sensitivity, lowered thresholds for activation, and prolonged and enhanced response to the stimulation [29]. These neuroplastic changes may explain why OA participants experience heightened pain sensitivity and spontaneous pain. In this study, traditional measures of self-reported knee OA pain, the WOMAC pain scale, did not correlate as consistently with the somatosensory measures tested. This is in contrast to some prior studies [10, 12, 30]. In particular, in a large systematic review, Fingleton et al. demonstrated there was greater pressure pain sensitivity in a high symptom severity group compared to a low symptomatic group [8]. In our study, there was some association noted between allodynia and WOMAC pain and some of the relationships between PPTs and WOMAC pain approached significance. It could be that with greater numbers of participants, these relationships would be more evident, and small size is a limitation of our study. Nevertheless, the strong association observed between spontaneous pain, PPT, and allodynia suggests that perhaps more descriptive characteristics and temporal characteristics of pain should be examined as markers of sensitization. Certainly these findings provide further support for a role for quantitative sensory assessments of pain as being distinct and complementary to subjective reports of pain ratings.

Our study has several limitations. We did not control for all potential confounders or comorbidities such as specific nervous system disorders or baseline medications, though we did exclude those subjects who had inflammatory arthritis, neuropathy, diabetes, or any lower extremity joint replacement. We did not have information on duration of disease. Some of our results are based on subgroup analyses that were not originally part of our original power calculations. We looked at one measure of sensory function, vibratory sense, and future studies may want to investigate other measures such as balance and proprioception. Although the question regarding "spontaneous pain" in our study is not necessarily a validated questionnaire tool, and it may be subject to variations in interpretation [31], it nonetheless appeared to be attested to frequently in the OA participants and appeared to separate them from controls. Future studies should look at additional ways to help detail characteristics of subjective pain in OA and how pain characteristics may be markers of central or peripheral sensitization.

Conclusions

In summary, vibratory acuity in knee OA appears to be associated with the presence of sensitization and pain sensitivity in OA, such that there is a generalized increase in sensitivity to cutaneous mechanical stimulation, including vibratory sense. This relationship between nociceptive sensory alterations and other somatosensory alterations in

OA had not previously been evaluated. The presence of spontaneous pain may be an indicator of the presence of sensitization in OA. An understanding of the relationships between spontaneous pain, stimulus-evoked pain, and somatosensory measures will be critical to fully understand pain processing in OA.

Abbreviations:
KL: Kellgren-Lawrence; MTP: Metatarsophalangeal joint; OA: Osteoarthritis; PPT: Pain pressure thresholds; VPT: Vibratory perception threshold; WOMAC: Western Ontario and McMaster Universities Arthritis Index

Authors' contributions
AD made substantial contributions to the conception and design of this manuscript, collection and assembly of data, analysis and interpretation of the data, drafting of the article, critical revision of the article for important intellectual content, final approval of the article; TN made substantial contributions to the conception and design of this manuscript, drafting of the article, analysis and interpretation of the data, critical revision of the article for important intellectual content, and final approval of the article; RM made substantial contributions to collection and assembly of data, administrative and logistic support, critical revision and final approval of the article; JB made substantial contributions to the analysis and interpretation of data, revision of the article for important intellectual content and final approval of the article; NS made substantial contributions to the conception and design of this manuscript, provision of study materials and patients, analysis and interpretation of the data, drafting of the article, critical revision of the article for important intellectual content, final approval of the article, and statistical expertise.

Competing interests
The authors declare that they have no competing interests.

Author details
¹Section of Rheumatology, University of Chicago, 5841 S Maryland Ave, MC0930, Chicago, IL 60637, USA. ²Section of Clinical Epidemiology Research and Training Unit, Boston University School of Medicine, Boston, MA, USA. ³Inventlv Health, Clinical, Abbvie, Chicago, IL, USA. ⁴Division of Rheumatology, Rush Medical College, Chicago, IL, USA.

References
1. Felson DT. The sources of pain in knee osteoarthritis. Curr. Opin. Rheumatol. 2005;17(5):624–8.
2. Szebenyi B, Hollander AP, Dieppe P, Quilty B, Duddy J, Clarke S, Kirwan JR. Associations between pain, function, and radiographic features in osteoarthritis of the knee. Arthritis Rheumatol. 2006;54(1):230–5.
3. Dray A, Read SJ. Arthritis and pain. Future targets to control osteoarthritis pain. Arthritis Res. Ther. 2007;9(3):212.
4. Lluch E, Torres R, Nijs J, Van Oosterwijck J. Evidence for central sensitization in patients with osteoarthritis pain: a systematic literature review. Eur J Pain. 2014;18(10):1367–75.
5. Deveza LA, Melo L, Yamato TP, Mills K, Ravi V, Hunter DJ. Knee osteoarthritis phenotypes and their relevance for outcomes: a systematic review. Osteoarthr Cartil. 2017;25(12):1926–41.
6. Lee YC, Nassikas NJ, Clauw DJ. The role of the central nervous system in the generation and maintenance of chronic pain in rheumatoid arthritis, osteoarthritis and fibromyalgia. Arthritis Res Ther. 2011;13(2):211.
7. Staud R. Evidence for shared pain mechanisms in osteoarthritis, low back pain, and fibromyalgia. Curr Rheumatol Rep. 2011;13(6):513–20.
8. Fingleton C, Smart K, Moloney N, Fullen BM, Doody C. Pain sensitization in people with knee osteoarthritis: a systematic review and meta-analysis. Osteoarthr Cartil. 2015;23(7):1043–56.
9. Loeser JD, Treede RD. The Kyoto protocol of IASP basic pain terminology. Pain. 2008;137(3):473–7.
10. Arendt-Nielsen L, Nie H, Laursen MB, Laursen BS, Madeleine P, Simonsen OH, Graven-Nielsen T. Sensitization in patients with painful knee osteoarthritis. Pain. 2010;149(3):573–81.
11. Bajaj P, Bajaj P, Graven-Nielsen T, Arendt-Nielsen L. Osteoarthritis and its association with muscle hyperalgesia: an experimental controlled study. Pain. 2001;93(2):107–14.
12. Imamura M, Imamura ST, Kaziyama HH, Targino RA, Hsing WT, de Souza LP, Cutait MM, Fregni F, Camanho GL. Impact of nervous system hyperalgesia on pain, disability, and quality of life in patients with knee osteoarthritis: a controlled analysis. Arthritis Rheum. 2008;59(10):1424–31.
13. Pai YC, Rymer WZ, Chang RW, Sharma L. Effect of age and osteoarthritis on knee proprioception. Arthritis Rheumatol. 1997;40(12):2260–5.
14. Shakoor N, Agrawal A, Block JA. Reduced lower extremity vibratory perception in osteoarthritis of the knee. Arthritis Rheumatol. 2008;59(1):117–21.
15. N S, Lee KJ, Fogg LF, Block JA. Generalized vibratory deficits in osteoarthritis of the hip. Arthritis Care Res. 2008;59(9):1237–40.
16. Maier C, Baron R, Tolle TR, Binder A, Birbaumer N, Birklein F, Gierthmuhlen J, Flor H, Geber C, Huge V, et al. Quantitative sensory testing in the German research network on neuropathic pain (DFNS): somatosensory abnormalities in 1236 patients with different neuropathic pain syndromes. Pain. 2010;150(3):439–50.
17. Giesecke T, Gracely RH, Grant MA, Nachemson A, Petzke F, Williams DA, Clauw DJ. Evidence of augmented central pain processing in idiopathic chronic low back pain. Arthritis Rheum. 2004;50(2):613–23.
18. Shakoor N, Lee KJ, Fogg LF, Wimmer MA, Foucher KC, Mikolaitis RA, Block JA. The relationship of vibratory perception to dynamic joint loading, radiographic severity, and pain in knee osteoarthritis. Arthritis Rheum. 2012;64(1):181–6.
19. Woolf CJ. Central sensitization: implications for the diagnosis and treatment of pain. Pain. 2011;152(3 Suppl):S2–15.
20. Altman R, Asch E, Bloch D, Bole G, Borenstein D, Brandt K, Christy W, Cooke TD, Greenwald R, Hochberg M. Development of criteria for the classification and reporting of osteoarthritis. Classification of osteoarthritis of the knee. Diagnostic and therapeutic criteria Committee of the American Rheumatism Association. Arthritis Rheumatol. 1986;29(8):1039–49.
21. Bellamy N, Buchanan WW, Goldsmith CH, Campbell J, Stitt LW. Validation study of WOMAC: a health status instrument for measuring clinically important patient relevant outcomes to antirheumatic drug therapy in patients with osteoarthritis of the hip or knee. J Rheumatol. 1988;15(12):1833–40.
22. Kellgren JH, Lawrence JS. Radiological assessment of osteo-arthrosis. Ann Rheum Dis. 1957;16:494–502.
23. Felson DT, Zhang Y, Hannan MT, Naimark A, Weissman BN, Aliabadi P, Levy D. The incidence and natural history of knee osteoarthritis in the elderly. The Framingham osteoarthritis study. Arthritis Rheumatol. 1995;38(10):1500–5.
24. Neogi T, Frey-Law L, Scholz J, Niu J, Arendt-Nielsen L, Woolf C, Nevitt M, Bradley L, Felson DT. Sensitivity and sensitisation in relation to pain severity in knee osteoarthritis: trait or state? Ann Rheum Dis. 2013;74(4):682–8.
25. Theiler R, Sangha O, Schaeren S, Michel BA, Tyndall A, Dick W, Stucki G. Superior responsiveness of the pain and function sections of the western Ontario and McMaster universities osteoarthritis index (WOMAC) as compared to the Lequesne-Algofunctional index in patients with osteoarthritis of the lower extremities. Osteoarthr. Cartil. 1999;7(6):515–9.
26. Stucki G, Sangha O, Stucki S, Michel BA, Tyndall A, Dick W, Theiler R. Comparison of the WOMAC (western Ontario and McMaster universities) osteoarthritis index and a self-report format of the self-administered Lequesne-Algofunctional index in patients with knee and hip osteoarthritis. Osteoarthr. Cartil. 1998;6(2):79–86.
27. Pincus T, Koch GG, Sokka T, Lefkowith J, Wolfe F, Jordan JM, Luta G, Callahan LF, Wang X, Schwartz T, et al. A randomized, double-blind, crossover clinical trial of diclofenac plus misoprostol versus acetaminophen in patients with osteoarthritis of the hip or knee. Arthritis Rheumatol. 2001;44(7):1587–98.
28. McGrory BJ, Harris WH. Can the western Ontario and McMaster universities (WOMAC) osteoarthritis index be used to evaluate different hip joints in the same patient? J Arthroplasty. 1996;11(7):841–4.
29. Bonica J. Applied anatomy relevant to pain. The management of pain. Philadephia: Lea&Febiger; 1990.
30. Wylde V, Palmer S, Learmonth ID, Dieppe P. Somatosensory abnormalities in knee OA. Rheumatology. 2012;51(3):535–43.
31. Bennett GJ. What is spontaneous pain and who has it? J Pain. 2012;13(10):921–9.

14

The impact of sarcopenic obesity on knee and hip osteoarthritis: a scoping review

Kristine Godziuk[1]*[iD], Carla M. Prado[2], Linda J. Woodhouse[3] and Mary Forhan[4]

Abstract

Background: The progressive, debilitating nature of knee and hip osteoarthritis can result in severe, persistent pain and disability, potentially leading to a need for total joint arthroplasty (TJA) in end-stage osteoarthritis. TJA in adults with obesity is associated with increased surgical risk and prolonged recovery, yet classifying obesity only using body mass index (BMI) precludes distinction of obesity phenotypes and their impact on surgical risk and recovery. The sarcopenic obesity phenotype, characterized by high adiposity and low skeletal muscle mass, is associated with higher infection rates, poorer function, and slower recovery after surgery in other clinical populations, but not thoroughly investigated in osteoarthritis. The rising prevalence and impact of this phenotype demands further attention in osteoarthritis treatment models of care, particularly as osteoarthritis-related pain, disability, and current treatment practices may inadvertently be influencing its development.

Methods: A scoping review was used to examine the extent of evidence of sarcopenic obesity in adults with hip or knee osteoarthritis. Medline, CINAHL, Web of Science and EMBASE were systematically searched from inception to December 2017 with keywords and subject headings related to obesity, sarcopenia and osteoarthritis.

Results: Eleven studies met inclusion criteria, with indications that muscle weakness, low skeletal muscle mass or sarcopenia are present alongside obesity in this population, potentially impacting therapeutic outcomes, and TJA surgical risk and recovery.

Conclusions: Consideration of sarcopenic obesity should be included in osteoarthritis patient assessments.

Keywords: Sarcopenic obesity, Body composition, BMI, Osteoarthritis, Arthroplasty

Background

Osteoarthritis is a chronic, progressive joint disease and leading cause of pain and mobility disability for over 27 million Americans [1] and 4 million Canadians [2]. Age, sex, genetics, joint trauma, and obesity all influence the development of this disease [3], and its progressive nature means advanced treatment options may be required in later stages to reduce pain, improve function and maintain quality of life. Surgical replacement of articular joint components, called a total joint arthroplasty (TJA), is currently the most effective treatment for severe pain and disability associated with end-stage knee or hip osteoarthritis that ceases to respond to other therapeutic interventions.

There has been a rapid and sustained increase in demand for TJA surgery around the world over the past two decades. TJA rates in the USA doubled from 336,000 patients in 1993 to 735,000 patients in 2005 [4], and are projected to top 4 million patients by 2030 [5]. In Canada, volumes are lower but the accrual rate tripled from 42,000 patients in 2000 [6] to 117,000 patients in 2016 [7], and similar persistent growth is apparent throughout Europe [8]. This increased demand is outpacing the supply of TJA, leading to longer wait times and pressure on health care systems to reduce delays in accessing care. To ensure timely and appropriate TJA access, optimization and prioritization of patient selection is critical. Clear, evidence-based guidelines for surgical appropriateness are lacking, resulting in a reliance on clinical judgement [9]. This has led to subjectivity in risk stratification, conflicting approaches and barriers or

* Correspondence: godziuk@ualberta.ca
[1]Faculty of Rehabilitation Medicine, University of Alberta, 8205 – 114 Street, 2-64 Corbett Hall, Edmonton, AB T6G 2G4, Canada
Full list of author information is available at the end of the article

delays in treatment access for patients with obesity due to evidence of increased surgical risk.

Two meta-analyses have found increased risk of superficial infections (OR 1.7–2.2) [10, 11] and deep infections (OR 2.4) [10] after total knee arthroplasty (TKA) in patients with obesity (defined as a body mass index/BMI ≥ 30 kg/m^2) compared to patients without obesity (BMI < 30 kg/m^2). Those with severe obesity (BMI ≥ 40 kg/m^2) appear to be at even higher risk, with four times the rate of infection after TKA compared to those without obesity [11, 12]. Increased infection after total hip arthroplasty (THA) is less clear [13]. Yet controversy exists around evidence of increased risk related to excess body weight. Methodological concerns regarding quality and comparability of studies have been raised, with underpowered sample sizes, BMI categorization/dichotomization, and absence of sub-classification by comorbidity status limitations in current evidence [14, 15].

Suggestions for establishing a BMI threshold for withholding TJA surgery have been made [11, 14, 16], while others argue against using BMI as an outright contraindication for TJA [17, 18]. Without clear guidelines, orthopaedic surgeons may decide to deny or delay surgery based on their interpretation of evidence of surgical risk. Of greater concern, many surgeons recommend that patients lose weight to reduce their BMI before returning for re-assessment of surgical eligibility [12, 14, 19]. This recommendation is in contrast to current evidence that suggests weight loss does not improve perioperative TJA risk. Lui et al. [20] found weight loss of $\geq 5\%$ of body weight in the year prior to TJA resulted in either no difference or an increased risk of deep infection (OR 3.8). Weight loss may inadvertently increase perioperative infection, as muscle lost concomitantly with fat may lower lean muscle reserves, which are critical to the wound healing process [21].

Reliance on BMI may result in misclassification bias and denial of surgery for patients with obesity. BMI is a poor indicator of individual health as it cannot discern individual body composition of muscle, bone or fat [22]. Significant deviations in body composition within BMI categories have been reported [22–24], including twofold differences in adiposity [25] and 30 kg differences in lean soft tissue [26] between patients who have the same BMI [27]. Relying on BMI as a screening tool for TJA ignores the influence body composition has on surgical risk, particularly in relation to the amount of skeletal muscle mass as shown in other clinical scenarios [28, 29]. A high BMI could disguise important skeletal muscle mass depletion, as in the condition of sarcopenic obesity [26, 30].

What is sarcopenic obesity?

Sarcopenic obesity is defined as the co-occurrence of high adiposity and sarcopenia, a term coined to describe

low skeletal muscle mass, strength and physical function originally diagnosed in the elderly [31], but present across the age spectrum [32, 33]. Sarcopenia is associated with physical disability, falls, extended hospital stays, infection and non-infection related complications, and increased overall mortality [34–36]. Importantly, sarcopenia is not restricted to people who appear thin or underweight. Aging is often paralleled by increased rates of muscle loss and concomitant gains in adiposity (both subcutaneous and intramuscular), which can culminate in sarcopenic obesity [37].

Compounding the effects of both sarcopenia and obesity, sarcopenic obesity is associated with poorer quality of life and greater disability, morbidity and mortality when compared with either obesity or sarcopenia alone [37–39]. Although the majority of studies to date have been conducted in elderly individuals, sarcopenia and sarcopenic obesity are not limited to this population. There are several clinical disorders where individuals are prone to muscle loss (with or without concurrent obesity), including diabetes, cancer, chronic obstructive pulmonary disease, HIV, cirrhosis, and arthritis [40]. The presence of sarcopenic obesity may be particularly important to consider when surgery is indicated. In addition to increased length of hospital stay and increased mortality associated with this condition [40], there is convincing evidence of its relationship with increased infection rates [28, 29, 41].

With obesity present in 26 to 38% of adults in Canada and the USA respectively [42], and an aging population with a longer life span, sarcopenic obesity may be a new epidemiological trend of current times [43]. Importantly, it cannot be identified by simply measuring body weight or calculating BMI [44].

Is sarcopenic obesity a concern in osteoarthritis?

Individuals with osteoarthritis may be at particular risk for sarcopenic obesity. The prevalence of osteoarthritis rises with age and obesity, and osteoarthritis-related pain can lead to inactivity and a decline in physical function. These factors in combination create a vicious cycle of inflammation, inactivity and aging-related muscle loss accompanied by aging-related gains in adiposity, giving rise and perpetuating the sarcopenic obesity phenotype [45–47] (Fig. 1). Chronic diseases associated with osteoarthritis [48], such as diabetes, metabolic syndrome, and hypertension, along with weight loss and subsequent re-gain (weight cycling), could exacerbate skeletal muscle loss, increase adiposity and contribute to the development of sarcopenic obesity [49]. Further, the development and progression of sarcopenia and osteoarthritis may occur through interrelated pathways [50, 51].

Body composition phenotypes of low skeletal muscle and high adiposity have been reported in patients with knee and hip osteoarthritis by Karlsson [52–54], Purcell

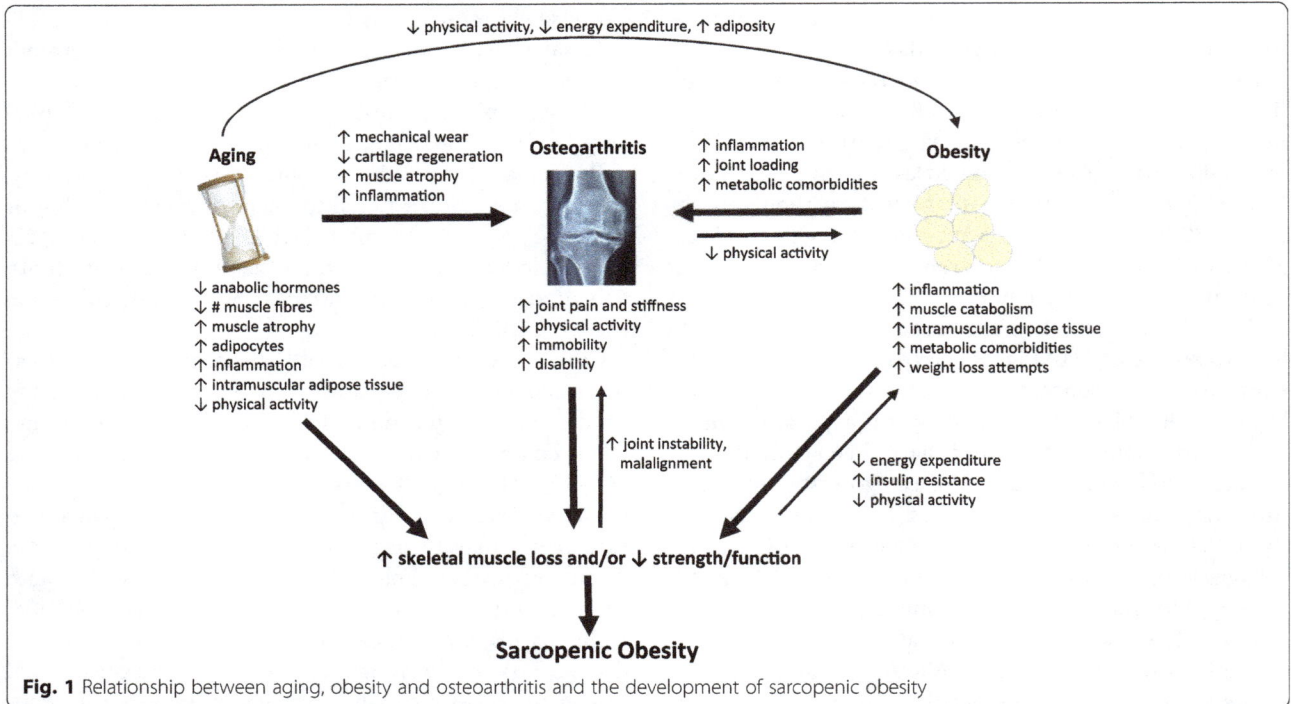

Fig. 1 Relationship between aging, obesity and osteoarthritis and the development of sarcopenic obesity

[55] and Visser [56], although sarcopenia or obesity were not specifically identified. Nevertheless, this is compelling evidence and may indicate that this condition is present in osteoarthritis but not recognized or identified as sarcopenic obesity.

To provide a more complete understanding of sarcopenic obesity in lower extremity osteoarthritis, a scoping review was conducted to determine the extent of reported prevalence and impact of low muscle mass, muscle weakness or sarcopenia in adults with obesity and knee or hip osteoarthritis. Scoping reviews enable a comprehensive and encompassing review of emerging literature on a topic [57], and can be preferable to systematic reviews when the research question is examining the breadth of evidence on a topic, as in this case. Scoping reviews utilize transparent processes and systematic search strategies much like systematic reviews, and while they don't typically include a grading system or formal quality assessment of included studies, a description of study limitations can be incorporated into the results.

Methods

This scoping review was conducted following the methodology of Arksey and O'Malley [58], including a systematic search of the published literature. Medline, CINAHL, Web of Science and Embase databases were searched from inception to December 2017 using MeSH terms and keywords related to osteoarthritis, obesity, and sarcopenia (including dynapenia, muscle weakness, muscle atrophy, low muscle mass, muscle loss, body

composition, body compartment, lean soft tissue, lean body mass, lean mass, fat free mass, muscle size or muscle mass). Inclusion criteria was determined by the authors prior to search initiation. Studies were to be included if they were primary or secondary analyses, and subjects had knee or hip osteoarthritis. Additionally, studies must have conducted group/subgroup analysis by obesity (identified using body mass index/BMI, waist circumference, fat mass or percent body fat), and examined muscle mass, muscle strength/weakness or sarcopenia. Studies on animal models and children were excluded, along with studies where participants did not have knee or hip osteoarthritis, or obesity, or if the study was an editorial, protocol or review article. Reference lists of relevant articles were hand searched to identify articles missed in the primary investigation. From each included study we extracted the author, publication year, study design, sample population, methodologies for assessing obesity and sarcopenia, study limitations and relevant findings. A summary of extracted information was tabulated and a descriptive analysis was conducted.

Results

A total of 796 articles were identified in the original search and 118 full text articles were screened for potential relevance (Fig. 2). Eleven studies met inclusion criteria [59–69], and a summary of study characteristics and key findings are presented in Table 1.

Publication dates ranged from 2005 to 2017, with the majority (n = 8, 73%) published in the last three years, potentially indicating a growing awareness and understanding of sarcopenic obesity. Ten of the eleven studies were cross-sectional [60–69], and one longitudinal [59]. Four studies (36.4%) were secondary analyses of the Korea National Health and Nutrition Examination Survey (KNHANES) population cohort [61, 63, 64, 68], two (18.2%) were secondary analyses of the North American Osteoarthritis Initiative (OAI) population cohort [59, 62], one (9%) was a secondary analysis of the French Knee and Hip OsteoArthritis Long-term Assessment (KHOALA) cohort [69], and the remaining four (36.4%) were independent studies with cohorts from Korea [60], Thailand [65], Japan [67] and the Netherlands [66]. Eight studies focused on osteoarthritis of the knee joint [59, 61–65, 67, 68], with two additional studies examining both knee and hip [60, 69], and one solely on hip osteoarthritis [66].

Discussion

This scoping review identified eleven studies with clear indications that muscle weakness, low skeletal muscle mass, or sarcopenia occur in conjunction with obesity in lower extremity osteoarthritis. The majority of included studies examined prevalence and association of the sarcopenic obesity phenotype with the presence of knee or hip osteoarthritis [60, 61, 63, 64, 67, 68], however others

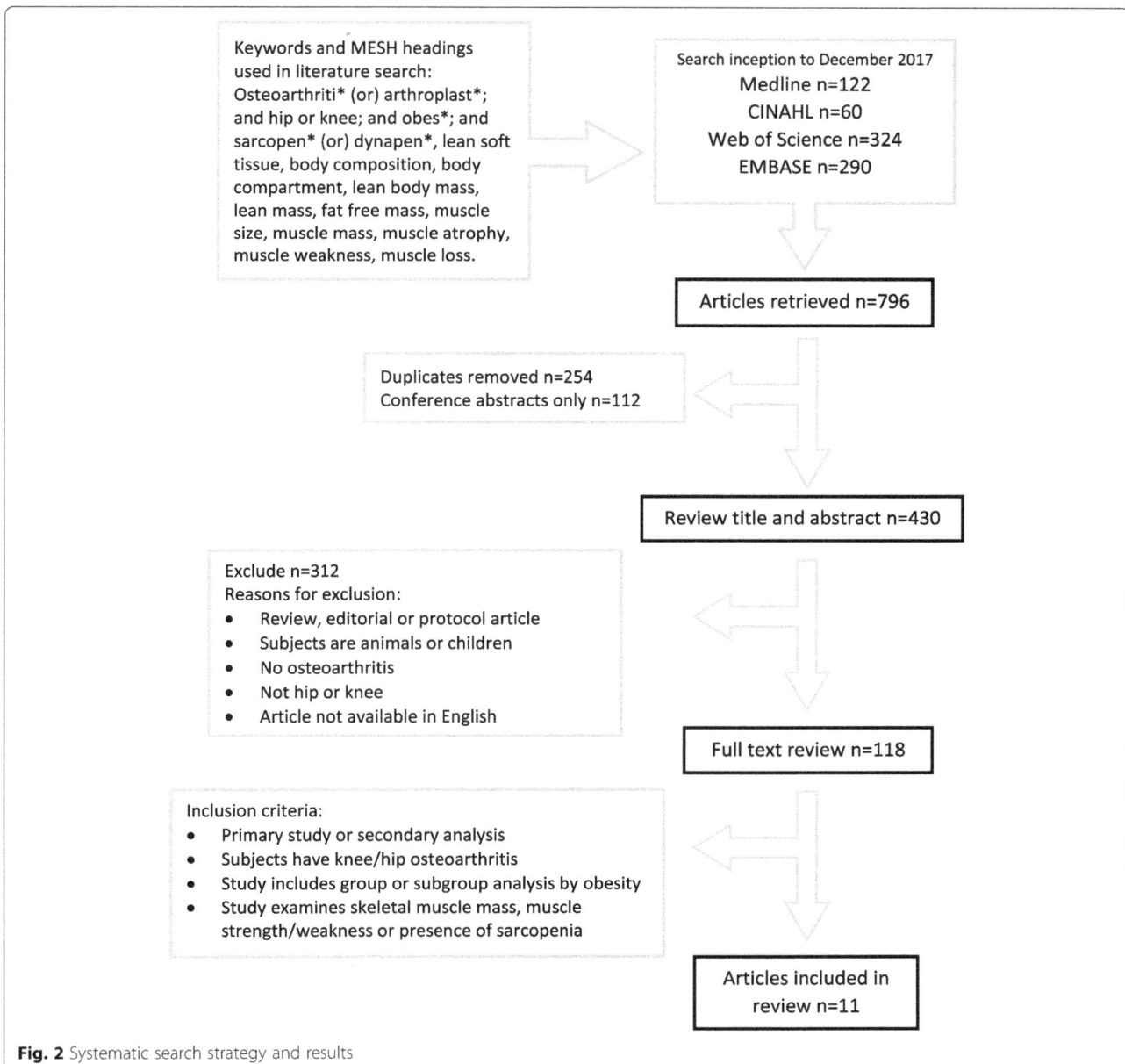

Fig. 2 Systematic search strategy and results

Table 1 Studies reporting low skeletal muscle mass and/or muscle weakness in adults with obesity and knee or hip osteoarthritis

Author, Year	Study purpose	Study design	Population	Definition of obesity	Body composition methodology	Definition of low muscle mass[a,b] or muscle weakness	Study limitations	Relevant findings
Batsis et al. [59], 2015	To describe the impact of dynapenic obesity on physical function in knee OA	Longitudinal,	North American population from OsteoArthritis Initiative (OAI), age ≥ 60 years, n = 526 in subgroup with knee OA, (rKOA),	BMI ≥30 kg/m²	NI	Lowest sex-specific tertile of knee extensor strength (dynapenia)	Secondary analysis of prospective data from longitudinal cohort. Excluded severe knee OA. No assessment of muscle mass or body composition	Prevalence of dynapenic obesity was 16%.
Clemence et al. [69], 2017	To analyze the association between low lean mass and clinical symptoms in knee and hip OA	Cross-sectional	French adults with hip and knee OA (KL grade ≥ 2) from KHOALA study, n = 358, age 63.4 ± 8.4 years	BMI ≥30 kg/m², or sex specific FM or WC cut-offs	DXA	ASM/BMI <0.789 for men and < 0.512 for women (FNIH cutoffs)	Secondary analysis of prospective data from longitudinal cohort. No information on exclusion criteria. No assessment of muscle strength or function	SO prevalence was 16.2%. Low lean mass was associated with pain and impaired function in subjects with normal BMI, but not with obesity (no significant differences between NSO and SO groups).
Ji et al. [60], 2016	To identify the prevalence of SO in knee and hip orthopedic surgery (OS) patients	Cross-sectional	Korean orthopedic surgery patients (hip or knee TJA or femoral fracture repair) (OS, n = 222) compared to control non-surgical outpatients (non-OS, n = 364)	BMI > 25 kg/m²	DXA	ASM/height², ASM/weight, and ASM/height and fat mass (residuals)	Retrospective analysis of data. No assessment of muscle strength or function	SO prevalence ranged from 1.3–35.4% in TKA and 0–18.4% in THA patients depending on definition used. SO rates were higher in OS patients compared to non-OS patients.
Jin et al. [61], 2017	To examine the associations between obesity, sarcopenia and OA in elderly	Cross-sectional	Korean population (KNHANES) age ≥ 65 years group with knee OA (K/L grade ≥ 2) (n = 1865) compared to lumbar spondylosis group (n = 1709)	BMI ≥25 kg/m²	DXA	ASM/weight, 2SDs below average of sex-matched young reference group	Secondary analysis of population survey data. No assessment of muscle strength or function	Results indicate correlation between SO and NSO with knee OA, but no relationship with lumbar spondylosis. Females with SO had increased OR for knee OA when adjusted for age and waist circumference (OR 1.80, CI 1.03–3.12).
Knoop et al. [62], 2011	To identify distinct clinical phenotypes and their impact in knee OA	Cross-sectional	North American population with knee OA (K/L grade 0–4) from OsteoArthritis Initiative (n = 842, age 63.2 ± 9.1)	BMI ≥30 kg/m²	NI	Low mean score of quadriceps and hamstring isometric strength	Secondary analysis of prospective data from longitudinal cohort. No assessment of muscle mass or body composition. No clear cut-off for defining weakness	Dynapenic obesity group ("obese and weak" phenotype) had higher pain and poorer physical function compared to "minimal joint disease", "strong muscle", and "non-obese and weak" phenotypes.
Lee et al. [63], 2016	To investigate association between lower limb muscle mass and knee OA	Cross-sectional	Korean population (KNHANES) age ≥ 50 years, n = 821 with knee OA (K/L grade ≥ 2), (n = 821), and control group without knee OA (n = 4103)	BMI ≥27.5 kg/m²	DXA	ASM/weight, 2SD below the mean in sex-matched young reference group (< 29.5% in men, < 23.2% in women)	Secondary analysis of population survey data. No assessment of muscle strength or function	SO prevalence was 5.2% in knee OA group compared to 1.8% in control group.
Lee et al. [64], 2012	To analyze the association between knee OA, sarcopenia	Cross-sectional	Korean population (KNHANES) with bilateral knee OA (K/L grade ≥ 2) age ≥ 50 years, n = 2893	BMI ≥27.5 kg/m²	DXA	ASM/weight, 2SD below the mean in sex-matched young reference	Secondary analysis of population survey data. No assessment of muscle strength or function	SO prevalence was 3% overall. When adjusted for age and sex, SO had stronger association with knee OA (OR 3.51, CI 2.15–5.75).

Table 1 Studies reporting low skeletal muscle mass and/or muscle weakness in adults with obesity and knee or hip osteoarthritis *(Continued)*

Author, Year	Study purpose	Study design	Population	Definition of obesity	Body composition methodology	Definition of low muscle mass[a,b] or muscle weakness	Study limitations	Relevant findings
	and obesity					group (<26.8% in men, <21% in women)		compared to NSO (OR 2.38, CI 1.80–3.15).
Manoy et al. [65], 2017	To assess association between leptin, vitamin D, muscle strength and physical performance in knee OA	Cross-sectional	Thailand knee OA patients (K/L grade <3) (n=208), age 65 ± 7 years	BMI > 25 kg/m²	BIA	ASM/weight < 30.4% in men and < 25.8% in women, and EWGSOP gait speed and grip strength cutoffs	Unclear if data collected retrospectively or prospectively. No description of sampling methods. Excluded severe knee OA	SO prevalence was 13.9%. Patients with SO had poorer performance on the timed up and go (TUG), sit to stand (STS) and 6 min walk tests (6MWT) compared to those with NSO or NO.
Oosting et al. [66], 2016	To determine the association of obesity and recovery after THA when stratified by muscle strength	Cross-sectional	Netherlands THA patients (n=297), age 69 ± 11 years	BMI > 30 kg/m²	NI	Maximal handgrip strength (< 20 kg for woman and < 30 kg for men)	Secondary analysis of prospective cohort. No assessment of muscle mass or body composition	Obesity and muscle weakness (dynapenic obesity) was associated with prolonged length of stay > 4 days (OR 3.59, CI 1.09–11.89) and delayed inpatient recovery (> 2 days to walk with gait aid) (OR 6.21, CI 1.64–23.65), but not in those with obesity alone.
Segal et al. [67], 2005	To analyze the impact of low limb lean mass in knee OA distinct from body weight	Cross-sectional	Japanese female orthopedic knee OA (K/L grade ≥ 2) patients age ≥ 45 years (n=341), compared to control group with fracture, sprains or back pain (n=604)	BMI > 24.9 kg/m²	BIA	Lower limb LST	Unclear if data collected retrospectively or prospectively. No clear cut-off for defining low LST. No assessment of muscle strength or function	Females with knee OA had 5–15% less lower limb LST compared to control groups across BMI categories, with significant 1.8 kg and 1.5 kg differences in overweight and obesity groups, respectively.
Suh et al. [68], 2016	To analyze the association between obesity, sex, and lower extremity lean mass in knee OA	Cross-sectional	Korean population (KNHANES) age ≥ 50 years with unilateral knee OA (K/L grade ≥ 2) (n=4246; 1829 men and 2417 women)	BMI ≥ 27.5 kg/m²	DXA	Lower extremity LST/weight, in lowest quartile	Secondary analysis of population survey data. No assessment of muscle strength or function	In females, obesity and low muscle mass was strongly association with knee OA (OR 2.31, CI 1.35–3.93) compared to obesity and normal muscle mass (OR 1.03, CI 0.26–4.02).

ASM appendicular skeletal mass, ASMI ASM/height², BIA bioelectrical impedance analysis, BMI body mass index, CI confidence interval, DXA dual-energy x-ray absorptiometry, EWGSOP European Working Group on Sarcopenia in Older People, FM fat mass, FFM fat free mass, FNIH Foundation for the National Institute of Health, KNHANES Korean National Health and Nutrition Examination Survey, K/L Kellgren/Lawrence radiographic osteoarthritis score, LST lean soft tissue, LSTI LST/height², NI not included in study design, NO normal body composition, NSO non-sarcopenic obesity, OA osteoarthritis, OR odds ratio, rKOA radiographic evidence of knee osteoarthritis, SD standard deviation, SO sarcopenic obesity, THA total hip arthroplasty, TJA total joint arthroplasty, TKA total knee arthroplasty, VAS visual analog scale, WC waist circumference, WOMAC Western Ontario and McMaster Universities Osteoarthritis Index

[a]Varied indices for identifying low muscle mass: LSTI, LST/weight, ASM, ASMI, ASM/weight, ASM/BMI, ASM relative to height and FM (residuals), and FM:FFM ratio [26]. Indices that consider LST or ASM relative to weight, BMI or FM may be most appropriate in adults with obesity [26], and relevant to identify clinically relevant weakness [76]

[b]Terms from included studies were adjusted for consistency and accurate representation of body composition compartment, and may differ from original reports

investigated the impact on pain, physical function, and quality of life [59, 62, 65, 69] or arthroplasty outcomes [66].

The prevalence of the sarcopenic obesity phenotype in adults with knee osteoarthritis may be as high as 35.4% [60], although a wide range was reported across included studies (prevalence of 3% [64], 13.9% [65], 16.2% [69], and up to 35.4% [60]). Differences in prevalence are likely related to varied obesity and sarcopenia classification criteria utilized in each study, a problem previously addressed elsewhere [26]. Obesity was classified by BMI (in kg/m^2) in all studies, but different cut-offs were used in Asian populations (either BMI ≥ 25 [60, 61, 65, 67] or ≥ 27.5 [63, 68]), and North American and European populations (BMI ≥ 30 [59, 62, 66, 69]), making it difficult to compare across study groups and populations. Prevalence also varied depending on the sarcopenia assessment method used in the study. Ji et al. [60] examined differences in sarcopenic obesity rates in hip and knee arthroplasty patients comparing low muscle mass (assessed with dual-energy x-ray absorptiometry/DXA) using three approaches: appendicular skeletal mass (ASM)/height^2, ASM/weight, and ASM relative to height and total fat mass, called the residual method [70]). They found prevalence of sarcopenic obesity differed between 1.3–35.4% in TKA patients and 0–18.4% in THA patients depending on the approach. Whether distinctions exist between low muscle mass present only in the lower extremities versus the whole body remains unclear [63, 67, 68]. Emerging evidence suggests that in patients with a larger body mass, the ratio between fat and muscle compartments (a metabolic load-capacity model) may be most relevant for identifying clinically important sarcopenic obesity [26].

There is currently no definitive diagnostic criteria established to identify sarcopenic obesity [71–73]. Several consensus papers on defining sarcopenia in the elderly have been published, including the European Working Group on Sarcopenia in Older Persons (EWG-SOP) [31], the European Society for Clinical Nutrition and Metabolism Special Interest Groups (ESPEN-SIG) [74], the International Working Group on Sarcopenia (IWGS) [75], and the Foundation for the National Institute of Health (FNIH) [76]. There is general agreement that the presence or absence of sarcopenia in the elderly should be based on a combined assessment of physical function (measurement of gait speed), muscular strength (measurement of handgrip or lower body strength), and body composition (to determine low skeletal muscle mass). However whether these measures are equally applicable to patients with concurrent chronic degenerative conditions remains to be explored.

Of the studies in this scoping review, seven used only body composition/low muscle mass for sarcopenia identification [60, 61, 63, 64, 67–69], three used only an assessment of muscle weakness (testing handgrip [66] or quadriceps strength [59, 62]), and only one study utilized a combined approach following EWGSOP consensus criteria [65] including assessment of physical function with gait speed in addition to muscle strength and body composition. Using gait speed as an assessment of physical function may create challenges in the osteoarthritis population. Osteoarthritis-related joint pain and stiffness may impact testing methods or may require alterations or alternatives to currently used criteria thresholds [77] or modifications to gait speed parameters. Additionally, risk of falls is high in those with moderate to severe osteoarthritis [78], which may increase the challenge of assessing physical function in this population.

The relationship between the sarcopenic obesity phenotype and knee osteoarthritis may be unique compared to other orthopedic and musculoskeletal conditions. In the included studies, no association was found between sarcopenic obesity and lumbar spondylosis [61], or in patients with fractures, sprains and back pain [67], or non-orthopedic hospital outpatients [60]. The development and progression of sarcopenic obesity may be interrelated with osteoarthritis development and progression. Lee et al. [63] found sarcopenic obesity was more prevalent in Korean adults with knee osteoarthritis compared to those without knee osteoarthritis (5.2% vs 1.8%, respectively). Batsis et al. [59] found rates of muscle weakness with obesity were higher in adults with clinically diagnosed knee osteoarthritis compared to those at risk for knee osteoarthritis (16% vs 6%, respectively). Sex specific differences may exist in this relationship. Suh et al. [68] found increased odds of knee osteoarthritis when low lower-extremity muscle mass was present in women with obesity (OR 2.31, CI 1.35–3.93), but not in men. Another study reported similar associations only in women over age 65 [61].

The findings of this scoping review support the theoretical impact of sarcopenic obesity on therapeutic outcomes for osteoarthritis, and surgical risk and recovery after joint arthroplasty. To date, only one study has investigated outcomes after TJA, with results showing obesity with muscle weakness was related to delayed independent walking (more than 2 days) and prolonged hospital stays (more than 4 days) compared to obesity alone [66].

It is reasonable to infer that reduced muscle strength or skeletal muscle mass would influence short and long-term recovery after arthroplasty and rehabilitation requirements to return to daily life. Muscle depletion is indicative of a reduction in physiologic protein reserves, which can contribute to impaired wound healing, increased risk of infections and longer recuperation after surgery [79]. A study by Kumar et al. [80] found that handgrip strength < 15 kg was associated with longer hospital stay after TJA, highlighting this potential relationship. Further, a study by Mau-Moller et al. [81] reported that low thigh muscle mass was a better predictor than BMI for loss of bone mineral density after TKA. This is important as loss of bone mineral density can lead to early prosthetic loosening after TKA and a need for revision surgery, suggesting that muscle mass may be more relevant than BMI for long term TKA outcomes.

Identifying sarcopenic obesity early in the continuum of care for osteoarthritis is critical to avoid inappropriate treatment recommendations. The current practice of recommending weight loss prior to TJA based on assessment of body weight or BMI [64] may need further consideration as weight loss attempts may also result in loss of skeletal muscle mass [40, 49], potentially exacerbating the sarcopenic obesity phenotype. Body composition measurement may be a critical assessment tool to distinguish between normal versus abnormal amounts of skeletal muscle mass and provide a more accurate assessment of adiposity [82], as anthropometric measures of obesity (using waist circumference, height, weight and BMI) may not differentiate between muscle and adipose tissue compartments. As previously discussed, body weight loss ≥5% in year preceding TJA was associated with increased surgical risk and higher readmission rates [20]. This may be a result of individuals with sarcopenic obesity losing weight, further reducing their already low muscle reserve, in turn impacting healing rates and perpetuating the vicious cycle of sarcopenia and obesity. Alternatively, it could suggest individuals with obesity and normal skeletal muscle mass (non-sarcopenic obesity) became sarcopenic post weight-loss (by losing more skeletal muscle mass without a substantial decrease in body weight to be considered non-obese) [40].

Study limitations

Every effort was made to comprehensively search and include all relevant studies in the literature, however there is a possibility that some were inadvertently missed. Further, while a limitation of scoping reviews is the lack of a formal risk of bias or study quality assessment, we have included a descriptive analysis of study design and limitations in Table 1 of the results section to enable assessment of level of evidence.

Conclusion

Sarcopenic obesity may be impacting therapeutic and surgical outcomes in osteoarthritis treatment approaches, yet this cannot be discerned until assessments for sarcopenic obesity are explored and regularly applied. There is a need to move beyond BMI and simple obesity diagnosis in osteoarthritis models of care, possibly including more sophisticated assessments of body composition. As gait speed and handgrip strength assessments to identify patients at risk

for sarcopenic obesity have not been well-tested in the osteoarthritis population, further research is required to clarify the effectiveness of these screening approaches in populations with physical function limitations. In the interim, incorporating clinical assessments for sarcopenic obesity through body composition may be essential to prevent misclassification bias and provide clarity on TJA surgical risk and recovery in adults with obesity.

Abbreviations
BMI: body mass index; CINAHL: Cumulative Index of Nursing and Allied Health Literature; DXA: dual-energy x-ray absorptiometry; EMBASE: Excerpta Medica dataBASE; MeSH: medical subject heading; THA: total hip arthroplasty; TJA: total joint arthroplasty; TKA: total knee arthroplasty

Funding
KG is supported by a Mitacs Accelerate internship in partnership with the Alberta Bone and Joint Health Institute. CMP is supported by a Canadian Institutes of Health Research (CIHR) New Investigator Salary Award and the Campus Alberta Innovation Program.

Authors' contributions
KG, CMP, LJW and MF contributed to the conception and design of the review. KG prepared the first draft, and KG, CMP, LJW and MF contributed to the manuscript revision and approval of the final version.

Competing interests
All authors declare they have no competing interests that would create a conflict of interest in connection with this manuscript. KG, CMP and MF have no disclosures; LJW has received funding from the Research Advisory Board of Focus on Therapeutic Outcomes Inc. (FOTO) and the American Physical Therapy Association Outcome Measures Registry.

Author details
[1]Faculty of Rehabilitation Medicine, University of Alberta, 8205 – 114 Street, 2-64 Corbett Hall, Edmonton, AB T6G 2G4, Canada. [2]Division of Human Nutrition, Faculty of Agricultural, Life and Environmental Sciences, University of Alberta, Edmonton, AB, Canada. [3]Department of Physical Therapy, Faculty of Rehabilitation Medicine, University of Alberta, Edmonton, AB, Canada. [4]Department of Occupational Therapy, Faculty of Rehabilitation Medicine, University of Alberta, Edmonton, AB, Canada.

References
1. Lawrence RC, Felson DT, Helmick CG, et al. Estimates of the prevalence of arthritis and other rheumatic conditions in the United States, part II for the National Arthritis Data Workgroup. Arthritis Rheum. 2008;58(1):26–35.
2. Bombardier C, Hawker G, Mosher D. The impact of arthritis in Canada : today and over the next 30 years. Arthritis Alliance of Canada. 2011;
3. Bastick A, Runhaar J, Belo J, Bierma-Zeinstra S. Prognostic factors for progression of clinical osteoarthritis of the knee: a systematic review of observational studies. Arthritis Res Ther. 2015;17(152):1–13.
4. Tian W, DeJong G, Brown M, Hsieh CH, Zamfirov ZP, Horn SD. Looking upstream: factors shaping the demand for postacute joint replacement rehabilitation. Arch Phys Med Rehabil. 2009;90(8):1260–8.
5. Bumpass DB, Nunley RM. Assessing the value of a total joint replacement. Curr Rev Musculoskelet Med. 2012;5(4):274–82.
6. Canadian Joint Replacement Registry. 2002 Report Total Hip and Total Knee Replacements in Canada.; 2002.
7. Canadian Institute for Health Information (CIHI). Hip and Knee Replacements in Canada: Canadian Joint Replacement Registry 2015–2016 Quick Stats.; 2017.
8. OECD/EU. Health at a Glance: Europe 2016 – State of Health in the EU Cycle. Paris; 2016.
9. Dowsey MM, Gunn J, Choong PFM. Selecting those to refer for joint replacement: who will likely benefit and who will not? Best Pract Res Clin Rheumatol. 2014;28(1):157–71.

10. Kerkhoffs GMMJ, Servien E, Dunn W, Dahm D, Bramer JAM, Haverkamp D. The influence of obesity on the complication rate and outcome of total knee arthroplasty. J Bone Jt Surg. 2012;94(20):1839–44.

11. Si H, Zeng Y, Shen B, et al. The influence of body mass index on the outcomes of primary total knee arthroplasty. Knee surgery, Sport Traumatol Arthrosc. 2015;23(6):1824–32.

12. Samson AJ, Mercer GE, Campbell DG. Total knee replacement in the morbidly obese: a literature review. ANZ J Surg. 2010;80(9):595–9.

13. American Academy of Orthopaedic Surgeons. Management of Osteoarthritis of the Hip: Evidence-Based Clinical Practice Guideline.; 2017.

14. Springer B, Parvizi J, Austin M, et al. Obesity and total joint arthroplasty. A literature based review. J Arthroplast. 2013;28(5):714–21.

15. Vaishya R, Vijay V, Wamae D, Agarwal AK. Is total knee replacement justified in the morbidly obese? A systematic review. Cureus. 2016;8(9):e804.

16. Springer BD, Carter JT, McLawhorn AS, et al. Obesity and the role of bariatric surgery in the surgical management of osteoarthritis of the hip and knee: a review of the literature. Surg Obes Relat Dis. 2016;1–8.

17. Kulkarni K, Karssiens T, Kumar V, Pandit H. Obesity and osteoarthritis. Maturitas. 2016;89:22–8.

18. Vasarhelyi EM, MacDonald SJ. The influence of obesity on total joint arthroplasty. J Bone Joint Surg Br. 2012;94(11 Suppl A):100–102.

19. Roth KC, Bessems G. Sorry, but you will have to lose weight before receiving your knee replacement. Erasmus J Med. 2013;3(2):54–7.

20. Lui M, Jones CA, Westby MD. Effect of non-surgical, non-pharmacological weight loss interventions in patients who are obese prior to hip and knee arthroplasty surgery: a rapid review. Syst Rev. 2015;4(1):121.

21. Demling RH. Nutrition, anabolism, and the wound healing process: an overview. Eplasty. 1954;9:65–94.

22. Prado CM, Gonzalez MC, Heymsfield SB. Body composition phenotypes and obesity paradox. Curr Opin Clin Nutr Metab Care. 2015;18(6):535–51.

23. Kuk JL, Lee S, Heymsfield SB, Ross R. Waist circumference and abdominal adipose tissue distribution: influence of age and sex. Am J Clin Nutr. 2005;81(6):1330–4.

24. Romero-Corral A, Somers VK, Sierra-Johnson J, et al. Normal weight obesity: a risk factor for cardiometabolic dysregulation and cardiovascular mortality. Eur Heart J. 2010;31(6):737–46.

25. Gallagher D, Heymsfield SB, Heo M, Jebb SA, Murgatroyd PR, Sakamoto Y. Healthy percentage body fat ranges: an approach for developing guidelines based on body mass index. Am J Clin Nutr. 2000;72(3):694–701.

26. Johnson Stoklossa C, Sharma A, Forhan M, Siervo M, Padwal R, Prado C. Prevalence of sarcopenic obesity in adults with class II/III obesity using different diagnostic criteria. J Nutr Metab. 2017;

27. Gonzalez MC, Correia MITD, Heymsfield SB. A requiem for BMI in the clinical setting. Curr Opin Clin Nutr Metab Care. 2017;20(5):1.

28. Nishigori T, Tsunoda S, Okabe H, et al. Impact of sarcopenic obesity on surgical site infection after laparoscopic total gastrectomy. Ann Surg Oncol. 2016:524–31.

29. Visser M, van Venrooij LMW, Vulperhorst L, et al. Sarcopenic obesity is associated with adverse clinical outcome after cardiac surgery. Nutr Metab Cardiovasc Dis. 2013;23(6):511–8.

30. Prado CM, Lieffers JR, McCargar LJ, et al. Prevalence and clinical implications of sarcopenic obesity in patients with solid tumours of the respiratory and gastrointestinal tracts: a population-based study. Lancet Oncol. 2008;9(7):629–35.

31. Cruz-Jentoft AJ, Baeyens JP, Bauer JM, et al. Sarcopenia: European consensus on definition and diagnosis. Age Ageing. 2010;39(4):412–23.

32. Prado CM, Siervo M, Mire E, et al. A population-based approach to define body-composition. Am J Clin Nutr. 2014:1369–78.

33. Cherin P, Voronska E, Fraoucene N, De Jaeger C. Prevalence of sarcopenia among healthy ambulatory subjects: the sarcopenia begins from 45 years. Aging Clin Exp Res. 2014;26(2):137–46.

34. Janssen I, Heymsfield SB, Ross R. Low relative skeletal muscle mass (sarcopenia) in older persons is associated with functional impairment and physical disability. J Am Geriatr. 2002;50:889–96.

35. Santilli V, Bernetti A, Mangone M, Paoloni M. Clinical definition of sarcopenia. Clin Cases Miner Bone Metab. 2014;11(3):177–80.

36. Metter EJ, Talbot LA, Schrager M, Conwit R. Skeletal muscle strength as a predictor of all-cause mortality in healthy men. J Gerontol: Biol Sci. 2002;57:B359 B365.

37. Roubenoff R. Sarcopenic obesity: the confluence of two epidemics. Obes Res. 2004;12(6):887–8.

38. Baumgartner RN, Wayne SJ, Waters DL, Janssen I, Gallagher D, Morley JE. Sarcopenic obesity predicts instrumental activities of daily living disability in the elderly. Obes Res. 2004;12(12):1995–2004.

39. Tian S, Xu Y. Association of sarcopenic obesity with the risk of all-cause mortality: a meta-analysis of prospective cohort studies. Geriatr Gerontol Int. 2016;16:155–66.

40. Prado CM, Wells JCK, Smith SR, Stephan BCM, Siervo M. Sarcopenic obesity: a critical appraisal of the current evidence. Clin Nutr. 2012;31(5):583–601.

41. Kallwitz ER. Sarcopenia and liver transplant: the relevance of too little muscle mass. World J Gastroenterol. 2015;21(39):10982–93.

42. Organization for Economic Cooperation and Development. Obesity Update, 2017.

43. Roubenoff R. Sarcopenic obesity: does muscle loss cause fat gain? Lessons from rheumatoid arthritis and osteoarthritis. Ann N Y Acad Sci. 2000;904:553–7.

44. Juby AG. A healthy body habitus is more than just a normal BMI: implications of sarcopenia and sarcopenic obesity. Maturitas. 2014;78(4):243–4.

45. Thijssen E, van Caam A, van der Kraan PM. Obesity and osteoarthritis, more than just wear and tear: pivotal roles for inflamed adipose tissue and dyslipidaemia in obesity-induced osteoarthritis. Rheumatology. 2015;54(4):588–600.

46. Zamboni M, Mazzali G, Fantin F, Rossi A, Di Francesco V. Sarcopenic obesity: a new category of obesity in the elderly. Nutr Metab Cardiovasc Dis. 2008;18(5):388–95.

47. Lee D, Drenowatz C, Blair SN. Physical activity and sarcopenic obesity: definition, assessment, prevalence and mechanism. Futur Sci. 2016;

48. Griffin TM, Huffman KM. Insulin resistance: releasing the brakes on synovial inflammation and osteoarthritis? Arthritis Rheumatol. 2016;68(6):1–30.

49. Cauley JA. An overview of sarcopenic obesity. J Clin Densitom. 2015;18(4):499–505.

50. De Ceuninck F, Fradin A, Pastoureau P. Bearing arms against osteoarthritis and sarcopenia: when cartilage and skeletal muscle find common interest in talking together. Drug Discov Today. 2014;19(3):305–11.

51. Papalia R, Zampogna B, Torre G, et al. Sarcopenia and its relationship with osteoarthritis: risk factor or direct consequence? Musculoskelet Surg. 2014;98(1):9–14.

52. Karlsson MK, Magnusson H, Coster M, Karlsson C, Rosengren BE. Patients with knee osteoarthritis have a phenotype with higher bone mass, higher fat mass, and lower lean body mass. Clin Orthop Relat Res. 2015;473(1):258–64.

53. Karlsson MK, Magnusson H, Coster MC, Vonschewelov T, Karlsson C, Rosengren BE. Patients with hip osteoarthritis have a phenotype with high bone mass and low lean body mass. Clin Orthop Relat Res. 2014;472(4):1224–9.

54. Karlsson MK, Karlsson C, Magnusson H, et al. Individuals with primary osteoarthritis have different phenotypes depending on the affected joint - a case control study from southern Sweden including 514 participants. Open Orthop J. 2014;8:450–6.

55. Purcell S, Thornberry R, Elliott SA, et al. Body composition, strength, and dietary intake of patients with hip or knee osteoarthritis. Can J Diet Pract Res. 2016;77:1–5.

56. Visser AW, de Mutsert R, Loef M, et al. The role of fat mass and skeletal muscle mass in knee osteoarthritis is different for men and women: the NEO study. Osteoarthr Cartil. 2014;22(2):197–202.

57. Levac D, Colquhoun H, O'Brien KK. Scoping studies: advancing the methodology. Implement Sci. 2010;5:69.

58. Arksey H, O'Malley L. Scoping studies: towards a methodological framework. Int J Soc Res Methodol. 2005;8(1):19–32.

59. Batsis JA, Zbehlik AJ, Pidgeon D, Bartels SJ. Dynapenic obesity and the effect on long-term physical function and quality of life: data from the osteoarthritis initiative. BMC Geriatr. 2015;15(1):118.

60. Ji HM, Han J, Jin DS, Suh H, Chung YS, Won YY. Sarcopenia and sarcopenic obesity in patients undergoing orthopedic surgery. Clin Orthop Surg. 2016;8(2):194–202.

61. Jin WS, Choi EJ, Lee SY, Bae EJ, Lee T, Park J. Relationships among obesity, sarcopenia, and osteoarthritis in the elderly. J Obes Metab Syndr. 2017:36–44.

62. Knoop J, Van Der Leeden M, Thorstensson CA, et al. Identification of phenotypes with different clinical outcomes in knee osteoarthritis: data from the osteoarthritis initiative. Arthritis Care Res. 2011;63(11):1535–42.

64. Lee S, Kim TN, Kim SH. Sarcopenic obesity is more closely associated with knee osteoarthritis than is nonsarcopenic obesity: a cross-sectional study. Arthritis Rheum. 2012;64(12):3947–54.

65. Manoy P, Anomasiri W, Yuktanandana P, et al. Elevated serum leptin levels are associated with low vitamin D, sarcopenic obesity, poor muscle strength, and physical performance in knee osteoarthritis. Biomarkers. 2017:1–22.

66. Oosting E, Hoogeboom TJ, Dronkers JJ, Visser M, Akkermans RP, NLU VM. The influence of muscle weakness on the association between obesity and inpatient recovery from total hip arthroplasty. J Arthroplasty. 2016;

67. Segal NA, Toda Y. Absolute reduction in lower limb lean body mass in Japanese women with knee osteoarthritis. J Clin Rheumatol. 2005;11(5):245–9.

68. Suh DH, Han KD, Hong JY, et al. Body composition is more closely related to the development of knee osteoarthritis in women than men: a cross-sectional study using the fifth Korea National Health and nutrition examination survey (KNHANES V-1, 2). Osteoarthr Cartil. 2016;24(4):605–11.

69. Clémence J, Bernard M, Lorraine B, Francis G, Anne-Christine R. Body composition and clinical symptoms in patients with hip or knee osteoarthritis: results from the KHOALA cohort. Semin Arthritis Rheum. 2017;

70. Newman AB, Kupelian V, Visser M, et al. Sarcopenia: alternative definitions and associations with lower extremity function. J Am Geriatr Soc. 2003; 51(11):1602–9.

71. Bosy-Westphal A, Müller MJ. Identification of skeletal muscle mass depletion across age and BMI groups in health and disease - there is need for a unified definition. Int J Obes. 2015;39(3):379–86.

72. Donini LM, Poggiogalle E, Migliaccio S, Aversa A, Pinto A. Body composition in sarcopenic obesity: systematic review of the literature. Med J Nutrition Metab. 2013;6(3):191–8.

73. Batsis JA, Barre LK, Mackenzie TA, Pratt SI, Lopez-Jimenez F, Bartels SJ. Variation in the prevalence of sarcopenia and sarcopenic obesity in older adults associated with different research definitions: dual-energy X-ray absorptiometry data from the National Health and nutrition examination survey 1999-2004. J Am Geriatr Soc. 2013;61(6):974–80.

74. Muscaritoli M, Anker SD, Argilés J, et al. Consensus definition of sarcopenia, cachexia and pre-cachexia: Joint document elaborated by Special Interest Groups (SIG) " cachexia-anorexia in chronic wasting diseases" and " nutrition in geriatrics.". Clin Nutr. 2010;29(2):154–9.

75. Fielding RA, Vellas B, Evans WJ, et al. Sarcopenia: an undiagnosed condition in older adults. Current consensus definition: prevalence, etiology, and consequences. International working group on sarcopenia. J Am Med Dir Assoc. 2011;12(4):249–56.

76. Studenski SA, Peters KW, Alley DE, et al. The FNIH sarcopenia project: Rationale, study description, conference recommendations, and final estimates. Journals Gerontol - Ser A Biol Sci Med Sci. 2014;69 A(5):547–558.

77. Ilich JZ, Kelly OJ, Inglis JE. Osteosarcopenic obesity syndrome: what is it and how can it be identified and diagnosed? Curr Gerontol Geriatr Res. 2016;

78. Tsonga T, Michalopoulou M, Malliou P, et al. Analyzing the history of falls in patients with severe knee osteoarthritis. Clin Orthop Surg. 2015;7(4):449–56.

79. Chernoff R. Protein and older adults. J Am Coll Nutr. 2004;23(6 Suppl): 627S–30S.

80. Shyam Kumar AJ, Beresford-Cleary N, Kumar P, et al. Preoperative grip strength measurement and duration of hospital stay in patients undergoing total hip and knee arthroplasty. Eur J Orthop Surg Traumatol. 2013;23:553–6.

81. Mau-Moeller A, Behrens M, Felser S, et al. Modulation and predictors of periprosthetic bone mineral density following total knee arthroplasty. Biomed Res Int. 2015.

82. Prado CM, Heymsfield SB. Lean tissue imaging: a new era for nutritional assessment and intervention. J Parenter Enter Nutr. 2014;38(8):940–53.

15

The epidemiology of MRI detected shoulder injuries in athletes participating in the Rio de Janeiro 2016 Summer Olympics

Akira M. Murakami[1]*, Andrew J. Kompel[1], Lars Engebretsen[2,3,4], Xinning Li[5], Bruce B. Forster[6], Michel D. Crema[1,7,8], Daichi Hayashi[1,9], Mohamed Jarraya[1,10], Frank W. Roemer[1,11] and Ali Guermazi[1]

Abstract

Background: To use Magnetic Resonance Imaging (MRI) to characterize the severity, location, prevalence, and demographics of shoulder injuries in athletes at the Rio de Janeiro 2016 Summer Olympic Games.

Methods: This was a retrospective analysis of all routine shoulder MRIs obtained from the Olympic Village Polyclinic during the Rio 2016 Summer Olympics. Imaging was performed on 1.5 T and 3 T MRI, and interpretation was centrally performed by a board-certified musculoskeletal radiologist. Images were assessed for tendon, muscle, bone, bursal, joint capsule, labral, and chondral abnormality.

Results: A total of 11,274 athletes participated in the Games, of which 55 (5%) were referred for a routine shoulder MRI. Fifty-three (96%) had at least two abnormal findings. Seven (13%) had evidence of an acute or chronic anterior shoulder dislocation. Forty-nine (89%) had a rotator cuff partial tear and / or tendinosis. Subacromial / subdeltoid bursitis was present in 29 (40%). Thirty (55%) had a tear of the superior labrum anterior posterior (SLAP).

Conclusion: Our study demonstrated a high prevalence of both acute and chronic shoulder injuries in the Olympic athletes receiving shoulder MRI. The high rates of bursal, rotator cuff, and labral pathology found in these patients implies that some degree of glenohumeral instability and impingement is occurring, likely due to fatigue and overuse of the dynamic stabilizers. Future studies are needed to better evaluate sport-specific trends of injury.

Keywords: MRI, Olympics, Shoulder, Injury

Background

The 2016 Rio de Janeiro Summer Olympic Games were held from August 5 to 21, 2016, bringing together 11,274 elite athletes from 206 different countries and a team of refugees. In this elite international competition, 8% of athletes incurred at least one injury during participation. Forty percent of these injuries resulted in loss of competition for at least 1 day, and 20% of the injuries resulted in loss of competition for greater than 7 days [1, 2].

Shoulder injuries constitute a small subset of all injuries at the Olympic Games, however the pain associated with even chronic conditions such as tendinosis can result in significant pain symptoms [3]. The relative lack of osseous restraint within the glenohumeral joint allows for the mobility and flexibility required for high level athletic performance. However, it also places a high physical demand on the static and dynamic stabilizers of the shoulder, particularly in athletes at this level. Overuse injuries to the rotator cuff and shoulder girdle muscles as well as to the labrum, joint capsule, and cartilage can result in instability and impingement of the joint, impeding performance [4].

Shoulder pain and injury has been particularly well documented in sports with repetitive overhead motions [3, 5–8]. While the overhead throwing athlete in particular seems most at risk, there are many Olympic sports in which similar demands are placed on the glenohumeral joint. High level athletes in contact sports such as rugby and American football can also sustain similar injuries

---
* Correspondence: akira.murakami@bmc.org
[1]Section of Musculoskeletal Imaging, Department of Radiology, Boston University School of Medicine, FGH Building, 3rd Floor, 820 Harrison Ave., Boston, MA 02118, USA
Full list of author information is available at the end of the article

even when overhead throwing motions are not inherent in their particular activity [9–11]. While various imaging modalities have been used for diagnosis, magnetic resonance imaging (MRI) has been the established imaging modality of choice in evaluating such conditions [4].

The aim of our study is to use MRI to characterize the severity, location, prevalence, and demographics of acute and chronic shoulder injuries observed at the Rio de Janeiro 2016 Summer Olympic Games, in order to better anticipate athlete diagnosis and care in future events of an elite caliber.

Methods

This is a retrospective analysis of the patient information from the International Olympic Commission (IOC) athlete database and imaging data from the Radiological Information System (RIS) and Picture Archiving Communications System (PACS) of the Rio 2016 Summer Olympics. The earliest imaging was performed 6 days prior to the opening ceremonies, and the last study was acquired 1 day after the closing ceremony. The assigned athlete accreditation number was used to query the IOC database for demographic information, which included age, gender, nationality, and sport. All information was treated with strict confidentiality, and our medical database was de-identified. The study was approved by the medical research ethics committee of the South-Eastern Norway Regional Health Authority (2011/388) and was exempt from Ethics Committee approval. Informed written consent was waived since all epidemiological data was anonymized and unidentifiable. The use of anonymized imaging and demographic data for publication was approved by the IOC. An additional Institution Review Board (IRB) was obtained from Boston University (#H-36593). The data was collected, stored, and analyzed with strict compliance to data protection and athlete confidentiality.

All patients were imaged at the official IOC polyclinic in the Olympic Village using either a 3 T Discovery MR750w or 1.5 T Optima 450MRw MRI scanner (General Electric, Waukesha, Wisc). MRI sequences consisted of 3 planes (axial, oblique coronal, oblique sagittal) of fluid sensitive T2-weighted or proton density (PD)-weighted fat-suppressed sequences. A coronal or sagittal T1-weighted sequence was also acquired. Neither intravenous nor arthrographic Gadolinium was utilized.

Image interpretation

A board certified, subspecialty radiologist (AM) with 8 years of musculoskeletal imaging experience including imaging of sports injuries, retrospectively reviewed all MRI examinations. The radiologist was blinded to the official imaging report. All data was recorded on a Microsoft Excel spreadsheet, and a descriptive statistical analysis was performed.

Osseous lesions were characterized based on location and bone marrow signal characteristics. Any bone marrow hyperintensity or edema pattern on either a T2 or PD-weighted fat-suppressed sequence was considered a bone contusion. Any bone marrow edema pattern associated with osseous fragmentation or a low linear signal on the T1-weighted sequence was considered an acute fracture [12]. Hill Sachs and osseous Bankart lesions were diagnosed based on their characteristic locations on the posterior superior humeral head and anterior inferior glenoid, respectively. A designation of either acute or chronic was based on the presence of a bone marrow edema pattern [13, 14].

Fluid within the subacromial / subdeltoid bursa and within the glenohumeral joint was assessed on the T2 or PD-weighted fat-suppressed sequences. Any region of hyper-intense subacromial or subdeltoid bursal thickening that was 2 mm or greater was considered a bursitis [4]. A glenohumeral joint effusion was characterized on a 4-point scale as reported by Schweitzer et al. Normal intra-articular fluid produces a thin intraarticular rim of hyperintense signal, but without distension of a joint recess. The presence of slight fluid distension of the subscapular recess, fluid within the biceps tendon sheath, or fluid within the axillary recess was considered a small glenohumeral joint effusion. Fluid distension of two of these recesses represented a moderate sized effusion. Fluid distension of all three structures represented a large effusion [15].

Each rotator cuff tendon was evaluated for the presence of tendinosis or tear. Tendinosis was diagnosed by the presence of signal hyperintensity on the PD and to a lesser extent T2-weighted images, and or in the presence of tendon thickening without fiber discontinuity [16, 17]. Any morphologic defect of the tendon fibers, either along the bursal surface, intrasubstance, or articular surface that was filled with fluid signal, particularly on the T2-weighted sequences, was considered a partial thickness defect. A full thickness tear was considered present if the morphologic defect in the tendon fibers extended from articular surface to bursal surface [18].

Any muscle injury of the deltoid or rotator cuff was characterized using an MRI-modified version of the Peetrons classification system [19, 20]; grade 1 – ill-defined hyperintensity on the fluid sensitive sequences indicating edema signal without architectural distortion of muscle fibers or macroscopic tear; grade 2 – architectural distortion of muscle fibers or well-defined hyperintensity on fluid sensitive sequences indicating partial muscle tear; and grade 3 – total muscle tear with retraction.

The severity of rotator cuff muscle atrophy was assessed using the Goutallier classification system, which has been validated for use in both CT and MRI [21, 22]; grade 1 – some fatty streaks; grade 2 – fatty infiltration, but more muscle than fat; grade 3 – moderate fatty infiltration but as much fat as muscle; and grade 4 – severe fatty infiltration with more fat than muscle.

The morphologic contour and signal of the labrum was assessed for the presence or absence of tears on the T2 or PD-weighted sequences with or without fat suppression. Diagnostic criteria for a tear included the presence of intrasubstance labral high signal, irregular labral margins, high intrasubstance signal that was non-parallel to the glenoid margin, high signal intensity either posterior to the long head of the biceps origin or inferior to the three o'clock position, or a separation of glenoid and labrum that was greater than 2 mm. A special distinction of labral tear in association with a Bankart lesion was made [23, 24].

The presence of joint capsule abnormality of the acromioclavicular (AC) joint or the anterior inferior glenohumeral ligament of the glenohumeral joint was evaluated. An acute capsular injury was diagnosed by the presence of either a frank capsular defect, or by the abnormal morphology and edema signal both within the capsule and along the extracapsular margin. A chronic capsular injury or abnormality was diagnosed by the observation of a scar thickened joint capsule or capsular defect but with an absence of extracapsular edema signal [23, 25].

Injuries of the long head of the biceps were characterized as involving either the extra-articular vertical portion or the intra-articular horizontal portion. The severity of injury was assessed by the presence of either tendinosis, partial tear, or rupture. Tendinosis was defined as biceps tendon thickening and /or high intrasubstance signal on the fluid sensitive sequences. A partial thickness tear was defined as any focal tendon caliber change or high intrasubstance signal approaching fluid intensity. A complete tear was defined as a complete discontinuity of the tendon [26].

Lastly, cartilage defects were evaluated using a modified Outerbridge classification system on fluid sensitive sequences [27, 28]; grade 1 – heterogeneous signal; grade 2 – shallow ulceration, fibrillation, or fissuring < 50% depth; grade 3 – deep ulceration, fibrillation, fissuring or chondral flap > 50% depth; grade 4 – full thickness loss and exposed subchondral bone.

Results

A total of 11,274 athletes which included 5089 women (45%) and 6185 men (55%) participated in the 2016 Olympic Games. The National Olympic Committees and Rio 2016 medical staff evaluated a total of 1101 acute and chronic injuries during the course of the games. Of these injured athletes, 55 (5%) were referred for MRI of

the shoulder for further evaluation of shoulder pain and injury. The 55 patients included 28 males (51%) and 27 females (49%) with an average age of 26 years, ranging from 18 to 34. The patients came from 20 different Olympic sports; of these, swimming (6), judo (6), boxing (5), gymnastics (5), volleyball (5), and athletics (track and field) (4) provided the most number of patients. Of all the MRIs, only 2 (4%) were considered completely normal. The remaining 53 (96%) MRI studies each had two or more abnormal findings.

Osseous abnormalities
Two patients presented with an acute fracture. This included an acute Hill Sachs deformity and one highly comminuted fracture of the scapula. Seven patients sustained a bone contusion by study criteria.

Anterior instability
Seven patients presented with evidence of an anterior shoulder dislocation. Boxing, taekwondo, rugby, athletics (track and field), judo, basketball, and wrestling were each represented. One of these patients sustained an acute Hill Sachs injury in combination with a soft tissue Bankart lesion (anterior inferior labral tear, Fig. 1) and acute capsular tear of the anterior inferior glenohumeral ligament. The six other patients had chronic Hill Sachs deformities as evidenced by the classic bony contour abnormality of the superior humeral head, but with a lack of bone marrow edema signal. Two of the patients also had an osseous Bankart deformity, while the remaining four patients had a purely soft tissue displaced anterior inferior labral tear.

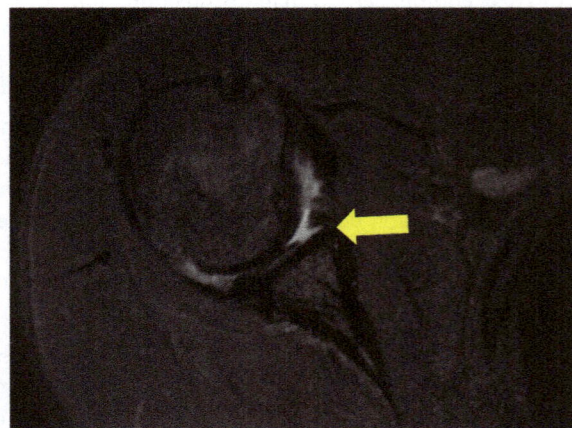

Fig. 1 Female rugby player in her late 20's: Axial T2-weighted fat-suppressed MRI demonstrates tear of the anterior inferior labrum (Bankart) lesion (arrow) and adjacent high grade chondral loss over the glenoid

Rotator cuff

Abnormalities of the rotator cuff were common in this sample, being observed in up to 49 patients (89%). Swimming, volleyball, judo, gymnastics, and track and field provided the most patients. The highest proportion of athletes per number of participants came from volleyball, judo, and gymnastics. Distribution of rotator cuff injury are listed by sport (Table 1).

Of the total patients, 22 presented with tendinosis only, while 27 had a partial thickness tear of the tendon (Fig. 2). There were no patients with either full thickness or complete rupture of a tendon. Nine patients demonstrated additional edema signal within the muscle and myotendinous junction of the rotator cuff which was interpreted as an acute, low grade muscle strain. The distribution of the rotator cuff tendons involved in either tendinosis (Fig. 3) or partial tear (Fig. 4) was similar.

Labrum

Tears of the superior labrum anterior posterior (SLAP), were relatively common, seen in 30 patients (55%). Thirteen of these SLAP tears were accompanied with abnormalities of the intra-articular long head of the biceps; seven patients had a partial thickness tear of the biceps with their SLAP tear, while 6 had at least tendinosis of the biceps. The distribution of SLAP tears are listed by

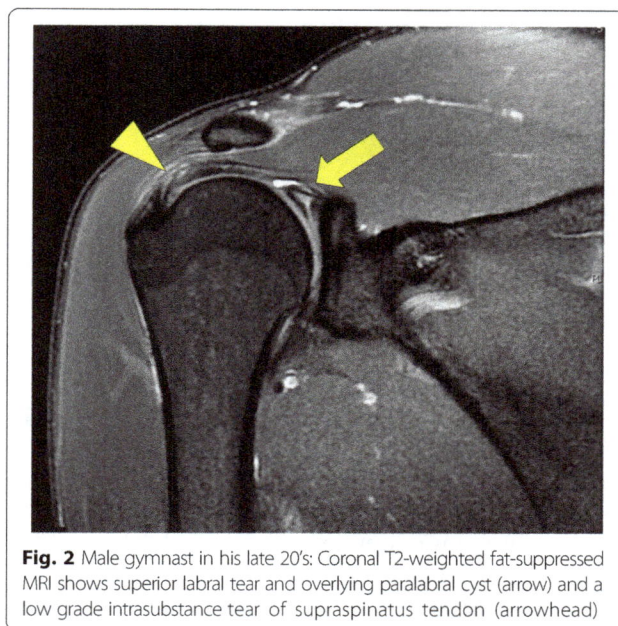

Fig. 2 Male gymnast in his late 20's: Coronal T2-weighted fat-suppressed MRI shows superior labral tear and overlying paralabral cyst (arrow) and a low grade intrasubstance tear of supraspinatus tendon (arrowhead)

sport (Table 2). Gymnastics had the highest proportion of SLAP tears relative to the total number of Olympic participants.

Long head of the biceps tendon

Abnormalities of the biceps tendon were present in 16 patients. Only 1 had involvement of the vertical portion, which presented as a partial tear. The remainder of these patients had involvement of the horizontal portion of the tendon. Thirteen of these patients (87%) were in association with a SLAP tear and are described in detail above. The remaining 2 patients had tendinosis.

Bursa

A subacromial / subdeltoid bursitis was present in 29 patients (40%).

Table 1 Distribution of rotator cuff abnormality by per sport

Sport	Patients	Total Number of Participants	Fraction of patients to the # of participants
Aquatics - Swimming	6	901	0.007
Volleyball	5	288	0.017
Judo	5	390	0.013
Gymnastics - Artistic	5	194	0.026
Athletics (Track and Field)	4	2367	0.002
Wrestling	3	349	0.009
Cycling - Road	3	211	0.014
Boxing	3	289	0.010
Tennis	2	199	0.010
Rugby	2	291	0.007
Handball	2	335	0.006
Weightlifting	1	256	0.004
Taekwondo	1	127	0.008
Hockey	1	384	0.003
Football	1	503	0.002
Field Hockey	1	384	0.003
Canoe - Sprint	1	248	0.004
Beach volleyball	1	96	0.010
Basketball	1	287	0.003
Aquatics - Water polo	1	258	0.004

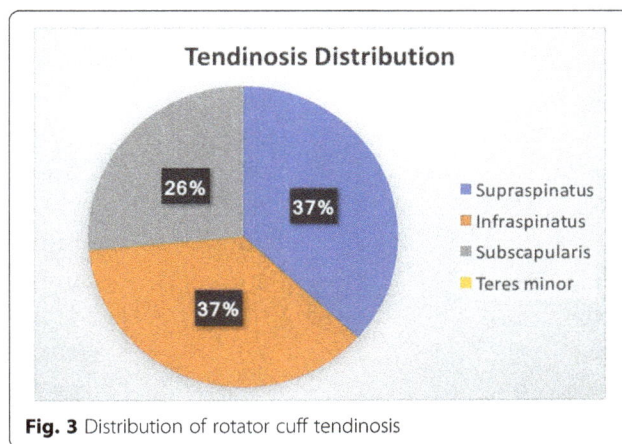

Tendinosis Distribution

- Supraspinatus 37%
- Infraspinatus 37%
- Subscapularis 26%
- Teres minor

Fig. 3 Distribution of rotator cuff tendinosis

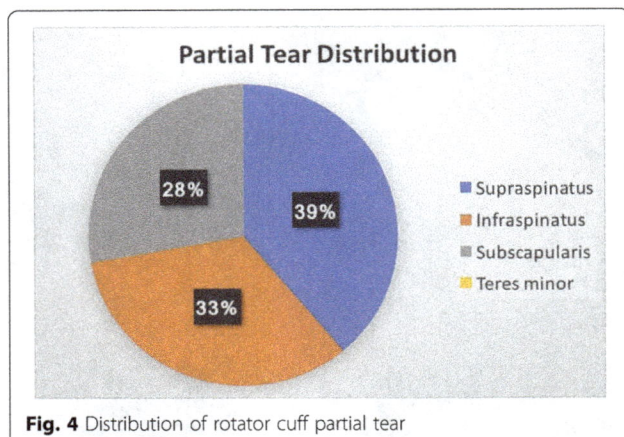

Fig. 4 Distribution of rotator cuff partial tear

Joints

A joint effusion was seen in 23 patients (42%). In all but three of these patients, the size was considered small.

Degenerative glenohumeral chondral loss was noted in 13 total patients (24%). Track and field (3) and gymnastics (2) provided the most patients. Of the total, 10 patients had chondral defects that were considered either an Outerbridge 3 or 4. Five of the patients (38%) with chondral loss had either a Hill Sachs deformity or osseous/soft tissue Bankart lesion or both. Nine of these patients (69%) with chondral loss also had a SLAP tear.

In regards to the AC joint, four patients demonstrated capsular defects, two acute and two chronic. Sixteen patients had evidence of either mild to moderate chondral loss of the AC joint.

Table 2 Distribution of superior labrum anterior posterior (SLAP) tears by sport

	Cases	Total Number of IOC Participants	Fraction
Judo	4	390	0.010
Gymnastics	4	194	0.021
Wrestling	3	349	0.009
Volleyball	3	288	0.010
Athletics (Track and field)	3	2367	0.001
Swimming	3	901	0.003
Tennis	2	199	0.010
Rugby	2	291	0.007
Cycling - Road	2	211	0.009
Football	1	503	0.002
Boxing	1	289	0.003
Basketball	1	287	0.003
Water polo	1	258	0.004

Discussion

Acute and chronic shoulder injuries are common problems in elite athletes. Sports with overhead throwing activities have been most frequently studied, with the prevalence of shoulder pain reported to be anywhere between 23 and 36% [7, 8]. This is ultimately attributed to the relatively unnatural and highly dynamic nature of the throwing movement. A strict balance of the dynamic and static stabilizers are needed to maintain a stable center of rotation [29], and loss or damage of these supporting structures can lead to shoulder pain as well as a decrease in performance. There are many additional sports in which repetitive overhead motion is inherent in competition, also leading to shoulder pain. For example, in elite, competitive swimmers, limiting shoulder pain has been reported to be between 40 and 90% [30–32]. In such cases, the etiology is most likely similar and backed by studies which have analyzed glenohumeral kinematics; With increasing rotator cuff fatigue, there is superior migration of the humeral head during arm elevations which leads to impingement and rotator cuff injury [33, 34].

Our findings are in line with this etiologic theory, given the high percentage of rotator cuff abnormalities and subdeltoid bursitis occurring in athletes involved in contact or overhead motion sports. In comparison to the general population, a review of the published literature performed by Teunis et al. [35] found that the prevalence of any rotator cuff abnormality (tendinosis or tear) is 9.7% in individuals less than 20 years, and 6.9% in those from 20 to 29 years. This is in contrast to our study patients, in which 89% demonstrated a rotator cuff abnormality (tendinosis or tear). The relatively even tendon distribution of the tears and tendinosis involving supraspinatus, infraspinatus, and subscapularis does slightly deviate from the previously described pathologic continuum of chronic subacromial impingement leading to predominantly supraspinatus tendinosis and tear [36]. However, the diversity of cuff involvement evident in these athletes may reflect the diversity of sports.

Labral injury, like rotator cuff injury, generally has a high prevalence in symptomatic and asymptomatic elite athletes. While the incidence is most commonly associated in sports with repetitive overhead motion or throwing, it has also been seen in contact athletes [4–6, 9]. For example, the incidence of SLAP tears in elite rugby players has been found to be as high as 83% [10, 11]. Our reported overall occurrence of SLAP tears at 55% is comparable to prior published studies on elite athletes. Also in keeping with the published data, the distribution of labral tears is mostly with sports with inherent overhead motion or contact.

Of patients with glenohumeral chondral loss, 85% had either evidence of anterior shoulder instability and prior dislocation and / or a superior labral tear. This is an entirely expected finding, as it is established that chronic shoulder instability can eventually lead to chondral loss. Previous studies have demonstrated that the incidence of chondral damage to be as high as 9.2% in patients with anterior shoulder instability [37] and up to 64% in patients undergoing arthroscopic Bankart repair [38].

Our study had several inherent limitations. As a strictly observational study, we did not analyze the medical record to correlate the clinical exam findings with the reason of study. Other than the clinical diagnosis of shoulder pain as an indication for MRI, we lacked detailed knowledge of clinical information that would better link our imaging findings to the clinical presentation. Our patient population inevitably included both acute injuries and pre-existing conditions. It is also possible that some of the observed imaging findings can be seen in asymptomatic individuals, and thus, establishing a direct cause and effect link is not possible given the retrospective study design and beyond the scope of this paper.

The overall prevalence of Olympic athletes in our study being evaluated for shoulder pain (5%) is certainly lower than prior reported values in overhead throwing athletes [7, 8]. This however, is likely a reflection of the diversity of Olympic sports as well as the selection bias geared toward a group of patients in which MRI imaging was indicated. We did not include other modalities that are routinely used to evaluate shoulder pain, which include ultrasound, radiograph, and computed tomography (CT). This means we likely have an underestimation of the overall athletes evaluated for shoulder pain. Thus, this study is a modality specific analysis rather than a study of overall injury prevalence.

In regards to our image interpretation, using one observer limited our ability to study intra-and inter-observer variability. It has also been shown that a higher MRI imaging matrix, stronger field strength, and intra-articular contrast (arthrography) increase the sensitivity of diagnosing labral tear [39–41]. In our study, both 3 T and 1.5 T MRI scanners were used and no arthrograms were performed. Thus, it is possible that our study lacked optimal sensitivity for labral tear detection. Furthermore, we do not know if any of these elite athletes underwent surgery for their shoulder pathology and their outcomes.

Conclusions

Our study demonstrates a high rate of bursal, rotator cuff, and labral pathology in Olympic athletes receiving MRIs at the 2016 Rio de Janeiro Summer Olympic Games. These findings imply that some degree of glenohumeral instability and impingement is occurring, likely due to fatigue and overuse of the dynamic stabilizers. Due to the diversity of Olympic sporting events, we lack sufficient numbers to draw any further sport-specific conclusions to the injuries exhibited here. More conclusive patterns may emerge by a combined analysis with future Olympic competitions. Since the cumulative effect of chronic injury and overuse syndromes in the elite athlete is an atypically higher rate of osteoarthritis [42], ultimately, it is our interest to continue understanding problems that affect those who have made such great sacrifices to represent their countries in international competition.

Abbreviations
AC: Acromial Clavicular; CT: Computed Tomography; IOC: International Olympic Commission; IRB: Institution Review Board; MRI: Magnetic Resonance Imaging; PACS: Picture archiving communications system; PD: Proton Density; RIS: Radiological Information System; SLAP: Superior Labrum Anterior Posterior

Acknowledgements
We would like to thank IOC members and all staff of Olympic Village imaging center and sports physicians/radiologists who provided clinical service.

Authors' contributions
AMM assessed the data, design of the analyses, wrote the first draft and revision of the manuscript. AJK data analysis and interpretation, and commented on all drafts of the manuscript. LE collected the data at the Olympics, commented on all drafts of the manuscript, and final approval of the version to be published. XL data analysis and commented on all drafts of the manuscript. BBF data analysis and commented on all drafts of the manuscript. MDC performed several examinations on site at the Olympics, contributed in the acquisition of the data and commented on all drafts of the manuscript. DH contribution to the conception of the work and commented on all drafts of the manuscript. MJ clean the data and data analysis and commented on all drafts of the manuscript. FWR interpretation of the data and commented on all drafts of the manuscript. AG conception of the work, analyses and interpretation of the data, commented on all versions of the manuscript, final approval of the version to be published and guarantor of accuracy and integrity of the data. All authors read and approved the final manuscript.

Competing interests
Ali Guermazi is the President of Boston Imaging Core Lab (BICL), LLC, and a Consultant to MerckSerono, AstraZeneca, Pfizer, GE Healthcare, OrthoTrophix, Sanofi and TissueGene. Frank Roemer and Michel Crema are shareholders of BICL, LLC. Lars Engebretsen is a consultant to Arthrex and Smith and Nephew. Bruce Forster has an equity position with a private MRI clinic in Vancouver. Akira Murakami, Andrew J. Kompel, Xinning Li, Daichi Hayashi, and Mohamed Jarraya have nothing to disclose.

Author details
[1]Section of Musculoskeletal Imaging, Department of Radiology, Boston University School of Medicine, FGH Building, 3rd Floor, 820 Harrison Ave., Boston, MA 02118, USA. [2]Medical and Scientific Department, International Olympic Committee, Lausanne, Switzerland. [3]Oslo Sports Trauma Research Center, Department of Sports Medicine, Norwegian School of Sport Sciences, Oslo, Norway. [4]Department of Orthopedic Surgery, Oslo University Hospital, University of Oslo, Oslo, Norway. [5]Department of Orthopaedic Surgery, Boston University School of Medicine, Boston, MA, USA. [6]Department of Radiology, University of British Columbia, Vancouver, BC, Canada. [7]Department of Sports Medicine, National Institute of Sports (INSEP), Paris, France. [8]Department of Radiology, Saint-Antoine Hospital, University Paris VI, Paris, France. [9]Department of Radiology, Stony Brook Medicine, Stony Brook, NY, USA. [10]Department of Radiology, Mercy Catholic Medical Center, Darby, PA, USA. [11]Department of Radiology, University of Erlangen-Nuremberg, Erlangen, Germany.

References

1. Guermazi AHD, Jarraya M, Crema MD, Bahr R, Roemer FW, Grangeiro J, Budgett R, Soligard T, Domingues R, Skaf A, Engebretsen L. Imaging-depicted sports-related stress injuries, fractures, muscle and tendon pathology at the Rio de Janeiro 2016 Summer Olympic games: retrospective analysis of utilization of diagnostic imaging services. Radiology. 2018;(287):922–32.

2. Soligard T, Steffen K, Palmer D, Alonso JM, Bahr R, Lopes AD, Dvorak J, Grant ME, Meeuwisse W, Mountjoy M, et al. Sports injury and illness incidence in the Rio de Janeiro 2016 Olympic summer games: a prospective study of 11274 athletes from 207 countries. Br J Sports Med. 2017;(51):1265–71.

3. Rodeo SA, Nguyen JT, Cavanaugh JT, Patel Y, Adler RS. Clinical and Ultrasonographic evaluations of the shoulders of elite swimmers. Am J Sports Med. 2016;44:3214–21.

4. Cowderoy GA, Lisle DA, O'Connell PT. Overuse and impingement syndromes of the shoulder in the athlete. Magn Reson Imaging Clin N Am. 2009;17:577–93. v

5. Abrams GD, Safran MR. Diagnosis and management of superior labrum anterior posterior lesions in overhead athletes. Br J Sports Med. 2010;44: 311–8.

6. Andrews JR, Carson WG Jr, McLeod WD. Glenoid labrum tears related to the long head of the biceps. Am J Sports Med. 1985;13:337–41.

7. Myklebust G, Hasslan L, Bahr R, Steffen K. High prevalence of shoulder pain among elite Norwegian female handball players. Scand J Med Sci Sports. 2013;23:288–94.

8. Andersson SH, Bahr R, Clarsen B, Myklebust G. Preventing overuse shoulder injuries among throwing athletes: a cluster-randomised controlled trial in 660 elite handball players. Br J Sports Med. 2017;51:1073–80.

9. Chambers CC, Lynch TS, Gibbs DB, Ghodasra JH, Sahota S, Franke K, Mack CD, Nuber GW. Superior labrum anterior-posterior tears in the National Football League. Am J Sports Med. 2017;45:167–72.

10. Funk L, Snow M. SLAP tears of the glenoid labrum in contact athletes. Clin J Sport Med. 2007;17:1–4.

11. Horsley IG, Fowler EM, Rolf CG. Shoulder injuries in professional rugby: a retrospective analysis. J Orthop Surg Res. 2013;8:9.

12. Palmer WE, Levine SM, Dupuy DE. Knee and shoulder fractures: association of fracture detection and marrow edema on MR images with mechanism of injury. Radiology. 1997;204:395–401.

13. Gyftopoulos S, Hasan S, Bencardino J, Mayo J, Nayyar S, Babb J, Jazrawi L. Diagnostic accuracy of MRI in the measurement of glenoid bone loss. AJR Am J Roentgenol. 2012;199:873–8.

14. Workman TL, Burkhard TK, Resnick D, Goff WB 2nd, Balsara ZN, Davis DJ, Lapoint JM. Hill-Sachs lesion: comparison of detection with MR imaging, radiography, and arthroscopy. Radiology. 1992;185:847–52.

15. Schweitzer ME, Magbalon MJ, Fenlin JM, Frieman BG, Ehrlich S, Epstein RE. Effusion criteria and clinical importance of glenohumeral joint fluid: MR imaging evaluation. Radiology. 1995;194:821–4.

16. Bachmann GF, Melzer C, Heinrichs CM, Mohring B, Rominger MB. Diagnosis of rotator cuff lesions: comparison of US and MRI on 38 joint specimens. Eur Radiol. 1997;7:192–7.

17. Rafii M, Firooznia H, Sherman O, Minkoff J, Weinreb J, Golimbu C, Gidumal R, Schinella R, Zaslav K. Rotator cuff lesions: signal patterns at MR imaging. Radiology. 1990;177:817–23.

18. Kassarjian A, Bencardino JT, Palmer WE. MR imaging of the rotator cuff. Magn Reson Imaging Clin N Am. 2004;12:39–60. vi

19. Ekstrand J, Healy JC, Walden M, Lee JC, English B, Hagglund M. Hamstring muscle injuries in professional football: the correlation of MRI findings with return to play. Br J Sports Med. 2012;46:112–7.

20. Peetrons P. Ultrasound of muscles. Eur Radiol. 2002;12:35–43.

21. Goutallier D, Postel JM, Bernageau J, Lavau L, Voisin MC. Fatty muscle degeneration in cuff ruptures. Pre- and postoperative evaluation by CT scan. Clin Orthop Relat Res. 1994:78–83.

22. Fuchs B, Weishaupt D, Zanetti M, Hodler J, Gerber C. Fatty degeneration of the muscles of the rotator cuff: assessment by computed tomography versus magnetic resonance imaging. J Shoulder Elb Surg. 1999;8:599–605.

23. Kompel AJ, Li X, Guermazi A, Murakami AM. Radiographic Evaluation of Patients with Anterior Shoulder Instability. Curr Rev Musculoskelet Med. 2017;10(4):425–33.

24. De Coninck T, Ngai SS, Tafur M, Chung CB. Imaging the glenoid labrum and labral tears. Radiographics. 2016;36:1628–47.

25. Alyas F, Curtis M, Speed C, Saifuddin A, Connell D. MR imaging appearances of acromioclavicular joint dislocation. Radiographics. 2008;28:463–79. quiz 619

26. Tadros AS, Huang BK, Wymore L, Hoenecke H, Fronek J, Chang EY. Long head of the biceps brachii tendon: unenhanced MRI versus direct MR arthrography. Skelet Radiol. 2015;44:1263–72.

27. Outerbridge RE. The etiology of chondromalacia patellae. J Bone Joint Surg Br. 1961;43-B:752–7.

28. Potter HG, Linklater JM, Allen AA, Hannafin JA, Haas SB. Magnetic resonance imaging of articular cartilage in the knee. An evaluation with use of fast-spin-echo imaging. J Bone Joint Surg Am. 1998;80:1276–84.

29. van der Hoeven H, Kibler WB. Shoulder injuries in tennis players. Br J Sports Med. 2006;40:435–40. discussion 440

30. Bak K, Magnusson SP. Shoulder strength and range of motion in symptomatic and pain-free elite swimmers. Am J Sports Med. 1997;25:454–9.

31. McMaster WC, Roberts A, Stoddard T. A correlation between shoulder laxity and interfering pain in competitive swimmers. Am J Sports Med. 1998;26:83–6.

32. Rupp S, Berninger K, Hopf T. Shoulder problems in high level swimmers--impingement, anterior instability, muscular imbalance? Int J Sports Med. 1995;16:557–62.

33. Maenhout A, Dhooge F, Van Herzeele M, Palmans T, Cools A. Acromiohumeral distance and 3-dimensional scapular position change after overhead muscle fatigue. J Athl Train. 2015;50:281–8.

34. Teyhen DS, Miller JM, Middag TR, Kane EJ. Rotator cuff fatigue and glenohumeral kinematics in participants without shoulder dysfunction. J Athl Train. 2008;43:352–8.

35. Teunis T, Lubberts B, Reilly BT, Ring D. A systematic review and pooled analysis of the prevalence of rotator cuff disease with increasing age. J Shoulder Elb Surg. 2014;23:1913–21.

36. Neer CS 2nd. Impingement lesions. Clin Orthop Relat Res. 1983:70–7.

37. Buscayret F, Edwards TB, Szabo I, Adeleine P, Coudane H, Walch G. Glenohumeral arthrosis in anterior instability before and after surgical treatment: incidence and contributing factors. Am J Sports Med. 2004;32:1165–72.

38. Krych AJ, Sousa PL, King AH, Morgan JA, May JH, Dahm DL. The effect of cartilage injury after arthroscopic stabilization for shoulder instability. Orthopedics. 2015;38:e965–9.

39. Gusmer PB, Potter HG, Schatz JA, Wickiewicz TL, Altchek DW, O'Brien SJ, Warren RF. Labral injuries: accuracy of detection with unenhanced MR imaging of the shoulder. Radiology. 1996;200:519–24.

40. Magee T. 3-T MRI of the shoulder: is MR arthrography necessary? AJR Am J Roentgenol. 2009;192:86–92.

41. Magee TH, Williams D. Sensitivity and specificity in detection of labral tears with 3.0-T MRI of the shoulder. AJR Am J Roentgenol. 2006;187:1448–52.

42. Gouttebarge V, Inklaar H, Backx F, Kerkhoffs G. Prevalence of osteoarthritis in former elite athletes: a systematic overview of the recent literature. Rheumatol Int. 2015;35:405–18.

16

Measure of activity performance of the hand (MAP-Hand) questionnaire: linguistic validation, cultural adaptation and psychometric testing in people with rheumatoid arthritis in the UK

Yeliz Prior[1]* (ID), Alan Tennant[2], Sarah Tyson[3], Ingvild Kjeken[4] and Alison Hammond[1]

Abstract

Background: Developed in the Norway, the Measure of Activity Performance of the Hand (MAP-Hand) assesses 18 activities performed using the hands. It was developed for people with rheumatoid arthritis (RA) using patient generated items, which are scored on a 0–3 scale and summarised into a total score range (0 to 54). This study reports the development and psychometric testing of the British English MAP-Hand in a UK population of people with RA.

Methods: Recruitment took place in the National Health Service (NHS) through 17 Rheumatology outpatient clinics. Phase 1 (cross-cultural adaptation) involved: forward translation to British English; synthesis; expert panel review and cognitive debriefing interviews with people with RA. Phase 2 (psychometric testing) involved postal completion of the MAP-Hand, Health Assessment Questionnaire (HAQ), Upper Limb HAQ (ULHAQ), Short-Form 36 (SF-36$_{v2}$) and Disabilities of the Arm Shoulder Hand (DASH) to measure internal consistency (Cronbach's alpha); concurrent validity (Spearman's correlations) and Minimal Detectable Difference (MDC^{95}). The MAP-Hand was repeated three-weeks later to assess test-retest reliability (linear weighted kappa and Intra-Class Correlations (ICC (2,1)). Unidimensionality (internal construct validity) was assessed using (i) Confirmatory Factor Analysis (CFA) (ii) Mokken scaling and (iii) Rasch model. The RUMM2030 software was used, applying the Rasch partial credit model.

Results: In Phase 1, 31 participants considered all items relevant. In Phase 2, 340 people completed Test-1 and 273 (80%) completed Test-2 questionnaires. Internal consistency was excellent ($\alpha = 0.96$). Test-retest reliability was good (ICC (2,1) = 0.96 (95% CI 0.94, 0.97)). The MAP-Hand correlated strongly with HAQ20 ($r_s = .88$), ULHAQ ($r_s = .91$), SF-36$_{v2}$ Physical Functioning (PF) Score ($r_s = -.80$) and DASH ($r_s = .93$), indicating strong concurrent validity. CFA failed to support unidimensionality (Chi-Square 236.0 (df 120; $p < 0.001$)). However, Mokken scaling suggested a probabilistic ordering. There was differential item functioning (DIF) for gender. Four testlets were formed, resulting in much improved fit and unidimensionality. Following this, testlets were further merged in pairs where opposite bias existed. This resulted in perfect fit to the model.

Conclusions: The British English version of the MAP-Hand has good validity and reliability in people with RA and can be used in both research and clinical practice.

Keywords: PROMS, Patient reported outcome measures, Hand activity performance, Hand function, Hand pain, Psychometric testing, Rasch analysis, Validity, Reliability

* Correspondence: y.prior@salford.ac.uk
[1]Centre for Health Sciences Research, University of Salford, Salford, UK
Full list of author information is available at the end of the article

Background

Rheumatoid arthritis (RA) is a chronic autoimmune disorder affecting joints and surrounding tissues [1]. Most commonly, RA results in swollen, hot and painful joints and generalised stiffness, which worsens with rest. The hands and wrists are the most commonly affected joints. Typically, metacarpophalangeal (MCP) and proximal interphalangeal (PIP) joints become swollen and painful. As a result, people struggle with daily activities requiring gripping, pinching and carrying. If unresolved, these difficulties may lead to activity limitation, participation restriction and loss of independence in later life [2]. Therefore, early recognition and rehabilitation of hand pain and problems may help to improve people with RA's future health and quality of life.

The National Institute for Clinical Excellence (NICE) Guidelines for the Management of Adults with RA [3] recommend that patients should have access to specialist occupational therapy if they have difficulties with hand function. To maintain or improve these abilities, occupational therapists need to effectively identify individual's difficulties and evaluate therapy outcomes. To this end, valid, reliable patient-informed Patient Reported Outcome Measures (PROMs) that are relevant to the interventions rheumatology occupational therapists provide are necessary, but there is only one appropriate measure is currently validated for use in the UK [4]. Several self-reported measures of hand function are available for use in RA [5–8] however these did not involve patients in their development [9]. It is increasingly recognised that patients should inform the development of such measurement tools [10] to ensure that issues most relevant and important to them are included.

The Measure of Activity Performance of the Hand (MAP-Hand) questionnaire is an 18-item PROM of hand activity performance, which was developed and rigorously tested in Norway. It has good evidence of reliability and validity in Norwegian people with RA (n = 134) [9]. To ensure items were representative of normal hand function, items were matched to the eight main handgrips using the Sollerman handgrip classification [11]. Rasch analysis was used to finalise the 18-itemstructure representing a range of item difficulty. The scale is unidimensional and has a high person separation index of 0.93. Test-retest reliability is good (ICC = 0.94) although only conducted with 34 people. The MAP-Hand significantly correlated with the AIMS$_2$ hand and finger function (r = 0.78) and arm scales (r = 0.66) [9]. Following testing the MAP-Hand was translated into North American English in accordance with the recommended translation procedures for scale development [9]. The MAP-Hand developers recommended further testing in different countries to establish its psychometric properties and cultural validity.

Linguistic translation of self-administered questionnaires for use in different cultural contexts is insufficient [12, 13]. Researchers must also ensure cross-cultural adaptation to establish items are relevant and understandable to the population of interest, and whether additional items need including to avoid systematic bias [12]. Once adapted, further psychometric testing is required to ensure content validity and reliability is retained across different cultures [12, 13]. Beaton et al. [12] published guidelines for cross-cultural adaptation of self-report measures to standardise this process. A decade following this, Consensus-based Standards for the selection of health Measurement Instruments (COSMIN) checklist was developed to evaluate the methodological quality of the studies reporting measurement qualities [14, 15]. More recently COSMIN methodology for evaluating the content validity of patient-reported outcome measures were proposed as a rating system to summarise the evidence of a PROM's content validity [16]. This is deemed to be more detailed, standardised, and transparent than earlier published guidelines, including the previous COSMIN standards [16].

The overall aim of this study was to develop a British English version of the MAP-Hand following the recommended linguistic and cultural adaptation guidelines and test its psychometric properties (internal consistency, construct and concurrent validity, test-retest reliability and minimal detectable difference) using both the classical testing theory and item response theory in a UK population of people with RA.

Method
Study setting
Participants were recruited from rheumatology and occupational therapy departments in 17 National Health Service (NHS) Hospitals across the UK.

Eligibility criteria
Within a test-retest design it is important to ensure participants' disease status is clinically stable at two time points to avoid risk of bias [14]. Therefore a recent change in medication may result in changes of the participant's hand function and/or physical and mental health status. Patients were screened at the rheumatology outpatient clinics by research nurses and occupational therapists using an eligibility checklist and excluded if they are about to or recently started (during the last 3-months) or increased dose of a biologic or disease modifying anti-rheumatic drugs (DMARDs), low dose oral steroids or received an intra-muscular steroid injection, had cognitive impairment affecting ability to understand and complete the study questionnaire; had another health condition(s) which is moderately to

severely affecting their ability to participate in activities and/or hand function; had mental health problem(s) or terminal illness and it was inappropriate to request participation; or were unable to provide informed, written consent. However, people with Fibromyalgia, Osteoarthritis or other conditions that is secondary to RA (e.g. heart disease) were not excluded from the study. Those who were aged 18 years and above: able to read, write and understand English, and diagnosed with RA by a rheumatology consultant were included in the study providing written informed consent was obtained.

Procedures

Phase 1: Cross-cultural adaptation

The linguistic validation and cross-cultural adaptation guidelines were followed [12–14]. As a North American English version of the MAP-Hand was already available from the Norwegian developers, backward translation was not required (Additional file 1). Two native British English speakers forward translated the MAP-Hand; one of whom was unfamiliar with health outcome measures and not involved in health care; and the other was a rheumatology health professional. Translators synthesised translations to resolve discrepancies and an Expert Panel reviewed translations to agree a pre-final British English MAP-Hand. The Expert Panel included health professionals (occupational therapists and a physiotherapist), native English speakers, a methodologist and a layperson with RA. The panel reviewed the MAP-Hand for semantic (i.e. do words mean the same thing?), idiomatic (e.g. presence of colloquialism or idioms), experiential and conceptual equivalence.

Cognitive de-briefing interviews

A purposive sample of participants with wide range of demographic characteristics and health status were identified from the past participants of the EDAQ [Evaluation of Daily Activity Questionnaire] study [17, 18] within five rheumatology outpatient departments in the North West of England. They were mailed an invitation letter, participant information sheet, reply form and a FREEPOST envelope. Upon receipt of a positive reply, they were telephoned by an occupational therapist to go through the eligibility checklist, explain what the study involves and provide an opportunity to answer any questions they may have prior to deciding to take part. Consenting participants were booked in to partake in a cognitive de-briefing interview and mailed the Phase 1 questionnaire booklet to complete at home, in their own time no sooner than 1 week prior to the arranged telephone or face-to-face interview. These semi-structured interviews were aimed to ascertain whether the participant found the MAP-Hand items relevant, understandable and comprehensive (i.e. did they adequately reflect the most common daily activity difficulties experienced when using their hands and whether any additional items should be included). Such interviews are recommended during PROM development to ensure participants' understanding of their content matches the intended use [12]. The interviewer used a five-point rating scale to assess the relevancy and ease of comprehension of each item in the MAP-Hand (relevancy was measured as 1 = not relevant to 5 = very relevant; and comprehension was measured as 1 = very easy to understand to 5 = very difficult to understand). Interviews were audio-recorded, transcribed and analysed to identify the need for recommended changes and/or the inclusion of new items. A summary of the findings was reviewed by the Expert Panel to decide whether further changes were required. Following this, a detailed report of the linguistic validation and the cross-cultural adaptation process taken place and the finalised British English MAP-Hand were submitted to the Norwegian developers for review and approval.

Phase 2: Psychometric testing

It is highly recommended that culturally adapted questionnaires should be further tested following the cross-cultural validation process to ensure the new version demonstrated the psychometric properties needed for the intended application [12]. Therefore Phase 2 consisted of psychometric testing of the British English MAP-Hand Questionnaire.

Participants

During Phase 2, participants were recruited from rheumatology outpatient clinics within 17 NHS hospitals across the UK. These included both rural and urban populations and a wide mix of socio-demographics.

Data collection

Participants were mailed a Test 1 questionnaire booklet, which included demographic and health data (e.g. age, gender, marital, educational and employment status, disease duration, medication) and following outcome measures: the (i) Health Assessment Questionnaire (HAQ) which includes ability to perform 20 daily activities rated on a 0–3 scale (0 = not at all difficult; 3 = unable to do) [19] and Upper Limb HAQ (ULHAQ)[7 Upper Limb HAQ items] [20]; the Medical Outcomes Survey 36 item Short-Form 36 (SF-36$_{v2}$) from which sub-scale of Physical Function was selected [21, 22]; British English Disabilities of the Arm Shoulder Hand (DASH) which consists of 30 items, measured using five-point Likert scales, 21 daily activity ability items, five symptom items, three participation items, and one of self-image [4]; and Symptom Numeric Rating Scales (NRS) from the EDAQ Part 1, rating hand and wrist pain and arthritis severity on a 10-point scale [17, 18].

Participants were mailed a repeat [Test 2] questionnaire booklet two to 3 weeks later to complete at home to conduct the test-retest reliability of the British English MAP-Hand. Test 2 questionnaire booklet only included brief items on basic demographics (i.e. date of birth, gender and postcode); two single items about current health status and functioning (i.e. "Considering all the ways that your condition affects you, how have you been over the past month?" and "Overall, how much your arthritis is troubling you now compared to when you last completed this questionnaire a few weeks ago?") and the British English MAP-Hand for repeat testing (Additional file 2).

Statistical analysis
Sample size
The sample size calculation suggested that, for Rasch analysis a sample size of 243 will give 99% confidence of the person estimate being within ±0.5 logits, irrespective of whether or not the scale is well targeted to the patients [23]. A minimum of 79 sets of repeated responses were required to demonstrate that a test-retest correlation of 0.7 differs from a background correlation (constant) of 0.45, with 90% power and 99% significance.

Unidimensionality
The MAP-hand is reported to be a unidimensional extant scale [9]. As such, confirmation of its structure from a classical test perspective would follow from a Confirmatory Factor Analysis (CFA), where a priori there is evidence that the item set constitutes one factor [24]. Although the Rasch model assumes unidimensionality, and this can be tested post-hoc, it can still be informative to examine the scale through a CFA, particularly as Mokken scaling also has this assumption. Following Kline, fit is determined by a non-significant chi square statistic [25]. Approximate (or ancillary) fit statistics include the Root Mean Square Error of Approximation (RMSEA) where a value less than 0.06 would be appropriate, the Comparative Fit Index (CFI), a comparison of final model and baseline model and the Tucker Lewis Index (TLI), another incremental fit Index which adds penalties for increasing the parameters. Both indices would suggest good fit with values above 0.95. Thus in the present study the item set is fit to a CFA model in Mplus using a polychoric correlation matrix [26].

Mokken scaling
The Mokken scale is a non-parametric probabilistic model that utilises Loevinger's H coefficient to determine the 'scalability' of a set of items. 'H' is a measure of the degree to which the score is able to discriminate between persons in the given sample [27]. It has been argued that Mokken scaling is a natural starting point for item analysis, and it is used here in that context, to identify if any items from the MAP-Hand display a level of discrimination inconsistent with the expectations of the Rasch model, as represented by low values (< 0.3) of H. In the present study Mokken scaling is examined through the *msp* procedure in STATA 13 [28].

Construct validity
The Rasch model is widely applied to PROMs to ascertain if a quantitative structure is present for the domain(s) measured [29]. A practical realisation of additive conjoint measurement, where data are shown to meet the model expectations, it allows the transformation of ordinal data into an interval level latent estimate [30–34]. The model expectations are associated with a series of assumptions, or requirements, including the stochastic ordering of items (or fit), unidimensionality and local independence [35]. Fit is evaluated by several fit statistics, including chi-square statistics for items and in total (which should be non-significant, Bonferroni adjusted), standardised item and person residuals (within a range ± 2.5), and summary residuals with a mean of zero and standard deviation of one where data have perfect fit to the model. Local response dependency can be examined through the residual correlation matrix [36]. When the local independence assumption is violated, items can be grouped into 'testlets' which absorb the dependency [37]. When data are made into testlets, this delivers a bi-factor solution for the latent estimate, where any unique non-error variance is discarded [38].

A post-hoc test of unidimensionality was also undertaken following the approach described by Smith [39]. Finally, within the Rasch model framework, emphasis is placed upon the invariance of comparisons between groups, such that *at the same level of the trait* being measured (e.g. hand function), the probability of response to an item should be equal across groups, otherwise Differential Item Functioning (DIF) is present and will require adjustment [40, 41]. Consequently the process of fitting data to the Rasch model, widely referred to as Rasch analysis, consists of a series of tests related to the assumptions of the model, and adjustments to accommodate deviations from those expectations. This process, in relation to the measurement of health outcomes, is described in detail elsewhere [42].

In the current application, emphasis is placed upon fit to the model expectations, and invariance by contextual group, in this case by age, gender, employment and marital status, duration of disease and magnitude of disability as expressed by the HAQ. The analysis used the RUMM2030 software utilising the partial credit parameterisation of the Rasch model [43, 44].

Concurrent validity

The MAP-Hand scores were compared with comparative health measures, specifically the HAQ-20 and ULHAQ [19]; SF-36$_{v2}$ (Physical Functioning Score Norm-Based; General Health and Physical Component) [21, 22]; British English DASH [4]; numeric rating scales of hand and wrist pain (i.e. pain in the hand and wrist past week) and arthritis severity (i.e. effect of arthritis in the past month; pain when resting; pain when moving) [17]. Concurrent validity was measured using Spearman's correlations between the MAP-Hand and these comparative health measures.

Reliability.

Internal consistency was measured using Cronbach's Alpha (α) and the Person Separation Index (PSI) which, should the data have a normal distribution, is equivalent to Cronbach's Alpha [45].

Test-retest reliability

Test-retest reliability of the MAP-Hand was assessed using linear weighted kappas from Test-1 and Test-2 items and at scale level using Rasch transformed estimates and Intra Class Correlations (ICC) (2,1). Analyses were conducted using IBM SPSS Statistics v20 and MedCalc Statistical Software.

Measurement Error.

Measurement error was assessed by transforming the MAP-Hand scores into logits and linearly transforming them to produce an interval-scale. Following this, Standard Error of Measurement (SEM) and the minimal detectable change (MDC$_{95}$) score were calculated [46, 47]. If $\geq$15% of responders achieved either the lowest or highest score, floor and ceiling effects were considered to be present [48, 49].

Results

Phase-1: Cross-cultural adaptation

Cognitive debriefing interviews were conducted with 31 participants. Participants' socio-demographic and health characteristics are detailed in Table 1.

Overall, the interviews showed that the MAP-Hand items were both understandable and relevant, and take 2

Table 1 MAP-Hand Study Participant Characteristics ($n = 340$)

Participant Characteristics	Cognitive debriefing [Phase-1] Participants ($n = 31$)	Psychometric testing [Phase-2] Participants ($n = 340$)
Age:(Mean (SD)	63.42 (12.04)	61.96 (12.09)
Gender (M:F)	5:26	89:251
Condition duration (years) (Mean (SD):	15.71 (12.61)	14.44 (11.73)
Marital status: n (%):		
Married/living with partner	23 (74%)	241 (71%)
Living status: n (%)		
Family/significant other	24 (77%)	245 (72%)
Children living at home	4 (13%)	36 (11%)
Employment status:		
Paid employment	3 (10%)	108 (32%)
Retired	22 (71%)	204 (60%)
Other	6 (19%)	28 (8%)
Education level (ISCED):		
Secondary education only	19 (61%)	182 (54%)
Current medication:		
Not on DMARDs	2 (6%)	34 (10%)
Monotherapy	10 (32%)	91 (27%)
Combination therapy	10 (32%)	190 (56%)
Biologic drugs	9 (29%)	25 (7%)

minutes to complete. Specific items that were highlighted as potentially problematic were:

(i) Item 10 (slicing bread using a knife); as participants often bought sliced bread, this item was not applicable to most ($n = 24$). However, most responded to the item by recalling the last time they sliced bread, such as baguettes, as it is instructed.

(ii) Item 16 (type on a computer) was not applicable to some participants ($n = 7$) as they didn't use computers. As the 'not applicable' option is not available in the response options, these participants either left this item blank or guessed their ability based on other activities require similar input (e.g. using a mobile phone to text) to answer.

Nevertheless, all items were deemed to be relevant by the participants and expert panel and therefore retained in the British English MAP-Hand. Cultural adaptations included making small changes in the wording of three items i.e. the item 7 was reworded as "opening screw top

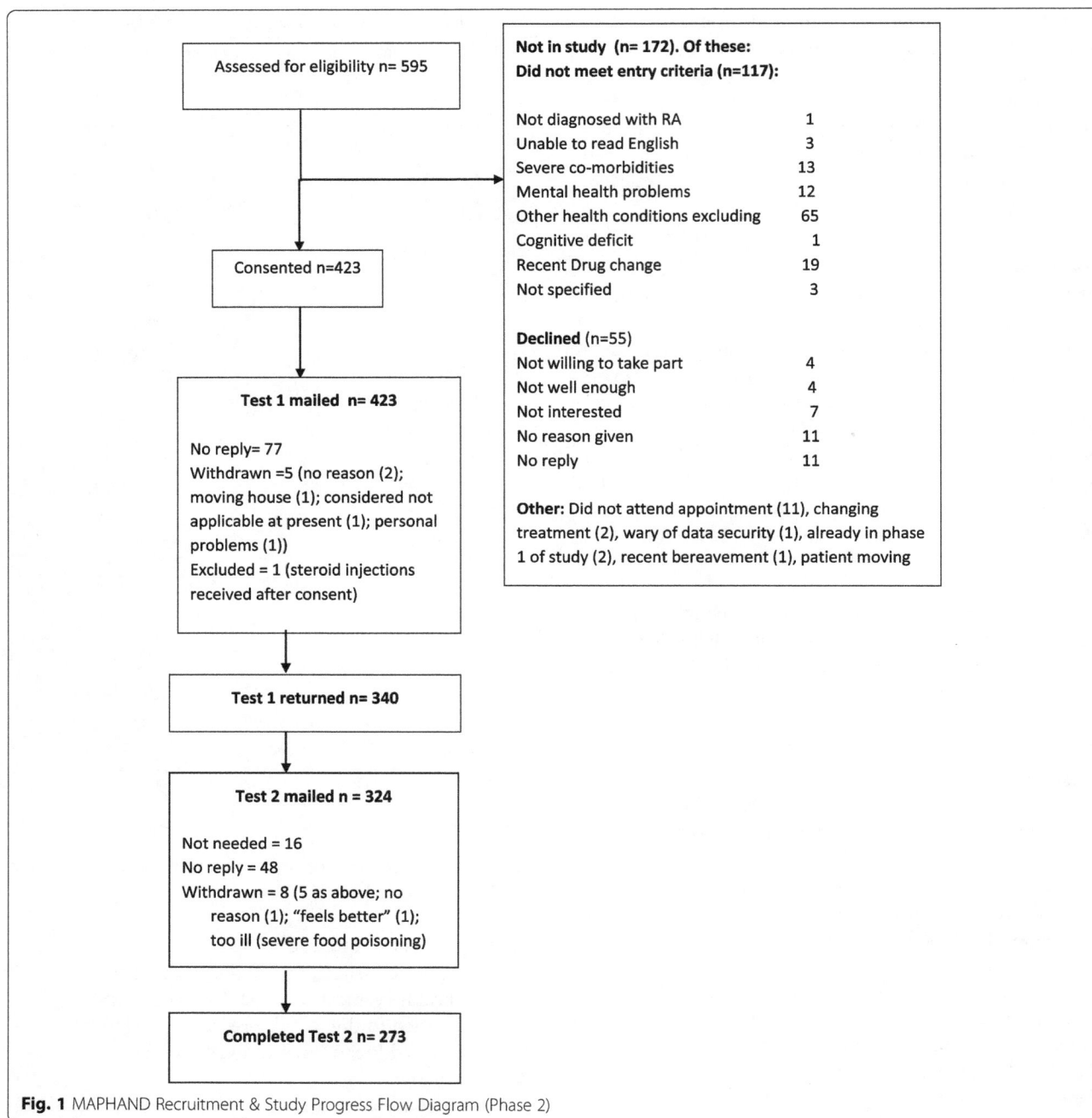

Fig. 1 MAPHAND Recruitment & Study Progress Flow Diagram (Phase 2)

bottles" instead of "opening bottle screw tops"; the item 8 was reworded as "opening cans (any type)" instead of "opening hermetic cans" and the item 12 was reworded as "stirring food in a pan" instead of "stirring food in a pot" (Additional file 2).

Phase 2: Psychometric testing

In Phase 2, 340 participants completed the Test 1 questionnaire and re-test was completed by the 80% ($n = 273$)

of the responders. The recruitment progress is summarised in Fig. 1 and the participants' socio-demographic and health characteristics are detailed in Table 1.

Construct validity (Mokken and Rasch models)

A CFA failed to support the unidimensional structure of the 18-item set of the British English MAP-Hand (Chi-Square 236.0 (df 120; $p < 0.001$). RMSEA was 0.53 (90%CI:0.43–0.63); CFI 0.995; TLI 0.994. Mokken scaling

Table 2 Rasch Analysis of the MAP-HAND (*n* = 340)

	Description	Chi-Square*	Df	P	Residual Item		Residual Person		Person Separation Index [PSI] Reliability	% tests > 5%	95%CI	N
					Mean	SD	Mean	SD				
1	MAP-HAND 18	113.17	72	0.001	−0.4073	1.4939	−0.2936	1.1725	0.95	13.4	11.0–15.7	340
2	Four testlet version	19.81	16	0.229	−0.197	2.6078	−0.4561	1.0624	0.92	5.36	3.0–7.8	340
3	Two testlet version	3.0	8	0.934	0.039	1.1792	−0.5832	0.8457	0.92	4.35	1.9–6.8	340
	Ideal Values			> 0.05*		< 1.4		< 1.4	> 0.70	< 5.0	LCI < 5.0	

*Bonferroni Adjusted

suggested that all 18 items showed a probabilistic ordering with a moderate scaling level of 0.61. Initial fit of the 18 items of the MAP-Hand to the Rasch model showed some misfit to the model (Table 2, Analysis 1), and a significant breach of the unidimensionality assumption. DIF was largely absent across all contextual factors, but was present for gender for the item 3 ' tying shoelaces', the item 7 'opening screw top bottles' and the item 18 'carrying heavy objects'. At any level of hand function, males were more likely to score higher (worse) than females for tying shoelaces, and females were more likely to score higher than males with opening screw top bottles. Reliability was high, but possibly inflated by the local dependency.

Clusters of locally dependent items could be observed. For example, button, socks and laces, any form of opening jars or cans and carrying bags or heavy objects. Consequently four testlets were formed from the item set

and the data refitted to the model. Here fit was much improved and the unidimensionality assumption held (Analysis 2). The average latent correlation between the four testlets was 0.91, and the amount of common non-error variance in the latent estimate was 0.97, meaning that just 3% of the non-error variance was discarded. This suggests the earlier breach of the unidimensionality assumption was caused by clusters of locally dependent items. Nevertheless, some gender DIF persisted. As earlier it was noted that some items favoured males, and others favoured females, the testlets were further merged in to pairs where opposite bias existed. This resulted in perfect fit to the model, and no DIF (Analysis 3). The scale and patients were slightly off-target in that the latter were more able (less difficulties) than the average of the scale (Fig. 2). However, the floor effect was minimal (5.6%). Table 3 provides the ordinal raw score-interval scale transformation.

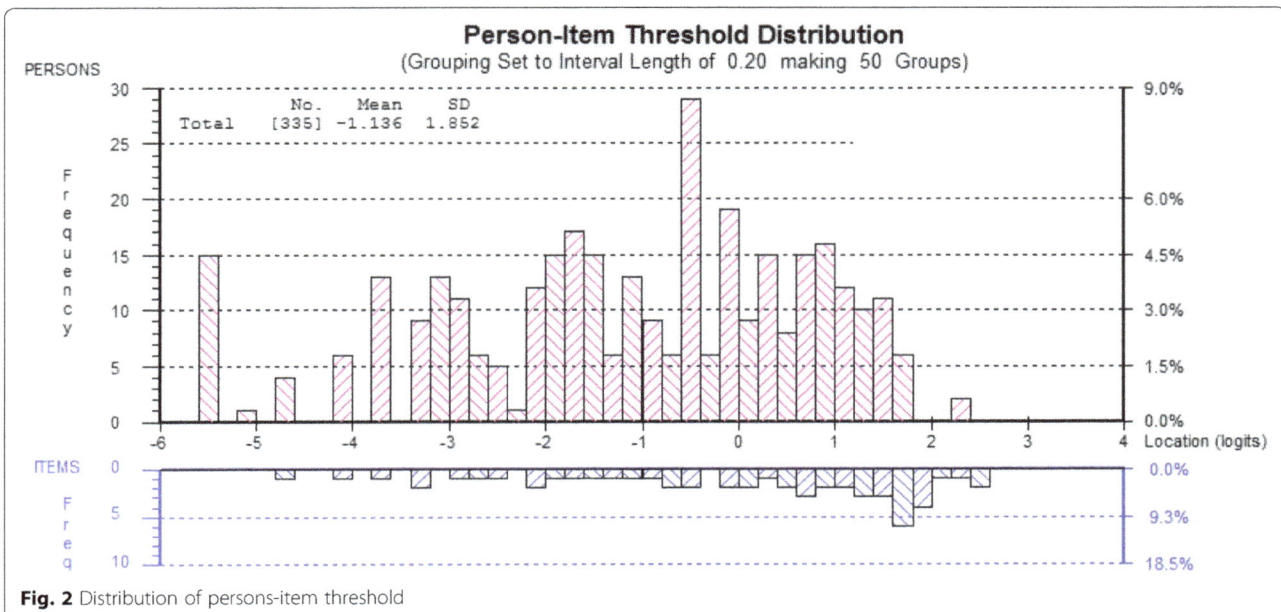

Fig. 2 Distribution of persons-item threshold

Table 3 Transformation of Raw score to Interval metric

0	0.0
1	4.9
2	8.4
3	10.9
4	12.9
5	14.6
6	16.1
7	17.5
8	18.8
9	20.1
10	21.4
11	22.6
12	23.7
13	24.9
14	26.0
15	27.0
16	28.0
17	29.0
18	29.9
19	30.8
20	31.7
21	32.5
22	33.3
23	34.1
24	34.8
25	35.5
26	36.2
27	36.8
28	37.4
29	38.0
30	38.6
31	39.1
32	39.6
33	40.1
34	40.6
35	41.0
36	41.5
37	41.9
38	42.2
39	42.6
40	43.0
41	43.3
42	43.6
43	44.0
44	44.3

Table 3 Transformation of Raw score to Interval metric *(Continued)*

45	44.7
46	45.1
47	45.5
48	46.0
49	46.6
50	47.3
51	48.1
52	49.3
53	51.1
54	54.0

A significant gradient of the transformed metric is seen across groups of functional limitation as defined by the HAQ (Table 4, Fig. 3) (ANOVA F = 217.1; $p < 0.001$). Females also showed more limitations in hand function than males (t-test; $t = 3.1$; $p = 0.002$). Duration of disease also showed a significant difference, mainly due to the group with duration over 21 years (ANOVA post-hoc tests). There was no significant difference by age group (ANOVA F = 0.254; p 0.851).

Concurrent validity

MAP-HAND correlated strongly with HAQ20 (r_s = .88), ULHAQ (r_s = .91), SF-36v2 (PF) Score (r_s = −.80) and DASH (r_s = .93), indicating strong concurrent validity (Table 5).

Internal consistency (reliability)

The Map-Hand showed a high Person Separation Index reliability (PSI), even after adjustment for local dependency (PSI range: 0.95–0.92). Reliability measured by Cronbach Alpha (α) was also excellent ($\alpha = 0.96$).

Test-retest reliability

Test-retest reliability was good: at item-level linear weighted kappa scores were good (range 0.61–0.75); at scale level, the ICC (2,1) score was 0.96 (95% CI 0.94, 0.97).

Table 4 MAP-hand metric across levels of the HAQ

HAQ	MAP-HAND
0–0.25	13.49
0.26–0.5	19.75
0.51–1.0	28.72
1.1+	37.28

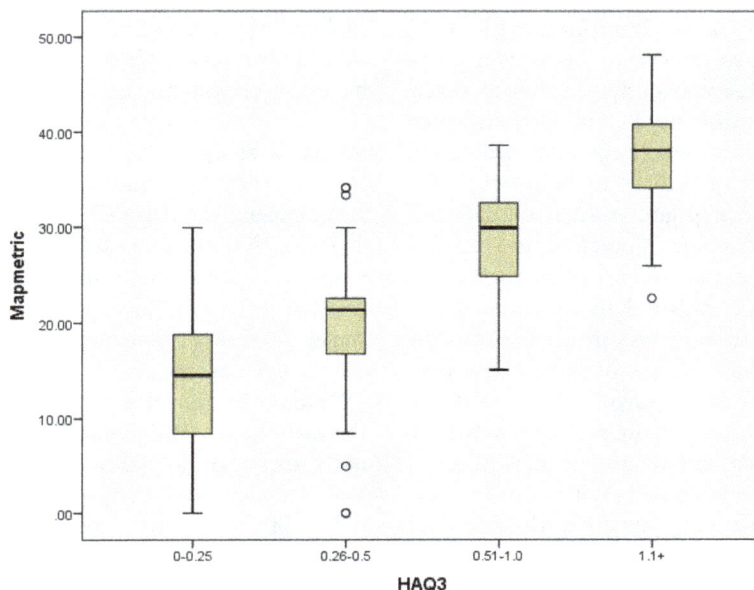

Fig. 3 Boxplot of MAP-hand Metric for HAQ groups (*n* = 340)

Measurement error

The SEM was 1.44 and the MDC$_{95}$ score was 3.99. There was no floor or ceiling effects present.

Summary of the results

The MAP-Hand questionnaire was linguistically validated and culturally adapted using the recommended guidelines [12–14] in a UK population of adults aged ≥18 years with RA [50]. The British English version of the MAP-Hand retained all original 18 items, with some changes to the phrasing of these and the instructions provided to make it easily understandable by British English speakers. The British English MAP-Hand was then psychometrically tested using both classical test theory and item response theory to provide quantitative assessments of the validity and reliability of this PROM in a UK population of adults with RA. The results of the analyses support the validity and the reliability of the British English Map-Hand [50, 51]. The raw score is a sufficient statistic for hand function, and an interval scale metric is provided on Table 3 [51].

Table 5 Concurrent validity of the British English MAP-Hand with quality of life measures

	HAQ20	Hand HAQ [ULHAQ]	DASH	SF36v2 Physical Function
MAP-Hand	0.88**	0.91**	0.93**	−0.80**

Key: Spearman's correlations; ** *p* <0.001

Discussion

The British English MAP-Hand is a brief, valid and reliable measure of hand activity performance, which can be completed in an average of 2 minutes by people with RA. Due to its ease of use and precision it is an ideal questionnaire to utilise in busy clinical environments, such as the NHS outpatient rheumatology and hand therapy clinics. As a psychometrically robust measure, it can be used to evaluate clinical outcomes, for research purposes, and to describe the patterns and extent of hand activity performance in people with RA in the UK.

Implications for clinical and research practice

The British English MAP-Hand correlated highly with the HAQ20 and ULHAQ [4]. Although these outcomes are measuring similar constructs, the MAP-Hand was developed using patient generated items and this is reflected in the way in which the functional limitation is defined and scores are calculated. For instance, the hand activity performance is measured in the MAP-Hand at a person-level functioning (activity) [52] with or without the use of aids and adaptations (i.e. gadgets). This means that the MAP-Hand functional limitation score does not increase when the responder appraise their ability to do an activity such as "Writing by hand" (item 15) as "No difficulty" due to their use of pen grip to reduce pain and ease function. People with RA are increasingly encouraged to self-manage their condition, which includes adherence to joint protection advice, that may require behavioural modifications and the use of aids and environmental adaptations [53]. In the hands PIP, thumb interphalangeal (IP) and Distal Interphalangeal (DIP) joints are most involved in executing tasks, hence the use of gadgets such as adapted cutlery, can and bottle opener, zip puller and button hooks are recommended by occupational therapists to encourage joint protection and decrease dependency on others to help with such activities (i.e. the need for help and assistance), decrease pain and prevent joint damage. Therefore use of aids and environmental adaptations are viewed as enablers of function and independence, rather than a marker of disability. Nevertheless, the scoring system used within the HAQ [21, 22] increases with the use of special device by 1 point, if the patient 'needs' help from others to do an activity by 2 points and if the patient usually needs both a special device and help from another person by 3 points [54]. Moreover, permanent adaptations of the person's environment (e.g. changing faucets in the bedroom or kitchen, using Velcro closures on clothing) are also counted as aids and devices [54]. This means, even if the responder has chosen to appraise their ability to do an activity as "without any difficulty" [scored 0] due to their use of aids and adaptations to enable function, their disability score will increase when they disclose the use of aids to help their functioning, unlike how the MAP-Hand is scored.

Another comparative scale that is commonly used in clinical and research practice and recently culturally validated for use in the UK is DASH [4]. DASH scores were also highly correlated with the MAP-Hand scores in this study (Table 6). DASH is a considerably larger, comprehensive scale of upper limb function, which also includes optional modules for assessing upper limb performance at work (WORKDASH) and measuring abilities and symptoms of athletes and performing artists (SPAMDASH). The optional modules are scored separately [4]. As the MAP-Hand, the DASH scores are calculated based on the responder's ability, regardless of how they do the task. However, unlike the MAP-Hand the DASH includes items measuring both activity limitation (person-level) and participation restriction (societal-level) and as well as the activities performed using hands, the arm and shoulder function is also measured. Although DASH is a comprehensive assessment including 30 items, QUICKDASH is available as a shorter version and consists of 11 items (6 daily activity ability; two symptoms (pain and tingling); and three participation) [4, 55]. Therefore, although the MAP-Hand and the DASH questionnaires appear to measure the same

construct at a first glance, their remits differ at conceptual and measurement level and clinicians and researchers should take these differences into consideration if they are having to choose the use of one measure over the other.

Statistical analysis

In this study the unidimensionality of the MAP-Hand was challenged by the CFA, but supported by the Rasch analysis. In both cases, substantial adjustments had to be made to accommodate the local dependency of the item set. The clusters of locally dependent items made clinical sense, grouping items with similar functional requirements, such as opening jars or cans.

Differential item function may also have contributed to the disturbance of dimensionality. The presence of DIF is not uncommon in health status measures of functioning [56]. The fact that, at any level of hand function males had more difficulty tying shoelaces may simply reflect that women are less likely to wear shoes with laces. Also that at any level of hand function, women have more problem opening jars may simply be a function of men having stronger grip. However at the scale level, the item DIF was cancelled out and, so as long as all 18 items are administered, the total score should remain unaffected.

In the analysis of the local independence, assumption took prominence, which was not reported in the original validation. This can inflate reliability, although in this case only marginally, and the level of reliability remained high, consistent with individual use. By using a testlet solution to absorb the local dependency, a satisfactory fit was achieved. The metric conversion that follows good fit will allow for an appropriate calculation of change scores, as well as aspects such as the minimal important difference, the calculations of which are invalid on ordinal scales [57].

Limitations

We only tested the British MAP-Hand in people with RA. Further testing of the British MAP-Hand in other conditions is needed to ensure the scale has validity and reliability for use in these conditions. In addition, further studies should consider longitudinal design with multiple follow-up points to test the British English MAP-Hand's ability to detect change in hand function over time (i.e. Responsiveness).

Conclusions

The British English version of the MAP-Hand has been linguistically and culturally validated, and found to be a

Table 6 Internal consistency and test-retest reliability of the British English MAP-Hand [Classical Testing]

	Cronbach's alpha	n for test-retest	Test 1 score Mean [SD]	Test 2 score Mean [SD]	ICC(2,1) (95% CI)
MAP-Hand	0.96	273	17.61 [11.65]	17.08 [11.53]	0.96 (0.94,0.97)

valid and reliable measure of hand function for people with RA in the UK. The British English MAP-Hand meets the COSMIN standards for evaluating the quality of PROM items [16] and can be used in both clinical practice and research.

Abbreviations
CFA: Confirmatory Factor Analysis; CFI: Comparative Fit Index; DASH: Disabilities of the Arm Shoulder Hand; DIF: Differential Item Functioning; DIP: Distal Interphalangeal; DMARDs: Disease Modifying Anti-Rheumatic Drugs; HAQ: Health Assessment Questionnaire; ICC: Intra-Class Correlations; MAP-Hand: The Measure of Activity Performance of the Hand; MCP: Metacarpophalangeal; MDC^{95}: Minimal Detectable Difference; NHS: National Health Service; NICE: The National Institute for Clinical Excellence; NRS: Numeric Rating Scales; PIP: Proximal Interphalangeal; PROMS: Patient Reported Outcome Measures; PSI: Person Separation Index; RA: Rheumatoid Arthritis; SD: Standard Deviation; SEM: Standard Error of Measurement; SF-36$_{v2}$: Short-Form 36; TLI: Tucker Lewis Index; UK: United Kingdom; ULHAQ: Upper Limb HAQ

Acknowledgements
The authors wish to thank all the study participants; Robert Peet and Kate Woodward-Nut, Centre for Health Sciences, University of Salford, for assistance with data collection and data entry; and all the Principal Investigators, rheumatology consultants, rheumatology and research nurses and occupational therapists assisting with participant recruitment and study support at the participating sites: Prof Terry O'Neill, Ann McGovern, Jennifer Green, Angharad Walker (Salford Royal Hospital); Prof Ian Bruce, Lindsey Barnes, Elizabeth Beswick, Sarah Evans (Manchester Royal Infirmary); Dr. Leena Dass, Dr. Sophia Naz, Lorraine Lock (North Manchester General Hospital); Dr. Chris Deighton, Alison Booth, Jo Morris (Royal Derby Hospital); Prof David Walsh, Debbie Wilson, Jayne Smith (Kings Mill Hospital, Sherwood Forest Hospitals NHS Foundation Trust); Dr. Chetan Mukhtyer, Loretta Dean, Susan Rowell (Norfolk and Norwich Hospitals); Dr. Bela Szenbenyi, Carol Gray (Diana Princess of Wales, Grimsby); Dr. Mike Green, Anne Gill, Lisa Carr (York Hospital); Dr. Kirsten Mackay, Julie Easterbrook, Liz Burnett (Torbay Hospital); Dr. Mike Green, Alison Miernik, Rachel Bailey-Hague (Harrogate District Hospital); Dr. Atheer Al-Ansari, Jayne Edwards, Julia Nicholas (Robert Jones & Agnes Hunt Hospital, Oswestry); Dr. Wendy Holden, Janet Cushnaghan, Angie Dempster, Hayley Paterson (Basingstoke and North Hampshire Hospital); Mr. David Johnson, Lindsey Barber, Jan Smith (Stepping Hill Hospital); Dr. Karen Douglas, Lucy Kadiki, Chitra Ramful, Daljit Kaur (Russell Hall Hospital, Dudley); Dr. Anca Ghiurlic, Christine Graver (Royal Hampshire Hospital, Winchester); Dr. Frank McKenna, Jane McConiffe (Trafford Hospitals); Dr. Sophia Naz and Lorraine Lock (Fairfield Hospital).

Funding
This paper presents independent research funded by the Arthritis Research UK [Grant No: 20031]. The views expressed of the authors are not necessarily of those of the NHS or Arthritis Research UK. The sponsor and the funding source (Arthritis Research UK) had no role in the design of this study, its execution, analyses, interpretation of the data, or decision to submit results, apart from study oversight.

Authors' contributions
AH conceived the study and was the Chief Investigator. AH, YP, AT and ST initiated the study design. AT, AH and YP conducted the statistical analysis. IK was an advisor and TSC member. All authors contributed to refinement of the study protocol and approved the final manuscript.

Competing interests
The authors declare that they have no competing interests.

Author details
^{1}Centre for Health Sciences Research, University of Salford, Salford, UK. ^{2}Swiss Paraplegic Research, Nottwil, Switzerland. ^{3}Division of Nursing, Midwifery & Social Work, University of Manchester, Manchester, UK. ^{4}Department of Occupational Therapy, Prosthetics and Orthotics, Oslo and Akershus University College of Applied Sciences, Oslo, Norway.

References
1. Imboden JB, Hellman DB, Stone JH. Current Dagnosis & Treatment Rheumatology. 3rd ed. USA: The McGraw-Hill Companies; 2013.
2. Hammond A, Prior Y. The effectiveness of home hand exercise programmes in rheumatoid arthritis: a systematic review. Br Med Bull. 2016:1–14. https://doi.org/10.1093/bmb/ldw024.
3. National Collaborating Centre for Chronic Conditions. In: Rheumatoid arthritis: national clinical guideline for management and treatment in adults. Royal College of Physicians; 2009. https://www.ncbi.nlm.nih.gov/pubmedhealth/PMH0009576/. Accessed 29 Mar 2018.
4. Hammond A, Prior Y, Tyson S. Linguistic validation, Validity and Reliability of the British English versions of the Disabilities of the Arm, Shoulder and Hand (DASH) questionnaire and QuickDASH in people with rheumatoid arthritis. BMC Musculoskelet Disord. 2018; 19–118 doi: https://doi.org/10.1186/s12891-018-2032-8. The British English DASH is available at: http://www.dash.iwh.on.ca/sites/dash/public/translations/DASH_English_UK.pdf Accessed 29 Mar 2018.
5. Durez P, Fraselle V, Houssiau F, Thonnard J-L, Nielens H, Penta M. Validation of the ABILHAND questionnaire as a measure of manual ability in patients with rheumatoid arthritis. Ann Rheum Dis. 2007;66:1098–105.
6. Duruoz MT, Poiraudeau S, Fermanian J, Menkes CJ, Amor B, Dougadoz M, et al. Development and validation of a rheumatoid hand functional disability scale that assesses functional handicap. J Rheumatol. 1996;23:1167–72.
7. Leeb BF, Sautner J, Andel I, Rintelen B. SACRAH: a score for assessment and quantification of chronic rheumatic affections of the hands. Rheumatology (Oxford, England). 2003;42:1173–8.
8. Chung KC, Pillsbury MS, Walters MR, Hayward RA, Arbor A. Reliability and validity testing of the Michigan hand outcomes questionnaire. J Hand Surg [Am]. 1998;23:575–87.
9. Paulsen T, Grotle M, Garratt A, Kjeken I. Development and psychometric testing of the patient-reported measure of activity performance of the hand (MAP-Hand) in rheumatoid arthritis. J Rehabil Med. 2010;42:636–44.
10. Kirwan JR, Hewlett SE, Heiberg T, Hughes RA, Carr M, Hehir M, et al. Incorporating the patient perspective into outcome assessment in rheumatoid arthritis: progress at OMERACT 7. J Rheumatol 2005; 32:2250–2256.
11. Sollerman C, Ejeskar A. Sollerman hand function test. A standardised method and its use in tetraplegic patients. Scand J Plast Reconstractive Surg Hand Surg. 1995;29:167–76.
12. Beaton DE, Bombardier C, Guillemin F, Ferraz MB. Guidelines for the process of cross-cultural adaptation of self-report measures. Spine. 2000;25(24):3186–91.
13. Acquadro C, Joyce CRB, Patrick DL, Ware JE, Wu AW. Linguistic validation manual for patient-reported outcomes (PRO) instruments. Mapi Res Trust. 2004; https://store.mapigroup.com/. Accessed 29 Mar 2018
14. Mokkink LB, Terwee CB, Patrick DL, Alonso J, Stratford PW, Knol DL et al. The COSMIN checklist for assessing the methodological quality of studies on measurement properties of health status measurement instruments: an international Delphi study. Qual Life Res 2010;19:539–549.
15. Mokkink LB, Terwee CB, Patrick DL, Alonso J, Stratford PW, Knol DL, Bouter LM, de Vet HCW. International consensus on taxonomy, terminology, and definitions of measurement properties: results of the COSMIN study. J Clin Epidemiol. 2010;63:737–45.
16. Terwee CB, Prinsen CAC, Chiarotto A, Westerman MJ, Patrick DL, Alonso J, Bouter LM, de Vet HCW, Mokkink LB. COSMIN methodology for evaluating the content validity of patient-reported outcome measures: a Delphi study. Qual Life Res. 2018; https://doi.org/10.1007/s11136-018-1829-0.
17. Hammond A, Tyson S. Prior Y, Hawkins R, Tennant a, Nordenskiold U, Thyberg I, Sandqvist G, Cederlund R. Linguistic validation and cultural adaptation of an English version of the evaluation of daily activity questionnaire in rheumatoid arthritis. Health Qual Life Outcomes. 2014;12(143)
18. Hammond A, Tennant A, Tyson A, Nordenskiold U, Hawkins R, Prior Y. The reliability and validity of the English version of the evaluation of daily activity questionnaire for people with rheumatoid arthritis. Rheumatology. 2015;54(9):1605–15.

19. Kirwan JR, Reeback JS. Stanford health assessment questionnaire modified to assess disability in British patients with rheumatoid arthritis. Br J Rheumatol. 1986;25(2):206–9.

20. Johnsson P, Eberhardt K. Hand deformities are important signs of disease severity in patients with early rheumatoid arthritis. Rheumatology. 2009;48:1398–401.

21. Ware JE Jr, Sherbourne CD. The MOS 36-item short-form health survey (SF-36). Conceptual framework and item selection. Med Care. 1992;30(6):473–83.

22. Ware JE Jr. SF-36 health survey update. Spine. 2000;25(24):3130–9.

23. Linacre JM. Sample Size and Item calibration stability. Rasch Meas Trans. 1994;7(4):328.

24. Brown TA. Confirmatory factor analysis for applied research: 2nd ed. London: Guildford Press; 2006.

25. Kline RB. Principles and practice of structural equation modeling third edition edn. New York: Guildford Press; 2011.

26. Muthén LK, Muthén BO. Mplus User's Guide. 6th ed. Los Angeles: Muthén & Muthén; 2011.

27. Christensen KB, Kreiner S. Monte Carlo tests of the Rasch model based on scalability coefficients. Br J Math Stat Psych. 2010;63:101–11.

28. StataCorp: Stata Statistical Software: Release 13. In. College Station: TX: StataCorp LP; 2013.

29. Leung YY, Png ME, Conaghan P, Tennant A. A systematic literature review on the application of Rasch analysis in musculoskeletal disease - a special interest group report of OMERACT 11. J Rheum. 2014;41(1):159–64.

30. Rasch G. Probabilistic models for some intelligence and attainment tests. Chicago: University of Chicago Press; 1960.

31. Luce RDTJ. Simultaneous conjoint measurement: a new type of fundamental measurement. J Math Psych. 1964;1:1–27.

32. Fischer GH, Molenaar IW. Rasch models: foundations, recent developments, and applications. New York: Springer; 1995.

33. Bond TG, Fox CM: Applying the Rasch Model. Fundamental Measurement in the Human Sciences. 2nd ed. Mahwah: University of Toledo; 2007.

34. Newby VA, Conner GR, Grant CP, Bunderson CV. The Rasch model and additive conjoint measurement. J Appl Meas. 2009;10(4):348–54.

35. Gustafsson JE. Testing and obtaining fit of data to the Rasch model. Br J Math Stat Psychol. 1980;33:205–33.

36. Marais I, Andrich D. Formalizing dimension and response violations of local independence in the unidimensional Rasch model. J Appl Meas. 2008;9(3):200–15.

37. Wainer HKG. Item clusters and computer adaptive testing: a case for testlets. J Educ Meas. 1987;24:185–202.

38. Andrich D. Cronbach's alpha in the presence of subscales. In: International conference on outcomes measurement. Maryland: Bathesda. p. 2010.

39. Smith EV Jr. Detecting and evaluating the impact of multidimensionality using item fit statistics and principal component analysis of residuals. J Appl Meas. 2002;3(2):205–31.

40. Tennant A, Penta, M., Tesio, L., Grimby, G., Thonnard, J-L., Slade, A. et al. Assessing and adjusting for cross cultural validity of impairment and activity limitation scales through differential item functioning within the framework of the Rasch model: the pro-ESOR project. Med Care 2004; 42(Suppl 1):37–48.

41. Terresi JA, Kleinman M, Ocepek-Welikson K. Modern psychometric methods for detection of differential item functioning: application to cognitive assessment measures. Stat Med. 2000;19:1651–83.

42. Tennant A, Conaghan PG. The Rasch measurement model in rheumatology: what is it and why use it? When should it be applied, and what should one look for in a Rasch paper? Arthritis Rheum. 2007;57(8):1358–62.

43. Masters G. A Rasch model for partial credit scoring. Psychometrika. 1982;47:149–74.

44. Andrich D, Sheridan BED, Luo G. RUMM2030: Rasch unidimensional models for measurement. Western Australia: RUMM. Laboratory. 2009;

45. Cronbach IJ. Coefficient alpha and the internal structure of tests. Psychometrika. 1951;16:297–333.

46. Stratford PW. Getting more from the literature: estimating the standard error of measurement from reliability studies. Physiother Can. 2004;56:27–30.

47. Donoghue D. Physiotherapy research and older people (PROP) group, stokes EK: how much change is true change? The minimum detectable change of the berg balance scale in elderly people. J Rehabil Med. 2009;41:343.

48. Terwee CB, Bot SDM, de Boer MR, et al. Quality criteria were proposed for measurement properties of health status questionnaires. J Clin Epidemiol 2007; 60:34–42.

49. Fitzpatrick R, Davey C, Buxton MJ, Jones DR. Evaluating patient-based outcome measures for use in clinical trials. Health Technol Assess. 1998;2(i-iv):1–74.

50. Prior Y, Hammond A, Tyson S, Tennant A. Development and testing of the British English measure of activity performance of the HAND (MAP_HAND) questionnaire in rheumatoid arthritis. Ann Rheum Dis. 2015;74(Suppl 2): 1324. https://doi.org/10.1136/annrheumdis-2015-eular.3404.

51. Prior Y, Tennant A, Hammond A, Tyson S. Psychometric testing of measure of activity performance in the hand (Map-Hand) questionnaire in rheumatoid arthritis: Rasch analysis. Clin Rehabil. 2015;29(10):1014.

52. International Classification of Functioning. Disability, and health. ICF. Geneva: World Health Organization; 2001.

53. Hammond A, Bryan J, Hardy A. Effects of a modular behavioural arthritis education programme: a pragmatic parallel-group randomized controlled trial. Rheumatology. 2008;47:1712–8.

54. The health assessment questionnaire (HAQ) disability index (di) of the Clinical health assessment questionnaire. https://www.niehs.nih.gov/research/resources/assets/docs/haq_instructions_508.pdf. Accessed 29 03 2018.

55. Kennedy CA, Beaton DE, Solway S, McConell S, Bombardier C. The DASH and QuickDASH outcome measure user's manual. 3rd ed. Institute for Work & Health: Toronto; 2011.

56. Randall M, Imms C, Carey LM, Pallant JF. Rasch analysis of the Melbourne assessment of unilateral upper limb function. Dev Med Child Neurol. 2014; 56(7):665–72.

57. Rouquette A, Blanchin M, Sebille V, Guillemin F, Cote SM, Falissard B, Hardouin JB. The minimal clinically important difference determined using item response theory models: an attempt to solve the issue of the association with baseline score. J Clin Epidemiol. 2014;67(4):433–40.

17

Burden of gluteal fibrosis and post-injection paralysis in the children of Kumi District in Uganda

Kristin Alves[1,6], Norgrove Penny[2], John Ekure[3], Robert Olupot[4], Olive Kobusingye[5], Jeffrey N. Katz[6] and Coleen S. Sabatini[7*]

Abstract

Background: The purpose of this study was to estimate the prevalence of postinjection paralysis (PIP) and gluteal fibrosis (GF) among children treated in a rural Ugandan Hospital.

Methods: We conducted a retrospective cohort study by reviewing the musculoskeletal clinic and community outreach logs for children (age < 18 yrs) diagnosed with either PIP or GF from Kumi Hospital in Kumi, Uganda between 2013 and 2015. We estimated the prevalence as a ratio of the number of children seen with each disorder over the total population of children seen for any musculoskeletal complaint in musculoskeletal clinic and total population of children seen for any medical complaint in the outreach clinic.

Results: Of 1513 children seen in the musculoskeletal clinic, 331 (21.9% (95% CI 19.8–24.1%)) had PIP and another 258 (17.1% (95% CI 15.2–19.0%)) had GF as their diagnosis. Of 3339 children seen during outreach for any medical complaint, 283 (8.5% (95% CI 7.6–9.5%)) had PIP and another 1114 (33.4% (95% CI 31.8–35.0%)) had GF. Of patients with GF, 53.9% were male with a median age of 10 years (50% between 7 and 12 years old). Of patients with PIP, 56.7% were male with a median age of 5 years (50% between 2 and 8 years old).

Conclusion: PIP and GF comprise over 30% of clinical visits for musculoskeletal conditions and 40% of outreach visits for any medical complaint in this area of Uganda. The high estimated prevalence in these populations suggest a critical need for research, treatment, and prevention.

Keywords: Gluteal fibrosis, Post-injection paralysis

Background

Approximately 12 billion intramuscular injections are administered annually worldwide for a wide range of conditions, with persons in limited-resource countries receiving an average two injections per year [1]. Over 70 % of these injections are estimated to be unnecessary [2]. Disabilities arising from injections include acute flaccid paralysis after injection due to sciatic nerve injury, also known as post-injection paralysis, and gluteal fibrosis [3–12]. Both of these entities have been reported among children in Uganda [4, 11].

When gluteal intramuscular injections are misdirected into the sciatic nerve or neurotoxic medications are delivered near the nerve, children may develop post-injection paralysis (PIP) acutely with loss of motor and sensory function of the sciatic nerve distal to the injection. The strong temporal association between the injections and subsequent neurologic findings argues for a causal relationship between injection and PIP. Children with post-injection paralysis present with varying degrees of the initial foot drop and the later acquired equino-varus foot deformities depending on timing of their presentation to the health care system [6–9, 11, 13, 14].

The etiology of gluteal fibrosis (GF) has not yet been determined; hypotheses range from a congenital collagen disorder to iatrogenic injection injury. The most

* Correspondence: Coleen.Sabatini@ucsf.edu
[7]University of California San Francisco Department of Orthopaedic Surgery, UCSF Benioff Children's Hospital Oakland, 747 52nd Street, OPC 1st Floor, Oakland, CA 94609, USA
Full list of author information is available at the end of the article

commonly reported hypothesis involves frequent gluteal intramuscular injections with the percentage of patients with gluteal fibrosis in the literature reporting a history of gluteal injections ranging from 51 to 100%. [3–5, 9, 10, 15, 16]. GF is characterized by hypertrophy of fibrotic tissue in the gluteal muscles that limits muscle excursion and therefore, hip range of motion. It was recognized and described in the 1970s [16, 17]. Patients with gluteal fibrosis present with difficulty with activities like squatting and sitting normally in a chair because they have limited excursion of the gluteal muscles causing external rotation and abduction when the hips are flexed actively or passively. On examination, patients are often found to have fixed abduction and external rotation with attempts at active or passive hip flexion. They have an awkward gait due to the deranged biomechanics raising concern for their risk of premature osteoarthritis [23]. The condition is usually bilateral and frequently diagnosed in school age children [3, 18, 19]. GF can limit the patient's ability to attend school and perform activities of daily living and community activities.

GF has been reported increasingly in Asia, Europe, Africa, and the USA [3–5, 9, 10, 12, 15–24]. However, few studies have assessed the prevalence of either PIP or GF in a particular, localized area. Published estimates for GF generally range between 1 and 2.5% in affected populations, with prevalence seen as high as 13.9% of the pediatric population in some districts of Taiwan [3, 12, 15, 18, 19, 22]. Both PIP and GF are seen commonly throughout Uganda, necessitating considerable care, yet the prevalence of these injuries in Uganda or elsewhere in East Africa has not been quantified, impeding efforts to estimate resource needs for these conditions [4, 8, 11]. Thus, our study aims to determine prevalence for GF and PIP in the pediatric population presenting for care in Kumi, a northeastern district of Uganda anecdotally known to have cases of GF and PIP.

Methods
Design
This was a retrospective cohort study of all pediatric children seen in Kumi Hospital's musculoskeletal clinic and in Kumi District's general medical outreach clinic logbooks between January 2013 and December 2015.

Setting
Kumi Hospital is a rural hospital located in Kumi District and serves the district's population through inpatient, outpatient and outreach services. Kumi Hospital has a musculoskeletal clinic located at the hospital for outpatients with musculoskeletal problems. The hospital also runs outreach programs held in outlying villages where patients are seen with a wide range of problems.

The study was approved by Makerere Institutional Review Board in Kampala, Uganda and the Uganda National Council for Science and Technology as well as the senior author's (CSS) institution.

Sample
The study sample included children (age ≤ 18 yrs) diagnosed with either PIP or GF from Kumi Hospital musculoskeletal clinic or Kumi District outreach medical visits between January 2013 and December 2015. Only children labeled as a new visit were recorded. PIP was diagnosed as initial acute flaccid paralysis after gluteal injection with later development of equinovarus foot deformity. GF was diagnosed as gluteal contractures causing limitation of hip range of motion, specifically obligate external rotation and abduction with hip flexion, with no other known cause.

Data sources and data elements
All patient information was obtained from written logbooks. The Kumi Hospital clinic logbooks included only patients seen in the clinic for musculoskeletal complaints (including pain, disability, deformity, or injury involving any extremity or the spine). The Kumi District Outreach visit logbooks included patients seen for any medical reason throughout Kumi District. For each set of logbooks, only patients ages 0–18 were collected for analysis. Data collected included patient's age, sex, village, diagnosis, and recommendation for treatment.

Reliability of data collection
Intraobserver reliability was assessed to ensure accuracy in data collection and data entry. KA selected 250 patients randomly and compared all variables entered into the database against the original log book entries; 100% of the variables matched initial entry. To determine interobserver reliability, a separate reviewer repeated the data abstraction process (from written logbook to Excel) on 100 randomly selected subjects. The two observers were in agreement on 99.7% of all data abstracted.

Furthermore, to ensure there was no overlap in patients seen with GF and PIP from the Kumi hospital clinic and Outreach logbooks, cross-checks between logbooks were performed. This process involved selecting groupings of GF and PIP patients seen in Outreach and cross checking Clinic logbooks to see if the same patient names showed up within a 3 month period after they were seen in Outreach. This process was performed for 200 patients with GF or PIP, with no evidence of children having been counted as a new patient for both Clinic and Outreach visits.

Data management

Once the logbook data was abstracted, patients' diagnoses and treatment recommendations were coded. Codes for diagnosis included: gluteal fibrosis, post-injection paralysis, both disorders, and other medical conditions. Codes for treatment recommendation included: surgery (only applicable for clinic visits), referral to surgeon (only applicable for outreach visits), physical therapy, assistive devices (i.e. ankle foot orthoses (AFOs)), and other recommendations (e.g. further testing including xrays, medications, etc.). The accuracy of these diagnosis codes was verified in a process in which the Principal Investigator examined the agreement between the diagnosis code and the actual diagnoses listed for every 4th patient entered in the database. The codes and original listed diagnosis agreed in 100% of the patients reviewed.

Statistical analysis

Statistical analysis was conducted using SAS 9.4 (SAS, Cary, NC, USA). For the clinic population, we estimated the prevalence of PIP, as a ratio of the number of children with a PIP diagnosis divided by the total population of children seen for any musculoskeletal complaint. For the community outreach population, we estimated the prevalence as the number of children with a PIP diagnosis divided by the total population of children seen for any medical complaint. The clinic and outreach prevalences of GF were estimated analogously. We used descriptive statistics (mean, median) to examine patient factors including sex, age, location and treatment recommendation. 95% confidence intervals were calculated assuming a binomial distribution. The median age of patients with PIP and those with GF were compared utilizing the Wilcoxon signed rank test. A p value of less than 0.05 was considered statistically significant. Treatment recommendations were determined and reported for each clinical setting.

Results

Of the 4852 total children, 1372 were diagnosed with gluteal fibrosis (28.3% (95% CI 27.0–29.6%)) and 614 were diagnosed with post-injection paralysis (12.7% (95% CI 11.8–13.6%)) (Table 1). Only 15 of these children were found to have both disabilities (0.3%). Of 1513 children seen in the musculoskeletal clinic, 331 (21.9% (95% CI 19.8–24.1%)) had PIP and another 258 (17.1% (95% CI 15.2–19.0%)) had GF as their diagnosis. Of 3339 children seen on outreach in the community for any medical complaint, 283 (8.5% (95% CI 7.6–9.5%)) had PIP and another 1114 (33.4% (95% CI 31.8–35.0%)) had GF as their diagnosis. The diagnosis of another fibrotic disease, quadriceps fibrosis (QF), was made in 46 children (1%).

Table 1 Demographic Distribution

	No (%)	Sex (% male)	Age (median, years) (25th – 75th percentile, years)
GF	1372 (28.3)	53.9	10 (7–12)
Outreach	1114	53.4	10 (7–12)
Clinic	258	55.8	10 (8–12)
PIP	614 (12.7)	56.7	5 (2–8)
Outreach	283	52.7	6 (3–9)
Clinic	331	60.1	4 (2–8)
Other	2881 (59.4)	54.6	6 (3–11)

Demographic distribution of Gluteal Fibrosis (GF) and Post-Injection Paralysis (PIP) in Kumi District, Uganda. Of note, 15 patients had GF and PIP diagnosis, 8 in outreach and 7 in clinic

For both GF and PIP, a larger proportion was male; this gender difference was greater in the clinic population (Table 1). The median age for the GF patients was 10 years (25th – 75th percentile 7–12 years) while the median age for the PIP patients was 5 (25th – 75th percentile 2–8 years) (Fig. 1). The prevalence of GF increased with age, peaking at age group 8–11. In contrast, PIP prevalence was highest in the younger children with a peak in 0–3 and declining thereafter (Fig. 1).

The majority of the children seen with GF were recommended to have release if seen in clinic (92.6%) and referral to a surgeon if seen on outreach visits (87.1%). In both the clinic and outreach settings, recommendations for PIP generally consisted of non-operative management including AFOs and physiotherapy (Table 2).

Discussion

This retrospective review of all pediatric patients seen over a 3-year span in a northeastern Ugandan musculoskeletal clinic and comprehensive community-based rehabilitation outreach program highlights the community burden of both PIP and GF. These disabilities were found to comprise over 30% of hospital clinic visits for musculoskeletal conditions and 40% of outreach visits for any medical complaint in this northeastern region of Uganda.

The slightly greater proportion of males with both diagnoses may reflect an increased propensity to seek care for male children, a trend noted in other cultures [3]. In this rural region of Uganda, traveling to clinic generally takes more time and resources than an outreach visit near the child's village. We found a correspondingly greater percent of children to be male in the clinic setting in comparison to the outreach setting.

The current hypothesis for the etiology of PIP and GF, and for the greater prevalence in this study than the 1–13.9% reported in other countries, revolves around the treatment of malaria [3, 15, 18, 19, 22]. Commonly in East Africa, infants and young children who develop high fevers are thought to be suffering from malaria.

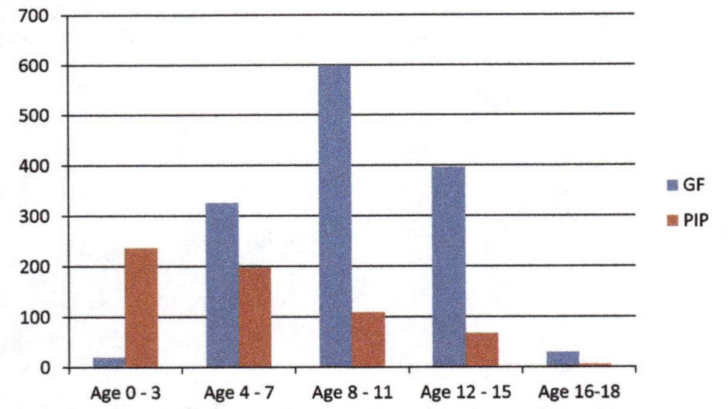

Fig. 1 Case Distribution by Age group. PIP was found more often in children under age 8 while GF more often found in children older than age 8. (*p-value < 0.0001 for association between age and diagnosis, Wilcoxon test)

averaged 10 years of age compared to 5 for children with PIP. Confirming the involvement of injections in the pathogenesis of GF, Ko et al. and Chung et al. note associations between intramuscular injections and gluteal fibrotic contractures in their case control studies with increasing odds of GF with increasing frequency of injections [3, 5]. The mechanisms of injury following injection have been hypothesized to include sterile abscesses, compartment syndrome caused by large volume injection, and muscle necrosis caused by toxic medications or toxic diluting solvents [12, 15, 21, 22]. Regardless of the cause, the common theory is that the fibrotic bands develop over time leading to clinical contracture at a later age.

Some authors further hypothesize a predisposing collagenous risk factor for gluteal fibrosis, with the intramuscular injection acting as a trigger mechanism [5, 16]. This intriguing theory finds some support in Uganda. While injection induced injuries (PIP) have been seen throughout the country, GF has been reported primarily in northeast Uganda, suggesting that an additional exposure may be acting as an effect modifier of the injections in this region. Further studies are underway to elucidate country wide prevalence and distribution of PIP versus GF, potential risks for development of these injection injuries to validate this claim and determine the focus of resources for prevention and treatment outcomes.

The current study demonstrates a large population of children in northeast Uganda suffering from PIP and GF with significant resource needs both for operative interventions and nonoperative (ie. AFOs and physical therapy) treatment. In addition to the significant proportion of children with PIP and GF, 46 children with quadriceps fibrosis were also seen, demonstrating even further potential injection-induced injuries and need for resources focused on injection induced disabilities and prevention education.

Our study must be interpreted in the context of methodologic limitations including retrospective data collection with a lack of data regarding potential sources of etiology of pathology, confirmation of and inclusion of only one region in Uganda. Another limitation of the

Patients' families seek care at various locations including local traditional healers, local clinics, hospitals, outreach clinics, pharmacies, etc. At one or another of these providers, children may receive a gluteal injection of medication and can develop acute PIP if the drug is neurotoxic or if the sciatic nerve is damaged directly. One prior assessment at Mulago Hospital in the capital of Uganda highlights this association, with 70% of the gluteal injections that resulted in PIP being administered for malaria or febrile illness. The medication quinine was involved in approximately 60% of those cases [8, 11]. Quinine is neurotoxic and can cause neural injury by being injected in the vicinity of the nerve [11]. It does not have to be injected into the nerve directly as it causes tissue necrosis. This neurotoxic intramuscular medication is presumably being given to children with suspected or diagnosed malaria although it is not recommended as a first line anti-malarial by the WHO [25].

While these practices help explain the potential cause of PIP in Uganda, little is known about the etiology and risk factors for gluteal fibrosis. The difficulty in determining the etiology of GF stems from the lack of a close temporal association with injections. Hang et al. and Napiontek et al. observed that GF developed two to 5 years after the damaging injections [9, 16]. This finding is consistent with our finding that children with GF

Table 2 Distribution of Treatment Recommendations

	No (%)	Surgery	Referral to Surgeon	Assistive Device	Physical Therapy	Other
Outreach Patients	3339					
GF	1114 (33.4)	n/a	970 (87%)	0	133 (12%)	11 (1%)
PIP	283 (8.5)	n/a	92 (33%)	109 (39%)	55 (19%)	27 (10%)
Clinic Patients	1513					
GF	258 (17.1)	239 (93%)	n/a	0	14 (5%)	5 (2%)
PIP	331 (21.9)	44 (13%)	n/a	151 (46%)	118 (36%)	18 (5%)

Distribution of treatment recommendations for Gluteal Fibrosis (GF) and Post-Injection Paralysis (PIP) in Kumi District, Uganda

study is the possibility of misdiagnosis as there are not confirmatory tests for these conditions outside the history and physical examination that are available in this environment. However, given the frequency of these conditions in the population, clinicians are very skilled at recognizing these findings on examination and when combined with relevant history questions, the diagnosis of PIP and GF can be confidently made. However, this study clearly demonstrates that a large proportion of pediatric patients seen for medical care are suffering from these disabilities in this region and supports the need for future research to determine the scope of the problem in Uganda. Further research should be focused on country-wide prevalence and incidence of GF and PIP, both quantitative and qualitative community-based studies to determine etiology and risk factors, as well as treatment studies to better understand how to care for children with these conditions.

While this study has focused on Uganda, prior studies have demonstrated sciatic nerve injury following injection in high and low resource countries alike [6, 7, 14]. To prevent further iatrogenic injuries it is imperative that countries begin to employ strict standards for injection education and delivery. In addition, it is important for orthopaedic surgeons to be aware of these diagnoses as noted by Scully et al. [10]. The unfamiliarity can lead to potential inaccurate diagnosis and treatment with children undergoing inappropriate operations with need for subsequent repeat surgery to correct the deformity. Resources for efforts to increase awareness and prevent further disability should be prioritized in addition to resources for the treatment of the current pediatric population suffering from these disabilities.

Conclusion

This study documents a concerning prevalence of PIP and GF in one area of Uganda and suggests an urgent need for more rigorous studies of country-wide prevalence, incidence, prevention and treatment outcomes. While population-based estimates of disease burden are sorely needed, the high estimated prevalence of these conditions in these clinical populations in Kumi, Uganda, suggest that substantial resources are needed to address these conditions currently. Simultaneously, appropriate policy and health systems changes are required to ensure appropriate health education and administration of injections to prevent further burden of injection-induced diseases in the pediatric population.

Abbreviations
GF: Gluteal Fibrosis; PIP: Post-injection paralysis

Funding
First author supported to perform research with NIH T32 grant: NIH 5T32AR055885-08.

Authors' contributions
All authors read and approved the final manuscript. Our list of authors and their individual contributions are as follows: KA performed data collection, data analysis, manuscript preparation. NP provided background information/context, manuscript preparation. JE provided background information/context, manuscript preparation. RO assisted in obtaining data for collection, manuscript preparation. OK helped with study design, assistance in obtaining Ugandan IRB, manuscript preparation. JK helped with study design, data analysis, manuscript preparation. CS helped with overall project oversight, study design, IRB preparation, obtained US & Ugandan IRB approval, data analysis, manuscript preparation.

Competing interests
The authors declare that they have no competing interests.

Author details
[1]Harvard Combined Orthopaedic Surgery Residency Program, Boston, MA, USA. [2]Department of Orthopaedic Surgery, University of British Colombia, Victoria, Canada. [3]Kumi Orthopaedic Center, Kumi, Uganda. [4]Kumi Hospital, Kumi, Uganda. [5]Makerere University School of Public Health, Kampala, Uganda. [6]Department of Orthopaedic Surgery, Brigham and Women's Hospital, Boston, MA, USA. [7]University of California San Francisco Department of Orthopaedic Surgery, UCSF Benioff Children's Hospital Oakland, 747 52nd Street, OPC 1st Floor, Oakland, CA 94609, USA.

References
1. World Health Organization. Safety of injections: a brief background. Fact sheet No. 231. Geneva: WHO; 1999.
2. World Health Organization. Unsafe injection practice and transmission of blood borne pathogens. WHO Bull. 1999;77:787–99.
3. Chung D, Ko Y, Pai H. A study on the prevalence and risk factors of muscular fibrotic contracture in Jia-dong township, Pingtung County, Taiwan. Gaoxiong Yi Xue Ke Xue Za Zhi. 1989;5:91–5.
4. Ekure J. Gluteal fibrosis. A report of 28 cases from Kumi hospital, Uganda. East and Central African Journal of Surgery. 2006;12:144–7.
5. Ko Y, Chung D, Pal H. Intramuscular-injection associated gluteal fibrotic contracture and hepatitis B virus infection among school children. Gaoxiong Yi Xue Ke Xue Za Zhi. 1991;7:358–62.
6. Mayer M, Romain O. Sciatic paralysis after a buttock intramuscular injection in children: an ongoing risk factor. Arch Pediatr. 2001;8:321–3.
7. Mishra P, Stringer M. Sciatic nerve injury from intramuscular injection: a persistent and global problem. Int J Clin Pract. 2010;64:1573–9.
8. Naddumba E, Ndoboli P. Sciatic nerve palsy associated with intramuscular quinine injection in children. East and Central African Journal of Surgery. 1999;4:17–20.
9. Napiontek M, Ruszkowski K. Paralytic drop foot and gluteal fibrosis after intramuscular injections. J Bone Joint Surg Br. 1993;75:83–5.
10. Scully W, White K, Song K, Mosca V. Injection-induced gluteus muscle contractures. diagnosis with the "reverse Ober test" and surgical management J Pediatr Orthop. 2015;35:192–8.
11. Sitati F, Naddumba E, Beyeza T. Injection-induced sciatic nerve injury in Ugandan children. Trop Dr. 2010;40:223–4.
12. Sun X. An investigation on injectional gluteal muscle contracture in childhood in Mianyang city. Zhonghua Liu Xing Bing Xue Za Zhi. 1990;11: 291–4.
13. Sharma S, Kale R. Post injection palsy in Chatisgarh region. Indian Pediatr. 2003;40:580–1.
14. Small S. Preventing sciatic nerve injury from intramuscular injections: literature review. J Adv Nurs. 2004;47:287–96.
15. Chen S, Chien C, Yu H. Syndrome of deltoid and/or gluteal fibrotic contracture: an injection myopathy. Acta Neurol Scand. 1988;78:167–76.
16. Hang Y. Contracture of the hip secondary to fibrosis of the gluteus maximus muscle. J Bone Joint Surg Am. 1979;61:52–5.
17. Valderrama J, Esteve de Miguel R. Fibrosis of the gluteus maximus: a cause of limited flexion and adduction of the hip in children. Clin Orthop Relat Res. 1981;(156):67–78.
18. Kotha V, Reddy R, Reddy M, et al. Congenital gluteus maximus contracture syndrome--a case report with review of imaging findings. J Radiol Case Rep. 2014;8:32 7.

19. Zhang K, Li P, Zhong-Ke L, et al. Treatment of gluteus contracture with small incisions: a report of 2518 cases. China Journal of Orthop Trauma. 2007;29:851–2.
20. Al Bayati M, Kraidy B. Gluteal muscle fibrosis with abduction contracture of the hip. Int Orthop. 2016;40:447–51.
21. Fu D, Yang S, Xiao B, et al. Comparison of endoscopic surgery and open surgery for gluteal muscle contracture. J Pediatr Orthop. 2011;31:e38–43.
22. Liu Y, Wang Y, Xue J, et al. Arthroscopic gluteal muscle contracture release with radiofrequency energy. Clin Orthop Relat Res. 2009;467:799–804.
23. Wang C, Gong Y, Li S, et al. Gluteal muscle contracture release for the treatment of gluteal muscle contracture induced knee osteoarthritis: a report of 52 cases. Zhongguo Gu Shang. 2011;24(7):594–6.
24. Zhang X, Ma Y, You T, et al. Roles of TGF-B/Smad signaling pathway in pathogenesis and development of gluteal muscle contracture. Connect Tissue Res. 2015;56:9–17.
25. Achan J, Talisuna A, Erhart A, et al. Quinine, an old anti-malarial drug in a modern world: role in the treatment of malaria. Malar J. 2011;10:144.

18

Is there a difference in joint line restoration in revision Total knee arthroplasty according to prosthesis type?

JuHong Lee, SungIl Wang and KiBum Kim*ⓘⒹ

Abstract

Background: The aim of this study is (1) to compare joint line (JL) restoration and clinical outcomes in revision TKA based on the contemporary prosthesis type and (2) to determine the restoration of posterior condylar offset (PCO) according to the use of a femoral offset stem.

Methods: Sixty knees that underwent revision TKA from April 2003 to December 2013 with a minimum of 1 year follow up were included. These were further subdivided into three groups according to prosthesis type: group I (2 mm offset), group II (4.5 mm offset), group III (2, 4, and 6 mm offset). The JL position change was defined as a change in the adductor tubercle distance, preoperatively versus postoperatively. We also collected the change of PCO in distal femur and clinical outcomes including range of motion (ROM) and knee scores at the preoperative and last follow-up periods.

Results: The JL elevation for group III was significantly lower than that of the other groups. Usage of the tibial and femoral offset stem in group III was more frequent than in the other groups. PCO in revision TKA with a femoral offset stem was significantly greater than in those with a femoral straight stem. The JL position in revision TKA with a femoral offset stem was less elevated than in those with a femoral straight stem.

Conclusions: More recent developed revision prosthesis with various sizes option of offset stem may be effective in restoring the native joint line as using the femoral offset stem more convenience in revision TKAs.

Keywords: Revision total knee arthroplasty, Joint line restoration, Offset stem, Posterior condylar offset

Background

Increasing numbers of total knee arthroplasties (TKAs) are being performed, with excellent clinical results [1]. Survivorship of primary TKA has been reported to be 90% or greater at 10 to 15 years of follow-up [2–5]. However, a small percentage of patients suffer from inevitable conditions such as infection, aseptic loosening, polyethylene wear, and instability requiring revision TKAs. Overall, orthopedic surgeons will be encountering an increase in the incidence of revision TKA [1].

Joint line (JL) restoration is essential for primary as well as revision TKAs. Unfortunately, there is a natural tendency of JL elevation during revision TKAs [6, 7]. Excessive JL elevation may result in decreased range of

motion (ROM) due to patella baja with impingement of the patella on the tibial component, anterior knee pain by increasing patellofemoral contact forces, increased component wear or extensor mechanism failure and mid flexion instability [7–9]. There are several recommendations to avoid JL elevation during revision procedures, including: (1) the size of the femoral component should be selected by medio-lateral remaining bone stock, not antero-posterior; (2) the flexion space should be kept as small as possible, as this results in a relatively larger flexion space after component removal and joint debridement, compared to the extension space; (3) a bone graft or metal augment should be used to reconstruct bone loss; (4) a constrained insert should be used in cases of extension-flexion gap mismatch [10]. Offset adapters, stem extensions and metal augments are commonly used to reconstruct the JL during revision TKA.

* Correspondence: tibikim@naver.com
Department Of Orthopaedic Surgery, Chonbuk National University Hospital, 20, Geonji-ro, Deokjin-gu, Jeonju 54907, South Korea

The restoration of posterior condylar offset (PCO) is also important in conjunction with restoring the JL to achieve a balance between the flexion and extension gaps [11]. Furthermore, the restoration of PCO improves clinical outcomes including ROM [12].

Although the above-mentioned surgical techniques are theoretically employed, JL restoration in revision TKAs is difficult to achieve due to the variability of metal augments and offset systems according to the implant manufacturer. To date, there is a paucity of studies comparing JL elevation according to the type of contemporary prosthesis depending on the variability of metal augments and offset system.

Therefore, we hypothesize that there is difference in JL elevation according to the type of contemporary prosthesis and this difference will affect the clinical outcomes. The aim of the present study is (1) to compare JL elevation based on the type of contemporary prosthesis in revision TKAs, (2) to determine the restoration of posterior condylar offset (PCO) according to the use of femoral offset stem, and (3) to determine the association between clinical outcomes and the amount of JL elevation.

Methods
Patients
We retrospectively reviewed case series of 75 knees that underwent revision TKA from April 2003 to December 2013 with approval from the Institutional Review Board of Chonbuk National University Hospital. All consecutive revision TKAs were performed by a senior surgeon (JHL). We excluded seven knees that had incomplete clinical and radiologic data due to loss of follow up, six knees using valgus-varus constraint polyethylene (PE) insert, 1 re-revision knee and 1 knee using the structural allobone graft in order to control for JL position bias. Finally, 60 knees with a minimum of 1-year of follow up were enrolled in the present study. The mean duration of follow-up was 62 months (ranging from 12 to 96 months). Of the 60 knees, 38 were of female patients and 22 were of male patients. Etiologies in this case series were periprosthetic joint infections (PJIs) (48 knees), aseptic loosening (9 knees), instability (2 knees), and PE wear (1 knee).

The revision TKAs were sequentially performed using three different revision prostheses. The PFC® Sigma knee system (Depuy, Warsaw, Indiana) was used in 17 knees from July 2004 to February 2006, the NexGen® LCCK system (Zimmer, Warsaw, Indiana) was used in 13 knees from May 2006 to November 2010, and the Legion® total knee system (Smith & Nephew, London, UK) was used in 30 knees from May 2011 to December 2013. The three revision systems used in this study differed in the size of metal augment, femoral offset and modularity (Table 1). Demographic datas including follow-up period of the three groups are presented in Table 2.

Operative technique
All revision TKAs for PJI were performed in two stages with the appropriate antimicrobial treatments, while surgeries for the other etiologies were performed in one stage. There was one re-revision case due to recurrence of PJI.

Similar to most revision TKAs, a standard medial parapatellar approach was performed in all procedures. When confronted with exposure difficulty due to tissue scarring or adhesion and patella baja, we conducted an additional procedure such as a rectus snip or tibial tubercle osteotomy. In this study, 5 cases required a rectus snip and 2 cases required a tibial tubercle osteotomy.

Femoral and tibial bone defects were assessed by the Anderson Orthopedic Research Institute (AORI) classification after removal of the original prosthesis [13]. Restoration of the native JL was the main goal with reconstruction of the tibia and femur by the prosthesis, including metal augments and offset systems. JL position was determined intraoperatively by measurement of the length from anatomical landmarks to the reconstructed JL. To obtain symmetry between the extension and flexion gaps, decreasing the flexion gap as much as possible was targeted by (1) using the larger femoral components unless an overhang of the mediolateral width of the remaining femoral bone stock was present, (2) a posterior translation of the femoral component whenever possible without notching the anterior femoral cortex.

Other intraoperative variables were also recorded such as grade of bone defects, thickness and constrained type of polyethylene, and whether bone grafts, metal augment and an offset stem of the tibia and femur were used or not. Finally, the prosthetic components were fixed with cement. The arthrotomy was closed in a routine manner. Identical post-operative management and rehabilitation protocol was conducted in all patients.

Clinical and radiologic evaluation
For clinical evaluation, clinical data such as ROM, Knee Society knee score (KSKS), Knee Society function score (KSFS), and Western Ontario and McMaster Universities Osteoarthritis (WOMAC) index score were collected at the preoperative period and the last follow-up visit. Radiologic parameters including adductor tubercle distance (ATD), PCO and tibiofemoral angle were measured with the standing long leg anterior-posterior (AP) view and 30-degree flexion true lateral views of the knee with completely overlapping femoral condyles. ATD was defined as the perpendicular distance between the adductor tubercle and the most distal point on the medial supracondylar slope of the femur and the JL was defined as the tangent to the most distal points of the medial and lateral femoral condyles [14]. Figure1-A PCO was defined as the maximal thickness of the posterior condyle projected posteriorly to the tangent of the posterior

Table 1 Characteristics of the revision prosthesis systemsd

	Group 1[a]	Group 2[b]	Group 3[c]
Femoral Offset	2 mm (Anterior or Posterior)	4.5 mm (360°)	2,4,6 mm (360°)
Tibial Offset	4 mm (360°)	4.5 mm (360°)	2,4,6 mm (360°)
Offset Adapter	x	x	o
Modularity[d] (piece)	3	2	3
Femoral Augments	4, 8, 12, 16 mm	5, 10, 15, 20 mm	5, 10, 15 mm
Tibial Augments	10, 15 mm	5, 10, 15, 20 mm	5, 10, 15 mm

[a]PFC® Sigma knee system (Depuy, Warsaw, Indiana)
[b]NexGen® LCCK system (Zimmer, Warsaw, Indiana)
[c]Legion® total knee system (Smith & Nephew, London, UK)
[d]The number of pieces in each femoral and tibial component after using the stem and offset adapter

cortex of the femoral shaft [15]. Figure 1-B To assess intra-observer reliability, the ATD and PCO were measured twice by one author (KBK), at a 1 month interval. To assess inter-observer reliability, a second author (SIW) measured the ATD and PCO.

In 56 cases with an unreplaced knee radiograph on the same or contralateral side, the change in JL position and PCO were defined as the difference between the ATD and PCO measured in the unreplaced knee radiograph and the postoperative ATD and PCO. Otherwise, in 4

Table 2 Preoperative characteristics of each group

	Group 1 ($n = 17$)	Group 2 ($n = 13$)	Group 3 ($n = 30$)	p-value
Age (years)	67.9 ± 4.5	66.4 ± 6.9	72.1 ± 7.6	0.07
Sex (M/F)	7/10	3/10	12/18	0.52
Cause of revision				0.6
PJI	14(82.4%)	9(69.2%)	24(80%)	
Aseptic loosening	2(11.8%)	3(23.1%)	5(16.7%)	
Instability	0	1(7.7%)	1(3.3%)	
PE wear	1(5.9%)	0	0	
Bone defect				
Femur				
I	0	2(15.4%)	1(3.3%)	0.14
IIA	2(11.8%)	1(7.7%)	0	
IIB	15(88.2%)	9(69.2%)	25(83.3%)	
III	0	1(7.7%)	4(13.3%)	
Tibia				
I	11(64.7%)	7(53.8%)	12(40%)	0.42
IIA	2(11.8%)	4(30.8%)	10(33.3%)	
IIB	4(23.5%)	2(15.4%)	8(26.7%)	
III	0	0	0	
Knee scores				
KSKS	46.5 ± 10.7	38.7 ± 8.6	43.2 ± 11.2	0.12
KSFS	39.4 ± 13.4	33.8 ± 10.8	41.7 ± 13.9	0.21
WOMAC	84.4 ± 14.4	88.8 ± 7.0	87.8 ± 8.2	0.87
Range of motion(°)	104.7 ± 15.5	105 ± 28.9	95.3 ± 27.7	0.54
Weight (kg)	61.1 ± 12.6	59.5 ± 9.3	59.8 ± 13.7	0.79
Height(m)	1.55 ± 0.09	1.52 ± 0.05	1.54 ± 0.12	0.6
BMI (kg/m^2)	25.3 ± 4.6	25.8 ± 3.0	25.2 ± 4.5	0.85
Follow up period (months)	66.1 ± 9.7	63.3 ± 10.3	60.7 ± 8.1	0.03

Data are presented as mean ± standard deviation or number (percentage), unless otherwise stated

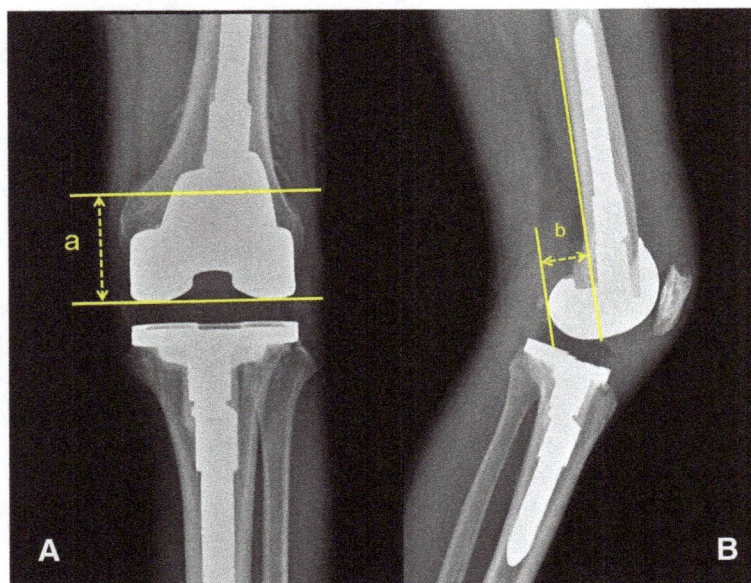

Fig. 1 Radiologic measurement of the adductor tubercle distance (a) and the posterior condylar offset (PCO) of the femur (b) in a standing anteroposterior view (**a**) and a 30-degree flexion lateral view (**b**), respectively

cases without an unreplaced knee radiograph on the same or contralateral side, the change in JL was defined as the difference between the preoperative ATD and PCO on the contralateral replaced knee radiograph and postoperative ATD and PCO on the operated side.

Overall, knees were divided into three groups based on the three different prosthesis types, prosthesis had difference of direction and size option of offset stem (Group I - PFC® Sigma knee system, Group II - NexGen® LCCK system, Group III - Legion® total knee system).

The JL elevation, change of PCO, and clinical outcomes such as ROM and knee scores were compared among the three groups. We analyzed the correlation between change of JL, PCO and intraoperative variables to answer the question ``which is the effect about the restoration of JL and PCO during revision TKAs? ``.

Statistical analysis

Repeatability and reproducibility of the radiologic measurements, such as ATD and PCO, were evaluated by calculating the intra-observer and inter-observer correlation coefficients. It was interpreted as poor if less than 0.4, marginal if greater than or equal to 0.4, but less than 0.75, and good when greater than 0.75. The difference in clinical outcomes after revision TKA was analyzed using a paired t-test. The radiologic and clinical variates among the three groups were analyzed by a Kruskal-Wallis test. The comparison of the change of JL and PCO according to the use of the femoral offset system was analyzed by a Mann-Whitney test. The correlation between change of JL, PCO and intraoperative

variables was analyzed by Pearson's correlation analysis. All statistical analyses were performed using SPSS for Windows, version 21.0 (SPSS, Chicago, Illinois). The level of significance was set at 5% ($p < 0.05$).

Results

There was significant improvement in clinical outcomes, including ROM and knee scores (KSKS, KFKS and WOMAC), at the last follow-up visit Table 3. The JL position based on the change of ATD had a mean elevation of 2.3 ± 2.8 mm (ranging from -3.92 mm to 9.92 mm). Fourteen knees (23.3%) were found to have a JL depression and 46 knees (76.7%) were found to have a JL elevation. Figure 2 Intraoperative variables among the three groups are delineated in Table 4. Both tibial and femoral stems were used more commonly in group III than in groups I and II. There was not a significant difference in the

Table 3 Clinical outcomes pre-operatively and at the last follow-up

	Pre-operative	Last follow-up	P-value
Tibiofemoral angle(°)	varus 0.2° ± 7.1°	valgus 4.6° ± 3.2°	0.00
Range of motion(°)	100.1 ± 25.2	108.8 ± 20.2	0.00
Flexion contracture(°)	6.6 ± 7.5	1.2 ± 2.5	0.00
Further flexion(°)	106.7 ± 21	109.9 ± 19.2	0.01
Knee scores			
KSKS	43.2 ± 11.2	86.7 ± 9.4	0.00
KSFS	39.3 ± 13.3	78.4 ± 9.7	0.00
WOMAC	87.1 ± 10.1	17.1 ± 7.5	0.00

Data are presented as mean ± standard deviation, unless otherwise stated

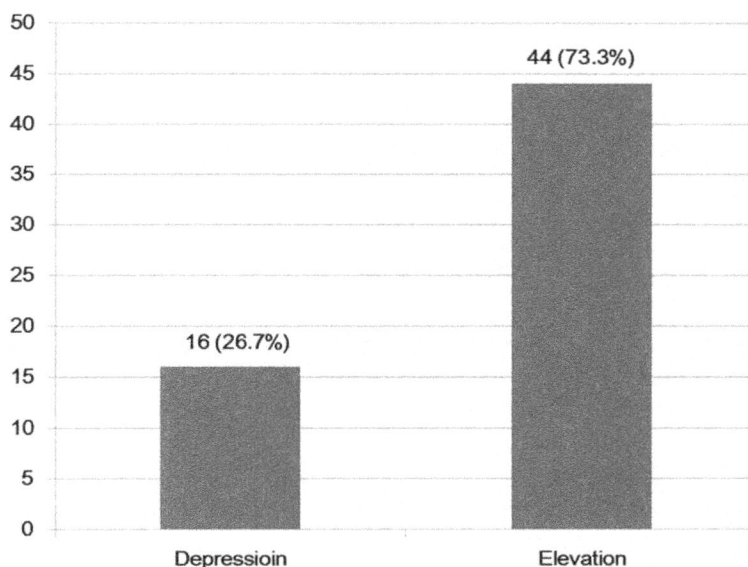

Fig. 2 The distribution of JL position after revision TKA in all case series (A) and by group (B)

utilization of tibial and femoral augments, with the exception of distal lateral femoral augments.

JL position was elevated in all three groups. JL elevation in group III (1.2 ± 2.8 mm) was significantly lower than that of the other two groups (group I: 3.6 ± 2.6 mm, group II: 3.4 ± 2.3 mm). However, there was no significant difference in knee scores (KSKS, KFKS and WOMAC) and ROM among the three groups. The postoperative PCO was restored or increased relative to preoperative PCO in all three groups.

The change in PCO was not significantly different between the three groups Table 5.

Size of femoral offset stem among the intraoperative variables had a statistical significant correlation with change of JL and PCO, respectively ($r = -0.29$, $r = 0.32$) Table 6. Based on these results, comparing the change of JL and PCO according to using femoral offset stem, the change of PCO in revision TKAs with a femoral offset stem was significantly greater than in those with a femoral straight stem. ($p = 0.03$) The JL position in revision

Table 4 Intraoperative variables, by group

	Group 1 (n = 17)	Group 2 (n = 13)	Group 3 (n = 30)	P-value
Femoral stem				
Offset/Straight (n)	9(53%) / 8(47%)	4(31%) / 9(69%)	29(97%) / 1(3%)	0.00
Size of offset (mm)	1.1 ± 1	1.4 ± 2.2	4.7 ± 1.7	0.00
Tibial stem				
Offset/Straight (n)	0(0%)/17(100%)	0(0%)/13(100%)	26(87%) / 4(13%)	0.00
Size of offset (mm)	0	0	3.7 ± 2.0	0.00
Metal Augments (n/size)				
Femoral Distal medial	16(94%) / 5.6 ± 2.5	9(69%) / 5 ± 4.1	26(87%) / 6 ± 3.3	0.16 / 0.38
Distal lateral	15(88%) / 5.4 ± 2.8	8(62%) / 4.6 ± 4.3	28(93%) / 6.5 ± 3.5	0.03 / 0.2
Posteromedial	17(100%) / 6.1 ± 2.1	11(85%) / 7.3 ± 3.9	24(80%) / 5 ± 3.2	0.15 / 0.08
Posterolateral	17(100%) / 6.1 ± 2.1	12(92%) /6.5 ± 3.2	24(80%) / 5.8 ± 4.0	0.11 / 0.49
Anterior	0 / 0	1(8%) / 0.4 ± 1.4	0 / 0	0.16 / 0.16
Tibial Medial	6(35%) / 4.1 ± 5.9	9(69%) / 5.8 ± 4.9	16(53%) / 4.5 ± 5.3	0.18 / 0.49
Lateral	4(24%) / 2.4 ± 4.4	2(15%) / 0.8 ± 1.9	8(27%) / 1.8 ± 3.6	0.72 / 0.67
Thickness of PE (mm)	15.9 ± 2.9	16 ± 2.6	14.9 ± 3.3	0.29

Data are presented as mean ± standard deviation or number (percentage), unless otherwise stated

Table 5 Comparison of the radiologic measurements and clinical outcomes between the three groups

	Group 1 (n = 17)	Group 2 (n = 13)	Group 3 (n = 30)	P-value
Change of ATD (mm)	3.6 ± 2.6	3.4 ± 2.3	1.2 ± 2.8	0.00
Change of PCO (mm)	0.5 ± 2.6	0.8 ± 3.0	1.3 ± 2.2	0.58
Knee scores				
KSKS	87.7 ± 4.7	86 ± 16.4	86.5 ± 7.4	0.32
KSFS	77.6 ± 7.3	78.5 ± 13.8	78.8 ± 9.1	0.65
WOMAC	20.1 ± 9.4	15.6 ± 7.5	16.1 ± 6.0	0.26
Range of motion(°)	112.1 ± 12.4	110.4 ± 24.2	106.22.2	0.62
Flexion contracture(°)	0.3 ± 1.2	1.2 ± 3.0	1.7 ± 2.7	0.14
Further flexion(°)	112.4 ± 12.0	111.5 ± 21.9	107.8 ± 21.5	0.75

Data are presented as mean ± standard deviation, unless otherwise stated

TKAs with a femoral offset stem was statistically significantly less elevated than in those with a femoral straight stem. ($p = 0.04$) Table 7.

More than 5 mm change of JL was 9 knees (15%) in our case series. However, there was no significant difference in clinical outcomes between knees with 5-mm or greater JL elevation or depression and the others. Table 8.

The intra-observer and inter-observer correlation coefficients were 0.94 and 0.88 for ATD and 0.89 and 0.83 for PCO, respectively, confirming good repeatability and reproducibility of the ATD and PCO measurements.

Discussion

The most important findings of the present study were that (1) the type of prosthesis used in group III was superior for restoring JL position although there was no significant difference in clinical outcomes between the three different types of prostheses, (2) using the femoral offset stem was beneficial for restoration of JL position by lessening the flexion gap, and (3) JL elevation or depression of 5 mm or greater did not deteriorate the clinical outcomes in this case series.

Table 6 Correlation coefficient (r) from Pearson's correlation analysis between change of JL, PCO and intraoperative variables

Size	Change of JL		Change of PCO	
	r	p	r	p
Femoral offset	−0.29	0.03*	0.32	0.01*
Femoral anterior augment	0.33	0.12	0.12	0.37
Femoral distal medial augment	−0.12	0.37	−0.02	0.86
Femoral distal lateral augment	−0.17	0.2	0.02	0.91
Femoral posterior medail augment	0.2	0.12	0.3	0.02*
Femoral posterior lateral augment	0.17	0.21	0.3	0.02*
Tibial medial augment	−0.07	0.59	−0.15	0.25
Tibial lateral augment	−0.05	0.71	−0.3	0.21

*: statistically significant

There are several methods available to determine JL position using plain radiographs. These methods typically use the distance between the JL and bony landmarks, such as the medial and lateral epicondyles, adductor tubercle, tibial tubercle and fibular head tip [16–18]. Various studies have reported the joint line position as an absolute value of these distances. However, recent studies have proposed that a ratio of these distances to the femoral width (the distance between the medial and lateral femoral epicondyles) has a theoretical advantage due to large variations between genders and different sized knees, making absolute values less useful [19, 20]. In revision TKA, bony landmarks are not always identified due to destruction by osteolysis and soft tissue scarring. In the present study, 57 of 60 knees were determined to have femoral bone defects greater than grade II and therefore the absolute value of the difference between the preoperative and postoperative ATD was inevitably used to determine the change of JL position.

The JL position in the present study was elevated by a mean of 2.3 mm and the PCO was enlarged by a mean of 1.0 mm after that revision TKA and clinical outcomes were comparable to previous studies of revision TKAs [21, 22]. These results were obtained using sufficient and appropriate metal augments (distal femoral augments in 55 (91.7%) of 60 knees, posterior femoral augments in 56 (93.3%) of 60 knees and femoral offset system in 42 (70%) of 60 knees). This resulted in restoration of PCO, and the JL position in group III was less elevated than in the two other groups.

We frequently encountered the difficult situations during revision TKAs and should solved these problems such as mismatch of metaphysis and diaphysis, unequal gap between extension and flexion space, asymmetry of mediolateral gap in flexion space to obtain stable and well functional reconstructed knee joint in revision TKAs [10, 23]. Offset stems were essential option to solve these problems in revision TKAs. Additionally, femoral offset stem had the theoretical advantages of restoration of PCO and JL [11]. In most revision TKAs,

Table 7 Comparison of the change of ATD and PCO, by use of a femoral offset stem, regardless of prosthesis type

	Offset stem (n = 42)	Straight stem (n = 19)	P-value
Change of ATD (mm)	2.0 ± 3.0	3.4 ± 2.1	0.04
Change of PCO (mm)	1.5 ± 2.4	−0.4 ± 2.2	0.03

Data are presented as mean ± standard deviation

We encountered the larger flexion gap than extension gap. To avoid the elevation of JL, We should be lessened the flexion gap by using larger femoral component and downward femoral offset stem. Unfortunately, we could not use the offset stem even if we had to use it in complex revision TKAs due to notching of anterior femoral cortex. We thought that revision knee prosthesis commonly used was not patient specific prosthesis. Therefore, various sizes and universal direction (360 degree) of offset stem in revision knee prosthesis is important to be able to cope with complex and difficulty situations. Interestingly, we found that usage of a femoral offset stem was more frequent in group III than in the other two groups. The prosthesis used in group III was the most recent contemporary prosthesis with more options in the offset system in terms of size and modularity. This prosthesis might allow surgeons to use the offset system more readily in complex revision TKAs. Likewise, a tibial offset stem was also used more frequently in group III than in the other groups, which supports our hypothesis. More frequent usage of femoral offset stems may also be associated with the less elevated JL position in group III, compared to the other two groups.

JL restoration following primary and revision TKAs has been shown to affect clinical outcomes and patient satisfaction. In particular, JL restoration in revision TKAs yields significantly better results than when it is left unrestored by more than 5 mm [24]. A JL elevation greater than 8 mm results in better knee society scores than that of less than 8 mm [7, 25].

Table 8 Comparison of the clinical outcomes between a 5-mm elevation or depression in JL position and the other else

	≥5-mm JL elevation or depression (n = 9)	The other else (n = 51)	P-value
Range of motion(°)	95.6 ± 25.8	111.1 ± 18.4	0.08
Flexion contracture(°)	1.7 ± 3.5	1.1 ± 2.3	0.77
Further flexion(°)	97.2 ± 22.7	112.2 ± 17.8	0.06
Knee scores			
KSKS	82.3 ± 19	87.5 ± 6.5	0.85
KSFS	73.9 ± 13.9	79.2 ± 8.7	0.35
WOMAC	21 ± 11	16.5 ± 6.7	0.24

Data are presented as mean ± standard deviation

There was no association between the level of JL elevation and clinical outcomes in the present study, namely no difference in clinical outcomes was observed between the knees with JL changes of 5 mm or greater and the others. The predominant cause of revision TKA in the present study was PJI (80%). Septic revision TKAs have been shown to have inferior clinical results compared to aseptic revisions [26]. We thought that large proportion of septic revision TKAs in our cases may be affect the similar clinical outcomes regardless of JL elevation and prosthesis type.

There were several limitations in the present study. First, a relatively small sample size in each group was retrospectively reviewed. Second, unfortunately the native JL level could not be identified in 4 (6.7%) cases due to the absence of an unreplaced knee radiograph. We thought that it was serious limitation of this study, however, we enrolled and analyzed the 4 cases because it occupied the relatively small proportion of our case series. Third, the cause of revision was heterogeneous with PJI being the most common. Fourth, we classified femoral and tibial bone defects according to the AORI grading system, although this classification has limitation regarding the severity of bony defects. In particular, in grade II, the AORI grading system does not distinguish between mild to severe defects. This may affect the results showing no association between the femoral bone defects classified by the AORI grading system and JL elevation. Finally, we inevitably compared the clinical outcomes among the three group at last follow up period that was inhomogeneous period. It seemed to have the bias to interpret our results, however, mean follow-up period was comparable even though there were difference of follow up period among the three groups.

Conclusion

More recent developed revision prosthesis with various sizes option of offset stem may be effective in restoring the native joint line as using the femoral offset stem more convenience in revision TKAs. Further studies with more patients and well-designed randomized controlled designs are required to confirm the results of the present study.

Abbreviations
ATD: adductor tubercle distance; JL: joint line; KSFS: Knee Society function score; KSKS: Knee Society knee score; PCO: posterior condylar offset; ROM: range of motion; TKA: total knee arthroplasty; WOMAC: Western Ontario and McMaster Universities Osteoarthritis

Funding
This paper was supported by Fund of Biomedical Research Institute and Chonbuk National University Hospital. The authors declare that they have no conflict of interest.

Authors' contributions

JHL collected data, performed the statistical analysis with interpretation and wrote the manuscript. SIW participated in the design of the study and coordination and helped to draft the manuscript. KBK participated in the design of the study and proofread the manuscript as the corresponding author. All authors read and approved the final manuscript.

Competing interests

The authors declare that they have no competing interests.

References

1. Kurtz S, Mowat F, Ong K, Chan N, Lau E, Halpern M. Prevalence of primary and revision total hip and knee arthroplasty in the United States from 1990 through 2002. J Bone Joint Surg Am. 2005;87(7):1487–97.
2. Abdeen AR, Collen SR, Vince KG. Fifteen-year to 19-year follow-up of the Insall-Burstein-1 total knee arthroplasty. J Arthroplast. 2010;25(2):173–8.
3. Parsch D, Kruger M, Moser MT, Geiger F. Follow-up of 11-16 years after modular fixed-bearing TKA. Int Orthop. 2009;33(2):431–5.
4. Roberts VI, Esler CN, Harper WM. A 15-year follow-up study of 4606 primary total knee replacements. J Bone Joint Surg Br Vol. 2007;89(11):1452–6.
5. Vessely MB, Whaley AL, Harmsen WS, Schleck CD, Berry DJ. The Chitranjan Ranawat award: long-term survivorship and failure modes of 1000 cemented condylar total knee arthroplasties. Clin Orthop Relat Res. 2006; 452:28–34.
6. Laskin RS. Joint line position restoration during revision total knee replacement. Clin Orthop Relat Res. 2002;404:169–71.
7. Partington PF, Sawhney J, Rorabeck CH, Barrack RL, Moore J. Joint line restoration after revision total knee arthroplasty. Clin Orthop Relat Res. 1999; 367:165–71.
8. Konig C, Sharenkov A, Matziolis G, Taylor WR, Perka C, Duda GN, Heller MO. Joint line elevation in revision TKA leads to increased patellofemoral contact forces. J Orthop Res. 2010;28(1):1–5.
9. Martin JW, Whiteside LA. The influence of joint line position on knee stability after condylar knee arthroplasty. Clin Orthop Relat Res. 1990;259: 146–56.
10. Bellemans J. Restoring the joint line in revision TKA: does it matter? Knee. 2004;11(1):3–5.
11. Mahoney OM, Kinsey TL. Modular femoral offset stems facilitate joint line restoration in revision knee arthroplasty. Clin Orthop Relat Res. 2006;446:93–8.
12. Clement ND, MacDonald DJ, Hamilton DF, Burnett R. Posterior condylar offset is an independent predictor of functional outcome after revision total knee arthroplasty. Bone Joint Res. 2017;6(3):172–8.
13. Engh GA, Ammeen DJ. Bone loss with revision total knee arthroplasty: defect classification and alternatives for reconstruction. Instr Course Lect. 1999;48:167–75.
14. Hofmann AA, Kurtin SM, Lyons S, Tanner AM, Bolognesi MP. Clinical and radiographic analysis of accurate restoration of the joint line in revision total knee arthroplasty. J Arthroplast. 2006;21(8):1154–62.
15. Bellemans J, Banks S, Victor J, Vandenneucker H, Moemans A. Fluoroscopic analysis of the kinematics of deep flexion in total knee arthroplasty. Influence of posterior condylar offset. J Bone Joint Surg Br Vol. 2002;84(1):50–3.
16. Iacono F, Lo Presti M, Bruni D, Raspugli GF, Bignozzi S, Sharma B, Marcacci M. The adductor tubercle: a reliable landmark for analysing the level of the femorotibial joint line. Knee Surg Sports Traumatol Arthrosc. 2013;21(12):2725–9.
17. Romero J, Seifert B, Reinhardt O, Ziegler O, Kessler O. A useful radiologic method for preoperative joint-line determination in revision total knee arthroplasty. Clin Orthop Relat Res. 2010;468(5):1279–83.
18. Havet E, Gabrion A, Leiber-Wackenheim F, Vernois J, Olory B, Mertl P. Radiological study of the knee joint line position measured from the fibular head and proximal tibial landmarks. Surg Radiol Anat. 2007;29(4):285–9.
19. Servien E, Viskontas D, Giuffre BM, Coolican MR, Parker DA. Reliability of bony landmarks for restoration of the joint line in revision knee arthroplasty. Knee Surg Sports Traumatol Arthrosc. 2008;16(3):263–9.
20. LaPrade RF, Engebretsen AH, Ly TV, Johansen S, Wentorf FA, Engebretsen L. The anatomy of the medial part of the knee. J Bone Joint Surg Am. 2007; 89(9):2000–10.
21. Peters CL, Erickson JA, Gililland JM. Clinical and radiographic results of 184 consecutive revision total knee arthroplasties placed with modular cementless stems. J Arthroplast. 2009;24(6 Suppl):48–53.
22. Hossain F, Patel S, Haddad FS. Midterm assessment of causes and results of revision total knee arthroplasty. Clin Orthop Relat Res. 2010;468(5):1221–8.
23. Abraham R, Malkani AL, Lewis J, Beck D. An anatomical study of tibial metaphyseal/diaphyseal mismatch during revision total knee arthroplasty. J Arthroplast. 2007;22(2):241–4.
24. Porteous AJ, Hassaballa MA, Newman JH. Does the joint line matter in revision total knee replacement? J Bone Joint Surg Br Vol. 2008;90(7):879–84.
25. Figgie HE 3rd, Goldberg VM, Heiple KG, Moller HS 3rd, Gordon NH. The influence of tibial-patellofemoral location on function of the knee in patients with the posterior stabilized condylar knee prosthesis. J Bone Joint Surg Am. 1986;68(7):1035–40.
26. Barrack RL, Engh G, Rorabeck C, Sawhney J, Woolfrey M. Patient satisfaction and outcome after septic versus aseptic revision total knee arthroplasty. J Arthroplast. 2000;15(8):990–3.

19

Ultrasound measures of muscle thickness may be superior to strength testing in adults with knee osteoarthritis: a cross-sectional study

Alfred C. Gellhorn[1]*⊙, Jordan M. Stumph[2], Hashem E. Zikry[3], Carly A. Creelman[1] and Rachel Welbel[1]

Abstract

Background: Evaluation of muscle strength as performed routinely with a dynamometer may be limited by important factors such as pain during muscle contraction. Few studies have compared formal strength testing with ultrasound to measure muscle bulk in adults with knee osteoarthritis (OA).

Methods: We investigated the muscle bulk of lower limb muscles in adults with knee OA using quantitative ultrasound. We analyzed the relationship between patient reported function and the muscle bulk of hip adductors, hip abductors, knee extensors and ankle plantarflexors. We further correlated muscle bulk measures with joint torques calculated with a hand held dynamometer. We hypothesized that ultrasound muscle bulk would have high levels of interrater reliability and correlate more strongly with pain and function than strength measured by a dynamometer. 23 subjects with unilateral symptomatic knee OA completed baseline questionnaires including the Western Ontario and McMaster Universities Arthritis Index (WOMAC) and Lower Extremity Activity Scale. Joint torque was measured with a dynamometer and muscle bulk was assessed with ultrasound.

Results: Higher ultrasound measured muscle bulk was correlated with less pain in all muscle groups. When comparing muscle bulk and torque measures, ultrasound-measured muscle bulk of the quadriceps was more strongly correlated with measures of pain and function than quadriceps isometric strength measured with a dynamometer.

Conclusions: Ultrasound is a feasible method to assess muscle bulk of lower limb muscles in adults with knee OA, with high levels of interrater reliability, and correlates negatively with patient reported function. Compared with use of a hand held dynamometer to measure muscle function, ultrasound may be a superior modality.

Keywords: Ultrasound, Osteoarthritis, Reliability, Strength

Background

Osteoarthritis (OA) is the most prevalent joint disease in the United States, with high levels of pain and functional disability in individuals affected by the disease. OA of the knee is particularly problematic, with the lifetime risk of developing knee OA estimated at 47% among women and 40% among men [1]. Conservative management strategies for knee OA frequently include therapeutic exercise, often with the guidance of a physical therapist to direct the specific exercise program. Muscular strength and neuromuscular control may modulate joint forces and this premise forms the basis for many physical therapy interventions in OA. Despite generally positive results from trials evaluating therapeutic exercise in adults with knee OA, there remains a lack of understanding about which muscle groups are most important in modifying joint forces, and, indeed, whether improvement in strength is the reason for the positive outcomes seen after such interventions.

* Correspondence: alg9109@med.cornell.edu
[1]Department of Rehabilitation Medicine, Weill Cornell Medicine, 525 E 68th Street, B16, New York, NY 10065, USA
Full list of author information is available at the end of the article

Joint forces are due to the bulk and composition of various muscle groups, the associated lever arm, and neural activation patterns that activate groups of muscles to produce joint motion. Measured strength as performed routinely with a dynamometer may be a useful indicator of the ability of muscle to affect force production upon a joint, but when tested at pathologic joints may be limited by important factors such as pain during muscle contraction. Pure muscle mass is another way to measure the theoretical ability of muscle to generate force; in situations where there is no pain during movement, muscle physiologic cross sectional area correlates strongly with muscle force generation [2]. Ultrasound has emerged as a safe and reliable method to evaluate muscle thickness, and these measurements correlate with muscle cross sectional area, [3] suggesting that ultrasound-measured muscle thickness may provide important information about muscle function.

While it is established that quadriceps muscle strength influences pain and function in knee OA, it is unknown whether similar associations exist for muscles at the hips and the ankles. Theoretically, as the primary knee extensors, the quadriceps are important in force modulation: the quadriceps are highly active during the majority of the gait cycle and slow the rapid knee flexion produced during initial contact when knee joint forces and the rate of loading are highest [4]. Hip abductors and hip adductors are also theoretically important given their role in controlling the position of the limb during gait. By determining the degree of limb adduction or abduction, these muscles will influence the ground reaction force vector relative to the center of the knee joint in the coronal plane [4]. Finally, the plantar flexors are important in many models of gait, and peak plantar flexor moments in adults with knee OA predict knee joint compressive forces [5]. Because of the possible importance of all of these muscle groups in influencing forces across the knee, an understanding of the relative importance of each muscle group on symptom generation would represent a positive advance.

Our primary aim in this preliminary study is to investigate the relationship between ultrasound measured bulk of the hip, knee, and ankle muscles and self-reported function in adults with knee OA. Secondarily, we aim to compare these relationships with strength as measured more conventionally using a hand held dynamometer.

Methods
Subjects and data collection
Subjects in this study included 23 adults with unilateral symptomatic knee osteoarthritis, recruited from the outpatient clinic of the primary investigator. Knee OA was diagnosed using American College of Rheumatology (ACR) guidelines [6] based on clinical and radiographic

findings. All subjects were screened by telephone for their suitability for enrollment based on ACR guidelines including pain in the knee and at least one of the following: age greater than 50 years, morning stiffness less than 30 min, and joint crepitus. Subjects were excluded from the study if they had any of the following: a prior corticosteroid injection into the knee within 4 weeks prior to enrollment, a prior diagnosis of a neuromuscular condition that affected lower extremity strength, or an alternative rheumatologic diagnosis explaining their knee pain. If subjects met these criteria, they received a weight bearing anterior-posterior and lateral radiograph of both knees. Based on ACR guidelines, the presence of osteophytes on the symptomatic knee was required for radiographic diagnosis of OA. Once subjects met clinical and radiographic inclusion and exclusion criteria, they were entered into the study. Data were collected by trained research assistants in a single in-person visit. The study was approved by the host institution's IRB and all patients provided written informed consent.

Variables
The Western Ontario and McMaster Universities Arthritis Index (WOMAC) was used to assess subjects' pain, stiffness, and physical functioning. The WOMAC questionnaire is well validated in adults with knee OA and includes 24 questions that measures the three dimensions of pain, disability and joint stiffness.

The Lower Extremity Activity Scale (LEAS) [7] was used to determine the level of daily physical activity in each patient. The LEAS is a self-administered 18-level questionnaire that has been validated in adults with knee OA.

Anthropomorphic measurements, including height and weight, were obtained to calculate joint torques and normalize muscle thickness measurements. Length of the lower limb was measured from the anterior superior iliac spine (ASIS) to the lateral malleolus, and the lower leg was measured from the lateral femoral condyle to the lateral malleolus. All lower limb measurements were performed by a trained research assistant with the subject supine using a flexible tape measure. The ASIS, lateral femoral condyle, and lateral malleolus were identified by palpation. The average of two separate measures was used for the calculating limb length based on previous reports of optimizing validity of this measurement method [8].

Kellgren Lawrence grading of the radiographic degree of osteoarthritis was performed for both knees by the primary investigator.

Ultrasound measurements
Muscle groups evaluated with ultrasound imaging included the knee extensor group (quadriceps femoris);

hip abductor group (gluteus medius and minimus); hip adductor group (adductor brevis, adductor longus, adductor magnus, and gracilis); and ankle plantarflexor group (gastrocnemius and soleus). Prior to obtaining ultrasound measures on study participants, we developed a standardized protocol for measuring muscle thickness using normal volunteers to ensure maximal interrater reliability. Two evaluators were trained to perform ultrasound scans following the same protocol. For each muscle studied, we used bony landmarks and surface markings to identify a location as close as possible to the mid-portion of the muscle belly. For the quadriceps and hip adductors, a skin mark was placed at half of the distance between the greater trochanter and the lateral condyle of the femur. This line was extended circumferentially across the anterior and medial leg to obtain consistent imaging of the quadriceps and adductors. Next, a mark was placed at 30% from the distal end of a line between the lateral femoral condyle and the lateral malleolus at the ankle. This corresponded to the mid-portion of the gastrocnemius and soleus. A final mark was placed at half the distance from the ASIS to the greater trochanter of the femur, corresponding to the mid-portion of the gluteus medius and minimus.

A Sonosite X-Porte (Bothell, WA) with a curvilinear 5–2 MHz transducer was used to obtain all ultrasound images. Subjects lay supine on an exam table. The transducer was placed perpendicular to the skin/musculature to minimize risk of sampling a muscle obliquely and to ensure repeatability. After the muscle was identified, the examiner slightly retracted the transducer so as to not compress the muscle; the image was considered to be optimized when a thin film of gel was present between the skin and the transducer indicating that no manual compressive forces were distorting the muscle. Once the ultrasound image was optimized, a still image was captured and the muscle thickness was measured with caliper-based tools included in the machine software (Fig. 1). The process was repeated three times for each muscle group and all three measurements were recorded. Once all images were obtained from one lower extremity, the same method was used for imaging of the other.

Strength measurements

A Lafayette Model 01165 hand-held dynamometer (Lafayette, IN) was used to measure peak force over a 3 s period, as per settings on the dynamometer. Anatomical markers were used for dynamometer placement to achieve accurate lever arm measurements. When obtaining measurements for the hip abductors, the subject was placed in the supine position, and the dynamometer was placed 5 cm proximal to the lateral malleolus on the

lateral side of the lower leg. The subject was cued to abduct the leg against the resisted pressure of the dynamometer. For the adductors, the subject was again supine, and the dynamometer was placed 5 cm proximal to the medial malleolus on the medial aspect of the lower leg, and instructed to adduct the leg against the resisted pressure of the dynamometer. Finally, for the quadriceps, the subject was seated and the dynamometer was placed in the midline at 5 cm proximal to the lateral malleolus. We chose these locations based on prior studies that indicated high levels of reliability and validity [9–11].

All of our strength tests were isometric "make tests", such that the subject pushed against the dynamometer while the examiner maintained the dynamometer as steadily as possible. For each test, the subject was allowed to have one warm-up (~ 50% maximum strength) to account for any habituation. The test was repeated three times for each muscle group. Each subject was given a 30 s rest period after each of the tests performed to avoid fatiguing the subject. All tests lasted 3 s as determined by the dynamometer. The settings on the machine itself were set to stop recording with an audible beep after this time period had elapsed. To initiate each test, the subjects were instructed to "go" then the examiner repeated "push, push, push" to signal the patient to push as hard as possible for the remaining 3 s of the test. After the dynamometer beeped, the examiner told the subject to "relax" to signal the end of the test. Maximal force attained during each attempt was recorded.

Based on prior studies regarding the ideal method of reporting strength in knee OA, we calculated joint torque as the product of the force measured by the dynamometer and the distance from the dynamometer to the axis of rotation of the joint [4]. Additionally, because strength varies with body size in adults with and without OA, [12] we calculated strength relative to body mass in kg.

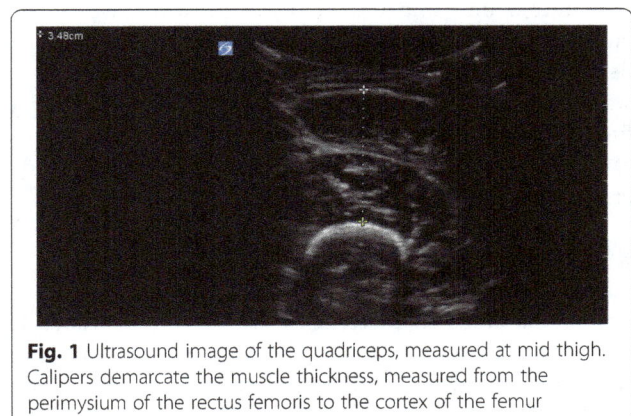

Fig. 1 Ultrasound image of the quadriceps, measured at mid thigh. Calipers demarcate the muscle thickness, measured from the perimysium of the rectus femoris to the cortex of the femur

Analysis

All analysis was performed using Microsoft Excel 15.1 (Redmond, WA) and STATA 14.1 (College Station, TX), with alpha level for hypothesis testing set at 0.05. Torque was calculated at each joint by multiplying the force obtained by dynamometry by the lever arm of the limb. For instance, knee extensor torque was calculated by multiplying the strength of knee extension by the length of the lower leg, and is reported in units of Newton meters (Nm).

Data were evaluated for normality using the Shapiro Wilk test and normal quantile plots. We used simple descriptive statistics to describe our cohort, and paired t-tests to evaluate for any differences in muscle parameters between symptomatic and asymptomatic limbs. Because some of the strength measures were not normally distributed, we used Spearman's rho to evaluate the correlation between baseline characteristics and muscle measures as well as between functional measures and muscle parameters. We considered r values < 0.3 to represent a weak association, 0.3–0.7 to represent a moderate association, and > 0.7 to represent a strong association [13].

To evaluate the relationship between muscle measures and WOMAC in more detail, we performed a simple linear regression analysis, with the total WOMAC score as the dependent variable, and muscle thickness or torque as the independent variable. To control for possible confounding, we performed a multivariable linear regression analysis using age and gender as covariates. We chose age and gender as possible confounders based on the conceptual model that muscle bulk and strength are correlated with both of these variables. In the multivariable analysis, we assessed how much the regression coefficient associated with the muscle measure changed after adjusting for each potential confounder. If the regression coefficient from the simple linear regression model changed by more than 10%, then the covariate was felt to represent a confounder, and was included in the final regression model [14].

To determine the reliability of measurements for both ultrasound thickness and muscle force, we calculated intra-class correlation coefficients (ICCs) (2,1), using a two-way mixed effects model [15]. ICC (2,1) was used because we were interested in generalizing findings beyond the two raters in the study. An ICC > 0.75 was considered good and ICC > 0.9 was considered excellent [16].

Results

Subject characteristics

Subject baseline characteristics are shown in Table 1. Subjects included 12 females and 11 males with average age of 63.8 years. The majority of patients had moderate osteoarthritis based on the Kellgren Lawrence scale, with

Table 1 Subject baseline characteristics, N = 23

	Mean (SD) or percent
Age	63.8 (9.3)
Gender, female	52%
Weight, kg	77.4 (14.5)
BMI	26.9 (3.7)
Pain level	4.1 (1.8)
Symptomatic side, right	52%
Symptom duration (months)	44.8 (62.1)
Symptomatic KL grade	
0	0
1	1
2	9
3	12
4	0
Asymptomatic KL grade	
0	8
1	7
2	7
3	0
4	0
WOMAC pain subscale (0–20)	4.6 (3.2)
WOMAC stiffness subscale (0–8)	3.1 (1.7)
WOMAC function subscale (0–68)	17.45 (13.3)
WOMAC total (0–96)	25.3 (17.4)

NRS Numeric Rating System, *BMI* Body Mass Index, *KL* Kellgren Lawrence, *WOMAC* Western Ontario and McMaster Arthritis Index

chronic painful symptoms due to OA and median symptom duration of 2 years. No subjects had grade 4 radiographic osteoarthritis. Some patients had radiographic osteoarthritis on the contralateral, asymptomatic knee, though radiographic osteoarthritis grade was less on the asymptomatic side. Symptoms as measured by the WOMAC index were mild to moderate, with a mean total WOMAC score of 25, on a scale from 0 to 96, where higher scores indicate worse symptoms. Functional daily activity as measured by the LEAS had a mean score of 13.1, on a scale of 1–18, where higher scores relate to greater daily functional activity.

Strength and muscle bulk measurements

Subject muscle characteristics are presented in Table 2. There were no significant differences in normalized measured strength (Nm/kg) between symptomatic and asymptomatic limbs. Similarly, there were no differences in muscle bulk of any of the investigated muscles between symptomatic and asymptomatic limbs.

Table 2 Subject muscle characteristics

	Symptomatic	Asymptomatic	Paired t-test
Strength measured as torque (Nm) normalized to body weight (kg)			
Knee extensor	96 (58.9)	95.2 (53.6)	0.84
Hip abductors	85.8 (27.1)	88.5 (29.1)	0.44
Hip adductors	90.4 (31.8)	91.9 (34.2)	0.72
Ankle plantarflexors	29.1 (11.1)	30.3 (11.7)	0.26
Muscle thickness (mm) normalized to weight (kg)			
Quadriceps	0.37 (0.12)	0.38 (0.12)	0.32
Hip abductors	0.42 (0.13)	0.42 (0.13)	0.72
Hip adductors	0.59 (0.18)	0.60 (0.18)	0.24
Ankle plantarflexors	0.56 (0.24)	0.56 (0.22)	0.98
Muscle thickness (mm) non-normalized			
Quad	28.4 (9.1)	29.2 (9.3)	0.27
Hip abductors	32.0 (10.9)	31.7 (10.2)	0.61
Hip adductors	44.7 (13.3)	45.4 (12.5)	0.34
Ankle plantarflexors	42.4 (17.5)	42.4 (16.2)	0.99

The terms in parentheses indicate standard deviations

Inter-rater reliability of ultrasound and strength measures

Intraclass correlation coefficients (ICCs) for ultrasound measurements were excellent for all ultrasound measures. ICC (2,1) was 0.95 for quadriceps, 0.92 for hip adductors, 0.91 for hip abductors, and 0.98 for ankle plantarflexors. ICC(2,1) for torque at the hip adductors was excellent (0.93), but only good at quadriceps (0.83), hip abductors (0.87), and ankle plantarflexors (0.77). Reliability was markedly better for ultrasound measures than torque measures at the quadriceps, hip abductors and ankle plantarflexors.

Correlations between baseline characteristics, muscle characteristics, and functional measures

Female gender was moderately associated with higher pain as measured by the WOMAC pain sub-scale. No other correlations between baseline characteristics and WOMAC or LEAS scales reached statistical significance.

Correlation of function, pain and muscle measures

Muscle bulk correlated negatively with pain scores such that greater muscle bulk was associated with lower pain scores (Table 3). This association was significant for the quadriceps and hip adductors but did not reach significance in other muscle groups. Quadriceps thickness was strongly correlated with function, with greater thickness associated with better function. Other muscle groups showed mild to moderate correlation with function, with significance seen in the symptomatic hip adductors. Symptomatic joint stiffness was not found to correlate with any measured muscle thickness. Age and symptom

duration were not correlated with muscle thickness in any muscle groups. Males showed higher values for muscle thickness than females for all muscle groups.

Similar to ultrasound-measured bulk, muscle torque generated by all muscle groups was negatively correlated with pain such that lower muscle torque was correlated with worse pain (Table 3). This correlation reached levels of significance for hip abductors, hip adductors, and plantarflexors on both limbs. Importantly, there was no significant correlation found between pain and quadriceps torque. Analyzing correlation with function, muscle torques were negatively correlated with function, with significant correlation seen in the hip abductors, adductors, and plantarflexors, but not quadriceps.

Regression analysis

In the simple linear regression analysis, quadriceps thickness was the only ultrasound measure significantly associated with the total WOMAC score. Conversely, dynamometer-measured strength of the quadriceps was not significantly associated with total WOMAC score, while strength of the abductors, adductors, and plantarflexors did show a significant association. When assessing for confounding by age and gender in the multivariable model, age did not change the regression coefficient by more than 10% for any of the strength or muscle thickness measures and was therefore deemed not a confounder. On the other hand, the addition of gender to the model resulted in a change in the regression coefficient by more than 10%, and so was considered a confounder and included in the final regression model. The full results of the multivariable regression analysis are presented in Table 4. In the final model, the unadjusted beta for symptomatic quadriceps thickness normalized to weight was − 67.2. In other words, for every 1 mm/kg increase in quadriceps thickness, the corresponding total WOMAC score decreased by 67.2. To place this in context, we calculated the minimum clinically important difference in WOMAC for this group as a 10% change in the mean WOMAC score, or 2.4 points. Using the above unadjusted beta, for a 70 kg adult, an increase in quadriceps thickness of 2.4 mm would be associated with an improvement of 2.4 on the WOMAC scale.

Discussion

This exploratory study identified a number of muscle characteristics that were associated with measures of pain and function in adults with knee OA. However, it is notable that muscle torque and ultrasound-measured muscle bulk did not always demonstrate the same degree of correlation with pain and function. Most notably, while quadriceps muscle bulk was strongly correlated with the WOMAC functional subscale and overall

Table 3 Unadjusted Spearman's rho correlations between muscle measures and functional measures

Muscle group	WOMAC pain	WOMAC stiffness	WOMAC function	WOMAC total	Age	Gender	BMI	Symptom duration
Muscle strength measures								
Symptomatic knee extension	−0.42	−0.18	−0.35	−0.36	−0.10	**0.49 ***	0.18	0.21
Asymptomatic knee extension	−0.31	−0.17	−0.29	−0.27	−0.02	0.41	−0.20	0.20
Symptomatic hip abduction	**−0.52 ***	−0.22	**−0.46 ***	**−0.47 ***	−0.25	0.17	0.01	0.11
Asymptomatic hip abduction	**−0.49 ***	−0.28	**−0.51 ***	**−0.51 ***	−0.22	**0.47 ***	0.04	0.10
Symptomatic hip adduction	**−0.52 ***	−0.13	**−0.44 ***	**−0.44 ***	0.02	0.36	−0.09	0.07
Asymptomatic hip adduction	**−0.51 ***	−0.25	**−0.54 ***	**−0.54 ‡**	0.10	0.28	−0.07	−0.08
Symptomatic ankle plantarflexion	**−0.46 ***	−0.06	**−0.49 ***	**−0.47 ***	**−0.43 ***	0.30	−0.09	0.19
Asymptomatic ankle plantarflexion	**−0.46 ***	−0.18	**−.042 ***	**−0.42 ***	−0.35	0.25	−0.04	0.27
Muscle thickness measures								
Symptomatic quadriceps thickness	**−0.48 ***	−0.09	**−0.62 ‡**	**−0.60 ‡**	−0.35	0.37	−0.04	0.15
Asymptomatic quadriceps thickness	−0.38	−0.22	**−0.54 ***	**−0.53 ***	−0.29	**0.51 ***	−0.01	0.15
Symptomatic hip abductor thickness	−0.13	−0.09	−0.14	−0.14	0.05	**0.41 ***	0.03	−0.10
Asymptomatic hip abductor thickness	−0.20	−0.02	−0.25	−0.22	−0.05	**0.43 ***	0.08	−0.10
Symptomatic hip adductor thickness	**−0.45 ***	−0.11	**−0.47 ***	**−0.44 ***	−0.02	**0.64 ***	−0.30	−0.06
Asymptomatic hip adductor thickness	**−0.45 ***	−0.10	−0.40	−0.38	−0.04	**0.58 ‡**	−0.27	−0.11
Symptomatic calf thickness	−0.39	−0.04	−0.39	−0.37	−0.14	**0.49 ***	−0.12	−0.05
Asymptomatic calf thickness	−0.37	−0.03	−0.37	−0.35	−0.15	**0.47 ***	−0.14	−0.08

WOMAC Western Ontario and McMaster Arthritis Index, *BMI* Body Mass Index
Strength measured in torque (Nm) normalized to body weight (kg), ie Nm/kg
Values indicated by * with bold text indicates significance at 0.05 level, ‡ with bold text indicates significance at 0.01 level

WOMAC score, quadriceps torque was not. This suggests that for some muscle groups, measuring torque alone may give an inadequate picture of the muscle's functional ability. In other words, muscle strength and muscle bulk do not provide the same information in adults with painful knee OA.

The divergence we observed between muscle torque and muscle bulk is not entirely surprising, since control at a joint is due to neural activation patterns as well as muscle bulk and fat infiltration. Neural activation patterns, in particular, are likely altered when activation of the muscle compresses a painful joint. Arthrogenic muscle inhibition is well described in painful knees, [17] wherein afferent discharge from neurons that innervate the knee joint have effects on spinal and supraspinal pathways to limit activation of the quadriceps muscle.

Therefore, measurement of quadriceps strength alone, as performed in many prior studies evaluating function in adults with knee OA [18–23] may provide an incomplete picture of the role of the quadriceps in predicting function. Indeed, a number of studies have attempted to account for the possibility of arthrogenic muscle inhibition using test techniques such as burst-superimposition, where electrical stimulation of muscle is superimposed on a muscle undergoing active contraction [23, 24]. While theoretically attractive, this type of testing is complex and painful.

We propose that ultrasound measured muscle bulk provides a complimentary method of determining muscle function in adults with knee OA, and our findings that quadriceps muscle thickness correlates significantly with function and overall WOMAC score supports this premise. The idea of an imaging biomarker that correlates with functional and pain measures is attractive and minimizes many of the above concerns about isometric strength testing to measure muscle function. Supporting this, a recent study showed that MRI measured change of quadriceps cross sectional area was both more sensitive to longitudinal change and correlated more strongly with disease progression when compared with isometric strength testing in a large cohort of patients with symptomatic knee OA [25]. While the costs and logistics of MRI preclude its use in a clinical setting to assess muscle function, ultrasound provides an appealing alternative that is likely feasible for most clinical and research settings.

Our use of quantitative ultrasound analysis to measure muscle bulk is based on data showing high levels of inter-rater, intra-rater, and inter-machine reliability when using a well described scanning protocol [26]. Furthermore, a strict scanning protocol enables even a novice ultrasound practitioner to achieve high levels of reliability with minimal training [26, 27], increasing the applicability of this technique. Importantly, our study had

Table 4 Summary of multivariable regression analysis for muscle characteristics predicting the total WOMAC score, controlled for gender

Predictor	Unadjusted beta	p-value
Muscle thickness measures (mm/kg)		
Symptomatic quadriceps	−67.2	0.009 *
Asymptomatic quadriceps	−60.5	0.031 *
Symptomatic hip abductors	−11	0.66
Asymptomatic hip abductors	−21.7	0.85
Sympatomatic hip adductors	−27.8	0.13
Asympatomatic hip adductors	−29	11
Symptomatic calf	−20.6	0.14
Asymptomatic calf	−19.9	0.19
Muscle torque measures (Nm/kg)		
Symptomatic knee extensors	−0.036	0.57
Asymptomatic knee extensors	−0.051	0.12
Symptomatic hip abductors	−0.197	0.08
Asymptomatic hip abductors	−0.138	0.27
Symptomatic hip adductors	−0.126	0.26
Asymptomatic hip adductors	−0.188	0.06
Symptomatic ankle plantarflexors	−0.65	0.05
Asymptomatic ankle plantarflexors	−0.56	0.05

* indicates p < 0.05

excellent levels of inter-rater reliability for all ultrasound measures, and were significantly better than measures of torque for the quadriceps, hip abductors and ankle plantarflexors. The ultrasound examination itself is well tolerated and rapid, with acquisition of images taking approximately 5 min, and measurement taking an additional 5–10 min, depending on the software included on the ultrasound unit.

By evaluating multiple muscle groups at once in the same subjects, we aimed to describe the relative importance of muscle strength at the knee, hip, and ankle in moderating symptoms of knee OA. A picture emerges of a beneficial effect of greater muscle strength in all muscle groups measured, though our data show that the strongest association between muscle function and symptoms is seen with the quadriceps. This is in line with many prior studies that have shown the importance of quadriceps strength [4] and that form the basis for many therapeutic exercise interventions. However, our data suggest that muscle evaluation and therapy should not be limited to quadriceps alone, and that the hip adductors, hip abductors, and ankle plantarflexors all contribute to improved lower limb function.

While we found moderate to strong correlations between muscle strength and WOMAC pain and function scales, we found no similar correlation between muscle strength and WOMAC stiffness subscale. While

the etiology of symptomatic joint stiffness in OA remains unclear, our results generally support the premise that joint stiffness is more related to intraarticular factors, especially synovitis [28].

This study does have some important limitations. It should be noted that our findings should be considered preliminary given the small sample size and the novelty of the assessments performed. A larger sample would enable a more accurate determination of the relative importance of each muscle group we studied in correlating with function. An additional limitation is the cross sectional nature of our study design. We are therefore only able to identify associations between various measures of muscle function and WOMAC scores, but we cannot draw any conclusions about the causality of these relationships. A longitudinal study design would enable us to better determine the predictive value of strength at the hips, knees, and ankles in functional measures in this type of cohort. Finally, because muscle strength at each joint tended to be collinear within individuals, it is possible that strength at each location measured is simply a proxy for a more gross measure of an individual's strength of the lower limb. While a more robust regression analysis would enable a clearer picture of each muscle group's importance as an independent predictor of symptoms, our findings of a stronger correlation between WOMAC and muscle function in the quadriceps than other muscle groups suggests at least some degree of independence in the function of these muscles in the symptomatic limb.

Conclusions

This study found that ultrasound determined muscle thickness had higher levels of measurement reliability than isometric torque testing in multiple muscle groups in the lower limbs of adults with knee OA. Additionally, muscle thickness of the hip abductors, hip adductors, knee extensors and ankle plantarflexors correlates with pain and function but not joint stiffness in adults with symptomatic knee OA. Weaker and thinner muscles in all locations were associated with worse symptoms, and the strongest correlation with symptoms was seen with quadriceps bulk. Future directions for study include a larger sample size to confirm these findings and allow for additional statistical adjustment, as well as a cohort that could be followed longitudinally with repeated strength measures following intervention such as formalized physical therapy. An optimized ultrasound protocol that would be suitable for routine clinical use would be a positive development in evaluating lower limb strength in this population.

Abbreviations
ACR: American College of Rheumatology; ASIS: Anterior superior iliac spine; ICC: Intraclass correlation coefficients; LEAS: Lower Extremity Activity Scale; OA: Osteoarthritis; WOMAC: Western Ontario and McMaster Universities Arthritis Index

Funding
This research was supported by the Internal Faculty Development Grant,
Department of Rehabilitation Medicine, Weill Cornell Medicine.

Authors' contributions
AG conceived of the study, performed analysis and interpretation of the
data, and drafted and revised the manuscript. JS contributed to study
conception and deisgn, data acquisition, and manuscript preparation. HZ
contributed to data acquisition, analysis and interpretation. RW contributed
to study conception and manuscript preparation. CC contributed to study
conception and data acquisition. All authors read and approved the final
manuscript.

Competing interests
The authors declare that they have no competing interests.

Author details
[1]Department of Rehabilitation Medicine, Weill Cornell Medicine, 525 E 68th
Street, B16, New York, NY 10065, USA. [2]Albert Einstein College of Medicine,
New York, NY, USA. [3]Icahn School of Medicine at Mount Sinai, New York, NY,
USA.

References
1.   Murphy L, Schwartz TA, Helmick CG, Renner JB, Tudor G, Koch G, et al.
     Lifetime risk of symptomatic knee osteoarthritis. Arthritis Rheum. 2008;59:
     1207–13.
2.   Brand RA, Pedersen DR, Friederich JA. The sensitivity of muscle force
     predictions to changes in physiologic cross-sectional area. J Biomech. 1986;
     19:589–96.
3.   Sanada K, Kearns CF, Midorikawa T, Abe T. Prediction and validation of total
     and regional skeletal muscle mass by ultrasound in Japanese adults. Eur J
     Appl Physiol. 2006;96:24–31.
4.   Bennell KL, Wrigley TV, Hunt MA, Lim B-W, Hinman RS. Update on the role
     of muscle in the genesis and management of knee osteoarthritis. Rheum
     Dis Clin N Am. 2013;39:145–76.
5.   Robon MJ, Perell KL, Fang M, Guererro E. The relationship between ankle
     plantar flexor muscle moments and knee compressive forces in subjects
     with and without pain. Clin Biomech (Bristol, Avon). 2000;15(7):522–27.
     http://doi.org/10.2307/41994847?refreqid=search-gateway:
     db4032910807ce6a4d16cff68530ffbd
6.   Altman R, Asch E, Bloch D, Bole G, Borenstein D, Brandt K, et al.
     Development of criteria for the classification and reporting of osteoarthritis.
     Classification of osteoarthritis of the knee. Diagnostic and therapeutic
     criteria Committee of the American Rheumatism Association. Arthritis
     Rheum. 1986;29(8):1039–49.
7.   Saleh KJ, Mulhall KJ, Bershadsky B, Ghomrawi HM, White LE, Buyea CM, et al.
     Development and validation of a lower-extremity activity scale. Use for
     patients treated with revision total knee arthroplasty. J Bone Joint Surg.
     2005;87:1985–94.
8.   Beattie P, Isaacson K, Riddle DL, Rothstein JM. Validity of derived
     measurements of leg-length differences obtained by use of a tape measure.
     Phys Ther. 1990;70:150–7.
9.   Martin HJ, Yule V, Syddall HE, Dennison EM, Cooper C, Aihie Sayer A. Is
     hand-held dynamometry useful for the measurement of quadriceps
     strength in older people? A comparison with the gold standard Bodex
     dynamometry. Gerontology. 2006;52:154–9.
10. Thorborg K, Petersen J, Magnusson SP, Hölmich P. Clinical assessment of
     hip strength using a hand-held dynamometer is reliable. Scand J Med Sci
     Sports. 2010;20:493–501.
11. Li RC, Jasiewicz JM, Middleton J, Condie P, Barriskill A, Hebnes H, et al. The
     development, validity, and reliability of a manual muscle testing device with
     integrated limb position sensors. Arch Phys Med Rehabil. 2006;87:411–7.
12. Jaric S. Role of body size in the relation between muscle strength and
     movement performance. Exerc Sport Sci Rev. 2003;31:8–12.
13. Taylor R. Interpretation of the correlation coefficient: a basic review. J Diagn
     Med Sonography. 2016;6:35–9.
14. Greenland S. Modeling and variable selection in epidemiologic analysis. Am
     J Public Health. 1989;79(3):340–49. https://doi.org/10.2105/AJPH.79.3.340
15. Shrout PE, Fleiss JL. Intraclass correlations: uses in assessing rater reliability.
     Psychol Bull. 1979;86:420–8.
16. Portney LG, Watkins MP. Foundations of clinical research: F.A. Davis; 2015.
17. Rice DA, McNair PJ. Quadriceps arthrogenic muscle inhibition: neural
     mechanisms and treatment perspectives. Semin Arthritis Rheum.
     2010;40:250–66.
18. Mizner RL, Petterson SC, Stevens JE, Vandenborne K, Snyder Mackler L. Early
     quadriceps strength loss after total knee arthroplasty. The contributions of
     muscle atrophy and failure of voluntary muscle activation. J Bone Joint
     Surg. 2005;87:1047–53.
19. Sharma L, Dunlop DD, Cahue S, Song J, Hayes KW. Quadriceps strength and
     osteoarthritis progression in malaligned and lax knees. Ann Intern Med.
     2003;138:613–9.
20. Ruhdorfer A, Wirth W, Hitzl W, Nevitt M, Eckstein F, Osteoarthritis Initiative
     Investigators. Association ofs thigh muscle strength with knee symptoms
     and radiographic disease stage of osteoarthritis: data from the osteoarthritis
     initiative. Arthritis Care Res. 2014;66:1344–53.
21. O'Reilly SC, Jones A, Muir KR, Doherty M. Quadriceps weakness in knee
     osteoarthritis: the effect on pain and disability. Ann Rheum Dis.
     1998;57:588–94.
22. Slemenda C, Brandt KD, Heilman DK, Mazzuca S, Braunstein EM, Katz BP,
     et al. Quadriceps weakness and osteoarthritis of the knee. Ann Intern Med.
     1997;127:97–104.
23. Stevens JE, Mizner RL, Snyder Mackler L. Quadriceps strength and volitional
     activation before and after total knee arthroplasty for osteoarthritis. J
     Orthop Res. 2003;21:775–9.
24. Lewek MD, Rudolph KS, Snyder Mackler L. Quadriceps femoris muscle
     weakness and activation failure in patients with symptomatic knee
     osteoarthritis. J Orthop Res. 2004;22:110–5.
25. Dannhauer T, Sattler M, Wirth W, Hunter DJ, Kwoh CK, Eckstein F.
     Longitudinal sensitivity to change of MRI-based muscle cross-sectional area
     versus isometric strength analysis in osteoarthritic knees with and without
     structural progression: pilot data from the osteoarthritis initiative. MAGMA.
     2014;27:339–47.
26. Gellhorn AC, Carlson MJ. Inter-rater, intra-rater, and inter-machine reliability
     of quantitative ultrasound measurements of the patellar tendon. Ultrasound
     Med Biol. 2013;39:791–6.
27. Bunnell A, Ney J, Gellhorn A, Hough CL. Quantitative neuromuscular
     ultrasound in intensive care unit--acquired weakness: a systematic review.
     Muscle Nerve. 2015;52:701–8.
28. Bonnet CS, Walsh DA. Osteoarthritis, angiogenesis and inflammation.
     Rheumatology (Oxford). 2005;44:7–16.

20

Postoperative function recovery in patients with endoprosthetic knee replacement for bone tumour: an observational study

Mattia Morri[1]*[iD], Cristiana Forni[1], Riccardo Ruisi[1], Tiziana Giamboi[1], Fabrizio Giacomella[1], Davide Maria Donati[2] and Maria Grazia Benedetti[3]

Abstract

Background: The objective of this study is to describe the rehabilitative pathway of patients undergoing endoprosthetic knee replacement surgery, build reference values of the functional results achieved, and identify possible prognostic factors.

Methods: Prospective observational study. All patients undergoing resection and knee replacement surgery using a modular prosthesis following bone tumor resection were consecutively recruited over the last 2 years. The patients were followed for a period of 1 year, the result values were collected at 3, 6 and 12 months.

Results: In total, 30 patients were enrolled. The median age was 19 years with 33% of patients being female. Median values recorded for knee flexion, quadriceps strength, Toronto Extremity Salvage Score, Time Up and Go and Six Minutes Walking Test showed an improvement of 16, 25, 18, 48 and 38% from 3 to 12 months, respectively. The level and width of the resection were correlated with the mobility of the knee and the strength of the quadriceps.

Conclusion: Patients undergoing knee replacement for bone tumors were able to achieve satisfactory functional outcomes from the first postoperative year. A specific assessment of outcomes can be conducted to facilitate the management of patient expectations. A very wide resection and interventions of the proximal tibia are risk factors for a poorer functional outcome.

Keywords: Bone tumors, Rehabilitation, Patient outcome assessment

Background

Bone tumors are rare pathologies; the Italian Association of Tumor Registries (AIRTUM) reported a rate of 0.8 per 100.000 inhabitants for osteosarcoma. Malignant bone tumors represent approximately 5 to 6% of all tumors in young people [1, 2]. These occur more frequently in the metaphysis of long bones, especially at the knee and the proximal humerus [3]. With the improvement of diagnostic techniques, chemotherapy treatments and reconstructive techniques, most of these patients can be treated with a modular prosthesis after bone resection [4]; furthermore, the 5-year survival rate

has improved from 20 to 85% [5, 6]. Because treatment and survival have improved, there is a need to manage residual impairment and disability in the medium and long term, bearing in mind that, being young, these patients will carry out very demanding motor activities. Indeed, several authors have underlined the achievement of good functional outcomes after surgery with modular prostheses [7–12], albeit with some physical limitations and a high rate of complications such as infections, mechanical failures and fractures of the implant [6]. In a study involving modular knee prostheses, Carty et al. [10] reported that at a mean follow up of 7.5 years (standard deviation, 5.1) the limitation of function and disability was correlated with the reduction of joint mobility and muscle strength. Moreover, balance was impaired, with greater difficulty in controlling posture in

* Correspondence: mattia.morri@ior.it
[1]Servizio di Assistenza Infermieristica, Tecnica e della Riabilitazione, IRCCS Istituto Ortopedico Rizzoli, Via Pupilli 1, 40136 Bologna, Italy
Full list of author information is available at the end of the article

an upright position, particularly when such control was required with closed eyes. During walking, a lateral instability and asymmetry was reported [13]. To our knowledge, no rehabilitation protocols or specific care pathways are defined in the literature that attempt to achieve and improve these results. Bekkering (2012) et al. [8] reported their results at up to two-years' follow-up with assessments at 3, 6, 9 12,18 and 24 months but rehabilitation methods in terms of intensity, type of exercises, and patient compliance with treatment are not well described. In addition, no predictive factors for recovery have been investigated. Only recently, Shehade et al. [14] attempted to describe and outline specific rehabilitation protocols for the different locations of the tumor. They concluded by advocating the use of standardized guidelines, as they can lead to an improvement in the final functional results. However, the paper does not report expected recovery times or whether good functional results can be achieved more quickly. The objective of the present study was to describe the rehabilitative pathway of patients undergoing knee replacement with modular prosthesis for bone tumour, as well as building reference values of the functional results achieved in the consecutive rehabilitative phases (3, 6, and 12 months) to identify possible prognostic factors.

Methods
Study design: Prospective observational study
Participants
Between September 2014 and January 2016, all patients, of varying ages, undergoing resection and knee replacement surgery using a modular prosthesis for a primary musculoskeletal tumor, were consecutively recruited. Patients were surgically treated at the Oncological Orthopaedic Surgery Unit and followed for physical rehabilitation during the period of postoperative chemotherapy at the Chemotherapy Unit of an orthopedic university hospital. The only exclusion criterion was patient refusal to participate in the study. Patients who, during the follow-up, showed complications such as local tumor recurrence, implant infection and/or complications related to the administration of the antiblastic drug, which made it impossible to continue the rehabilitation process, were excluded from the study. Conversely, patients able to continue the study were re-evaluated at the next follow-up period. All patients provided written consent and the study protocol received formal approval from the Institute's Ethics Committee (n. 0032914). The study variables included age, sex, diagnosis, resection level and length of resection. The patients were followed for the period of 1 year, with periodical assessment at 3, 6 and 12 months.

Outcome measure
During monitoring, an evaluation grid was used, based on the available literature and clinical experience. The aim of the grid was to obtain a summary of the patient's main motor skills and it outlined 5 main result measures:

- Knee flexion/extension range of motion (ROM) of the knee [15], measured with a manual articular goniometer with the patient placed in the supine position. The patient was asked to flex and extend the knee as far as possible and then the physiotherapist applied further light pressure until the patient's pain threshold was reached.
- The maximal strength of the quadriceps with the scale of the Medical Research Council [16]. In a sitting position, the patient was asked to extend the knee actively against the force of gravity and, where possible, against increasing pressure applied by the physiotherapist. This test was repeated for the healthy limb. The score ranged from 0, no muscular contraction, to 5, marked extension against manually applied pressure.
- The level of autonomy gained and perceived by the patient in everyday life according to the Toronto Extremity Salvage Score (TESS) [17] which is a self-administered patient questionnaire consisting of 30 items concerning the patient's motor skills when performing daily life activities. Each item receives a minimum score of 1 to a maximum score of 5. The overall score is then expressed as a percentage; a greater percentage indicates greater autonomy.
- Motor performance, measured by Time Up and Go (TUG) [18]. This test was performed with the patient in a sitting position with hands on legs. The patient was asked to stand up, walk 3 m, turn around and come back. The test ended when the patient was sitting down again.
- Walking endurance, measured by the 6 minutes walking test (6mWT) [19]. The patient was asked to walk as far as possible in 6 min at a preferred speed.

Rehabilitation program
Patients were followed for rehabilitation in the Surgical Unit immediately after the intervention, and at each admission to the Chemotherapy Unit. Postoperative chemotherapy treatment consisted of a series of in-patient hospital admissions and the administration of 2–6-day continuous infusions for, in most cases, a total duration of about 6 months [20]. The rehabilitation program consisted of two daily sessions of therapy lasting at least 45 min each until patient discharge. The aim of the treatment was to guide the patient in the recovery process in order to minimize the disabling effects of

surgery and to obtain the best possible recovery of residual abilities. The rehabilitation process was divided into two phases: in the initial phase, patients were prescribed a partial loading of the limb (15–20%) and then progressive loading during the second phase, up to complete weight bearing on the treated limb. The exact timeframe for increasing the load on the limb was decided by the orthopaedic surgeon according to the x-rays taken at 1, 3, and 6 months after surgery.

Partial weight-bearing phase (1st-2nd month) The treatment was mainly aimed at recovering basic lower limb function such as walking, increasing knee mobility and strengthening the quadriceps. Passive and active knee flexion-extension and quadriceps strengthening exercises, with particular focus on the last degrees of extension were performed in a supine position with the use of a ball, following the indications in the literature [10]. In this initial phase proprioceptive exercises were performed in a sitting or standing position aimed at controlling the leg with the use of various aids such as a ball and rubber bands. For patients treated by proximal tibia resection, the use of a rigid knee brace was not recommended in the first 40 days, as it does not allow the mobilization of the knee. This period was necessary to obtain an adequate healing of the patellar tendon and entailed a delayed start to the knee mobilization exercises. During this initial phase, it was important to stimulate the patient's proprioception of the treated limb by increasing the patient's confidence with the

prosthesis, in particular with the mechanical extension limitation.

Progressive weight-bearing phase (2nd-6th month) From the time the patient was allowed 50% loading on the operated limb, the rehabilitative treatment included specific exercises in the standing position. Patients were asked to shift the load onto the limbs while maintaining a correct body alignment. Motor control of the treated knee might have been stimulated by a slight knee flexion or by the use of external resistance such as an elastic band. Exercises for two-leg standing were progressively made more challenging by modifying the support surface or using increasingly unstable surfaces and even the use of Freeman balance boards. To make the task even more challenging, closed-eye training or dual task exercises, such as throwing a ball and standing in an unstable position were introduced. Once full weight-bearing was allowed, the same exercises were carried out in the one-leg stance. Examples of the exercises are shown in Fig. 1 [21].

Use of the Wii-fit balance board The Wii Balance Board was used as part of the physiotherapy treatment to test the shifting of load onto the lower limbs of a patient and assess the balance. The Balance Board is able to measure the distribution of body weight on the lower limbs of a player, according to changes in weight distribution under the sole of the foot. The player receives feedback from the exercise and the game they are playing. At the end of each game the console shows the

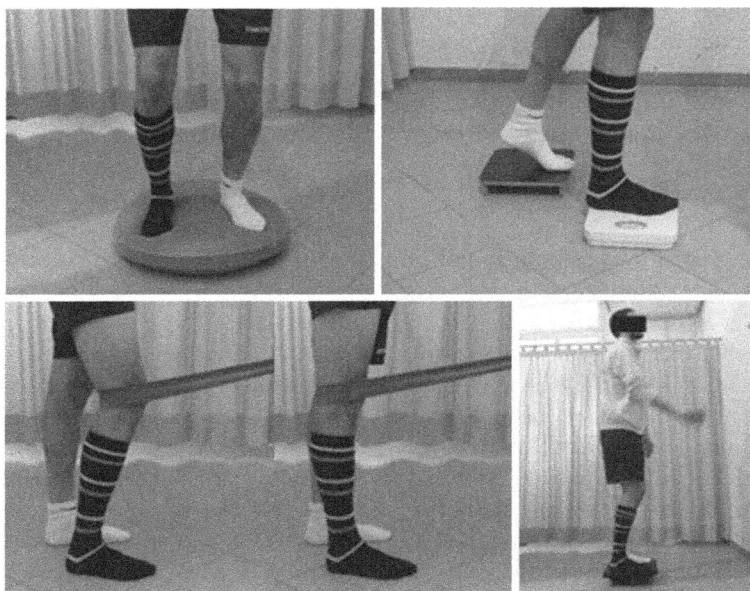

Fig. 1 Exercises for patients with endoprosthetic knee replacement

score. The Wii Balance Board was used in one of the two scheduled rehab sessions every day throughout hospitalization for chemotherapy for at least 20 min using the exercises/games the console is equipped with. Exercises required patients to hold the center of gravity in an upright position and shift loads in the latero-medial, anterior-posterior and multidirectional direction, as described by Fung et al. [22]. The choice of games was left up to the patient and the lowest score achieved was the one recorded.

Sample size

Bone tumors are rare [1]. Therefore, since it was not possible to define the number of cases necessary for the study as suggested by the usual statistical rules for observational studies, we arbitrarily decided to enroll all patients consecutively until a minimum number of 30 was reached.

Statistical analysis

Statistical analysis was performed using IBM SPSS Statistics v. 21. Because the number of patients was small, all continuous data were expressed as median and the relative quartile (25th and 75th), categorical variables were expressed as proportions or percentages. Data concerning the outcomes measured at the various follow-ups were summarized in radar-type graphs. These graphs are a tool that can be used in clinical practice to compare the performance of new patients undergoing knee replacement with modular prosthesis. The Mann Whitney test was used to perform an analysis on subgroups of the main variables collected, such as age, sex, diagnosis, length of resection and level of resection and the functional outcome measured 1 year after surgery. In the absence of information in the literature concerning the length of resection, a cut-off of 20 cm was established from the observation of the data collected in the present study. $P < 0.01$ was considered statistically significant.

Results

In total, 30 patients were eligible for the study, and all were consecutively enrolled. At the 3rd, 6th and 12th month of follow up it was possible to evaluate 26, 21 and 22 patients, respectively. A description of the sample and its basic characteristics is shown in Table 1. The median age was 19 years with 33% of patients being female. At the 12-month follow up, 6 patients (20%) did not complete the 6-month rehabilitation program after surgery: 3 decided to continue the chemotherapy at another hospital, and 3 did not complete rehabilitation due to complications. The flow chart of patients leaving the study and patients evaluated at various times is shown in Fig. 2. The description of the recovery of patients over

Table 1 Patient characteristics, variables and functional results

Patient characteristics	$N = 30$
Median Age, years (min-max)	19 (9–66)
Female, n. (%)	10 (33.3)
Morphology, n. (%)	
Osteosarcoma	25 (83.3)
Ewing	5 (16.7)
Site of the tumor, n. (%)	
Femur	19 (63.3)
Tibia	11 (36.7)
Median resection of bone length, cm (min-max)	14.5 (11–30)
Median number of chemotherapy cycles, (min-max)	10.5 (5–15)
Complications, n (%)	9 (30%)
Infections	5
Mechanical failures	2
Intervention for pulmonary metastases	1
Chemo side effects	1

time is summarized in Fig. 3. The knee ROM extension level was not reported in the graphs or tables. No patient had limitations in this direction of movement. Data of the present study gathered at each follow up were summarized in a radar-type chart. All the functional measures taken into consideration showed an improvement in the three subsequent follow-ups. Median values recorded for knee flexion, quadriceps strength, TESS score, TUG and 6mWT showed an improvement of 16%, 25%, 18%, 48% and 38 between 3 and 12 months, respectively. Table 2 shows a comparison between the data found in the literature and the data of the present study. A median knee flexion of 110 degrees (41.3), a quadriceps strength of 4.0 (1.6), a TESS score of 85% (13.3), a TUG of 7.1 s (1.8) and 6mWT of 450 m (47.5) were in line with the values found in the literature [7–11]. The analysis of subgroups showed that the level of resection made a difference in the knee flexion range of motion, having a p-value of 0.04, and the length of resection made a difference in quadriceps strength, having a p-value of 0.03. The data set is summarized in Table 3.

Discussion

Patients undergoing knee replacement with modular prostheses for musculoskeletal tumors can progressively achieve better functional levels during the first postoperative year. Knee resection entails a wide loss of bone and muscle structures resulting in a marked sensory-motor shock that has severe repercussions on the neuromotor control of the knee and balance, as documented by de Visser [13]. The choice of exercises in the patient's recovery process is aimed at training the patient's neuromotor control system from the initial postoperative

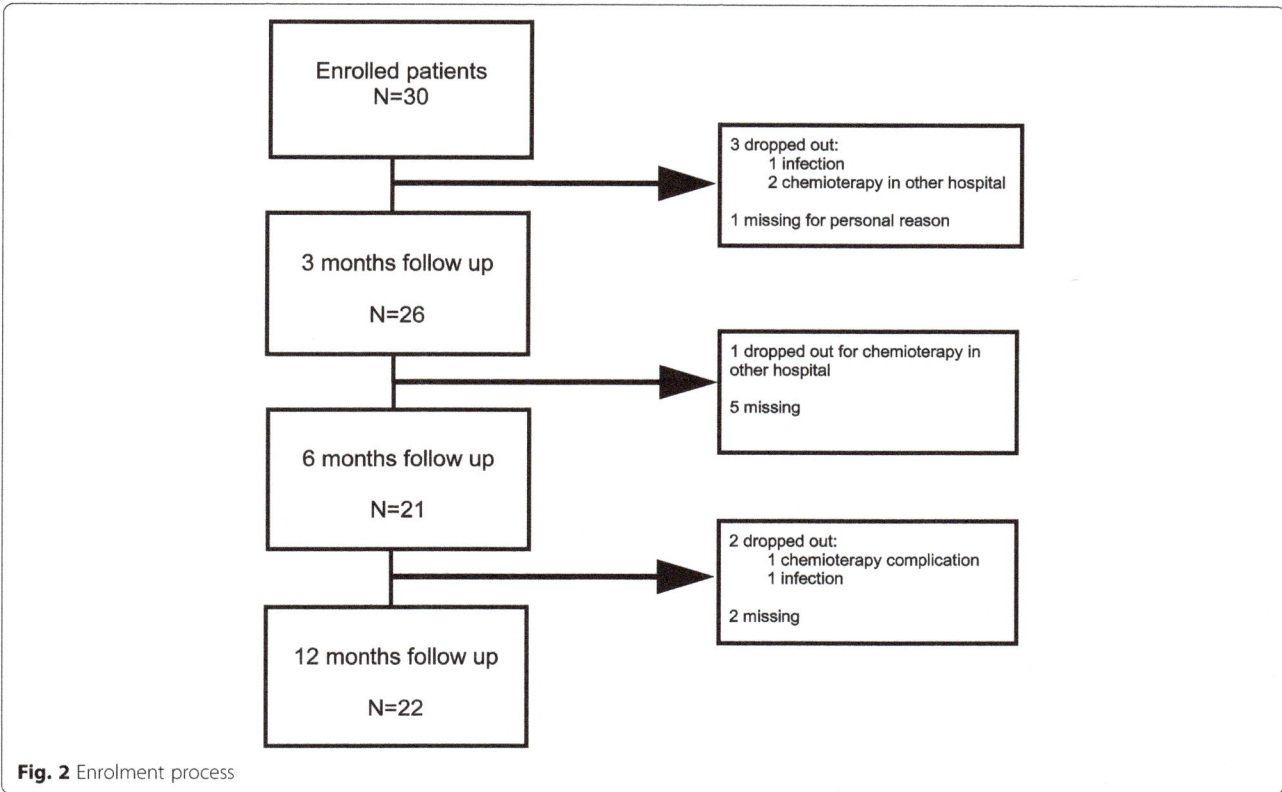

Fig. 2 Enrolment process

phase. The results achieved by the population in the present study are in line with those of most previous studies [7–11] both in terms of the evaluation of disability and motor performance (Table 2). However, it should be noted that comparison with other studies must take into account the type of intervention patients were subjected to, and the timing of follow-up. Whereas the main studies report findings at a follow up of more than 2 years, patients analyzed in the present study were able to reach a similar functional outcome at 1 year of follow-up. Further studies are needed in order to understand if this result might be determined by the rehabilitation program implemented and if a prolonged treatment beyond a year can further improve outcomes. Benedetti et al. [23] highlighted the need to continue the rehabilitation of these patients for more than a year after surgery. In comparison with the paper by Bekkering [8], the only study to report the functional outcome data 1 year after the intervention, we observed the same level of autonomy achieved. In particular, we observed a TESS score of 85%

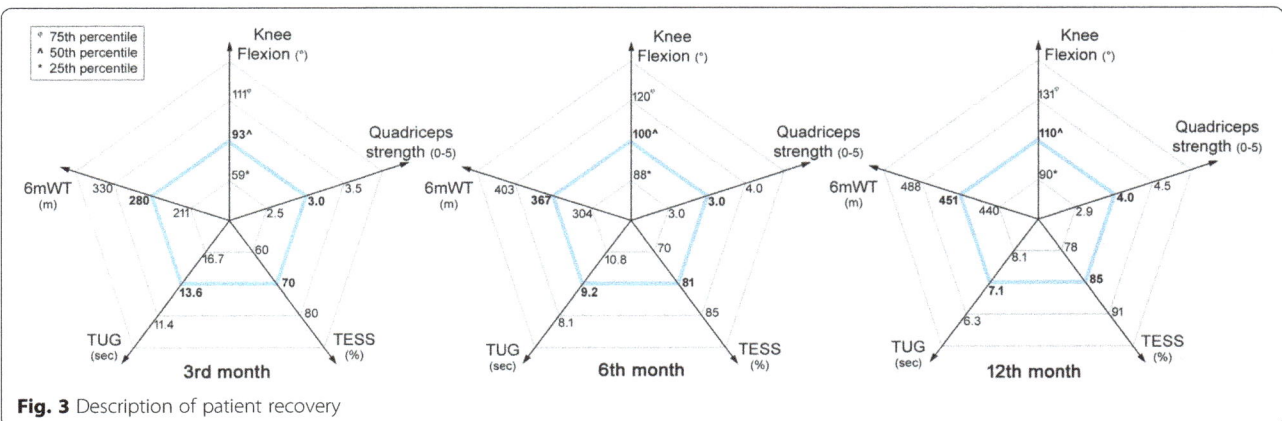

Fig. 3 Description of patient recovery

Table 2 Comparison of the results obtained between different studies

Authors (year)	N	Surgery	Follow-up (yr)	Flex (°)	Strength (0–5)	TESS (%)	TUG (sec)	6mWT (m)
Ginsberg, 2007 [7]	41	Limb sparing femur	4.29 (2.98)			86.4 (9.9)	6.6 (2.1)	
	24	Limb sparing tibia				88.1 (9.3)	6.0 (1.2)	
Henderson, 2012 [11]	12	Distal femur	4 (2–12)	98 (36)				
	3	Proximal tibia		105 (18)				
Carty, 2009 [10]	20	Limb salvage	7.5 (5.1)	125 (80–140)	4.15 (2–5)	86 (3.5)		
Bekkering, 2011 [9]	15	Knee endoprosthesis	2.3 (1.5)				7.2 (1.6)	471 (75)
Bekkering, 2012 [8]	4	Limb salvage and ablative	1			85 (2.4)		430 (18)
Current Study	*22*	*Knee endoprosthesis*	*1*	*110 (70–150)*	*4.0 (1.5–5.0)*	*85 (11.3)*	*7.1(1.8)*	*450 (47.5)*

and a similar distance walked during the 6mWT: 430 and 450 m, respectively. However, it should be noted that in Bekkering's study [8] the functional data presented were not stratified by type of intervention; instead, patients treated with limb salvage and amputation were grouped together. It is important to underline the importance of iterative evaluation at 3–6-12 months to evaluate the progress of the patient's recovery correctly by highlighting which skills are most deficient and which later on make functional recovery. In the field of oncology one of the tasks of rehabilitation is to guide the recovery of the patient and to address their expectations correctly [24]. The graphs presented in this study should be used as clinical tools able to provide indications on the progress of recovery, both for health care staff and patients. Sub-group analysis shows that when a resection of greater than 20 cm is made, a lower recovery of muscle strength with a median of 3.5 (IQR 1.9) is expected. Conversely, with resections below 20 cm, the median recovered force is 4.5 (IQR 1). This difference was not significant, having a more conservative p-value ($p = 0.01$). Regarding knee flexion, there is a difference between patients treated by distal femur resection (median 110° - IQR 40), compared to patients treated by tibia resection (median 90° - IQR 40). This difference may be the result of the immobilization period following

the proximal tibia resection, necessary for the reconstructed patellar tendon to heal. Therefore, with regard to functional recovery in terms of force and mobility of the knee, two fundamental elements must be taken into consideration: the width of the resection greater than or less than 20 cm and the proximal tibia or distal femur resection.

Limitation

The study has some limitations. First of all, the small sample size; bone tumors are rare and we collected all the patients admitted to our hospital over more than 1 year. Second, the arbitrary choice of 20 cm in the resection length. In the absence of information in the literature concerning the length of resection; that cut-off was established from the observation of the data collected in the present study. Finally, the lack of a control group.

Conclusion

Patients undergoing knee replacement with modular prostheses for bone tumors are able to achieve satisfactory functional outcomes starting from the first postoperative year. A specific assessment of outcomes can be performed to facilitate the management of patient expectations and to help clinicians analyze the results achieved. A very wide

Table 3 Multiple sub-group comparisons of the outcomes evaluated at 12 months

Variables		N	Flex °	Strenght	TESS	6mWT	TUG
Age	≤18y	9	110 (58)	3.4 (2.3)	87.5 (15.3)	450 (34)	7.5 (2.0)
	>18y	13	100 (28)	4 (1)	81.4 (12)	451 (108)	7.0 (1.8)
Sex	Men	17	110 (35)	4 (2)	83.6 (13.6)	450 (55)	7.4 (1.8)
	Women	5	90 (48)	4.5 (1.5)	87.5 (16.1)	468 (115)	6.9 (3.4)
Diagnosis	Osteosarcoma	18	110 (29)	3.75 (2)	85 (12.6)	449 (64)	7.5 (1.8)
	Ewing	4	112.5 (64)	4.5 (0.8)	85.3 (17.0)	459.5 (57)	6.3 (1.1)
Resection level	Femur	15	110 (40)	4 (1.5)	83.6 (13.1)	470 (80)	7.2 (1.9)
	Tibia	7	90 (40)	3.2 (1.5)	84.9 (14.1)	449 (25)	7.0 (1.6)
Resection amplitude	≤20 cm	16	105 (38)	4.5 (1)	91.9 (33.2)	449 (70)	7.3 (1.9)
	> 20 cm	6	115 (43)	3.5 (1.9)	82.7 (9.5)	469 (84)	6.8 (2.6)

resection and interventions of the proximal tibia might be risk factors for the functional outcome.

Abbreviations
6mWT: Six minutes walking test; IQR: Interquartile range; ROM: Range of motion; TESS: Toronto Extremity Salvage Score; TUG: Time Up and Go

Acknowledgements
We would like to thank Chemotherapy Department of Instituto Ortopedico Rizzoli.

Funding
This work was supported by Nurse Research Center and Physical Medicine and Rehabilitation Department of Istituto Ortopedico Rizzoli.

Authors' contributions
MM study conception and design, analyzed and interpreted the patient data, wrote the manuscript; FC study conception and design, analyzed and interpreted the patient data; RR collected data and built data set; GT collected and interpreted the data; FG collected data and built data set; DMD analyzed and interpreted the patient data, revised the paper critically for important intellectual content; MGB analyzed and interpreted the patient data, revised the paper critically for important intellectual content. All authors read and approved the final manuscript.

Competing interests
The authors declare that they have no competing interest.

Author details
[1]Servizio di Assistenza Infermieristica, Tecnica e della Riabilitazione, IRCCS Istituto Ortopedico Rizzoli, Via Pupilli 1, 40136 Bologna, Italy. [2]Clinica Ortopedica e Traumatologica III a prevalente indirizzo Oncologico, IRCCS Istituto Ortopedico Rizzoli, Bologna, Italy. [3]Servizio di Medicina Fisica e Riabilitativa, IRCCS Istituto Ortopedico Rizzoli, Bologna, Italy.

References
1. AIRTUM Working Group, Busco S, Buzzoni C, Mallone S, et al. Italian cancer figures--Report 2015: The burden of rare cancers in Italy. Epidemiol Prev. 2016;40(1 Suppl 2):1–120 Erratum in: Epidemiol Prev. 2016 Mar-40(2):83.
2. Stiller CA, Bielack SS, Jundt G, Steliarova-Foucher E. Bone tumours in European children and adolescents, 1978-1997. Report from the Automated Childhood Cancer Information System project. Eur J Cancer. 2006;42: 2124e35.
3. Picci P, Manfrini M, Fabbri N, Gambarotti M, Vanel D. Atlas of Musculoskeletal Tumors and Tumorlike Lesions: The Rizzoli Case Archive 2016. Springer International Publishing. https://doi.org/10.1007/978-3-319-01748-8.
4. Asavamongkolkul A, Waikakul S, Phimolsarnti R, Kiatisevi P, Wangsaturaka P. Endoprosthetic reconstruction for malignant bone and soft-tissue tumors. J Med Assoc Thail. 2007;90(4):706–17.
5. Gosheger G, Gebert C, Ahrens H, Streitbuerger A, Winkelmann W, Hardes J. Endoprosthetic reconstruction in 250 patients with sarcoma. Clin Orthop Relat Res. 2006;450:164–71.
6. Qadir I, Umer M, Baloch N. Functional outcome of limb salvage surgery with mega-endoprosthetic reconstruction for bone tumors. Arch Orthop Trauma Surg. 2012;132(9):1227–32.
7. Ginsberg JP, Rai SN, Carlson CA, Meadows AT, Hinds PS, Spearing EM, Zhang L, Callaway L, Neel MD, Rao BN, Marchese VG. A comparative analysis of functional outcomes in adolescents and young adults with lower-extremity bone sarcoma. Pediatr Blood Cancer. 2007;49(7):964–9.
8. Bekkering WP, VlietVlieland TP, Koopman HM, et al. A prospective study on quality of life and functional outcome in children and adolescents after malignant bone tumor surgery. Pediatr Blood Cancer. 2012;58(6):978–85.
9. Bekkering WP, Vliet Vlieland TP, Koopman HM, Schaap GR, Bart Schreuder HW, Beishuizen A, Jutte PC, Hoogerbrugge PM, Anninga JK, Nelissen RG, Taminiau AH. Functional ability and physical activity in children and young adults after limb-salvage or ablative surgery for lower extremity bone tumors. J Surg Oncol. 2011;103(3):276–82. https://doi.org/10.1002/jso.21828.
10. Carty CP, Dickinson IC, Watts MC, Crawford RW, Steadman P. Impairment and disability following limb salvage procedures for bone sarcoma. Knee. 2009;16(5):405–8.
11. Henderson ER, Pepper AM, Marulanda G, Binitie OT, Cheong D, Letson GD. Outcome of lower-limb preservation with an expandable endoprosthesis after bone tumor resection in children. J Bone Joint Surg Am. 2012;94(6):537–47. https://doi.org/10.2106/JBJS.I.01575.
12. Yalniz E, Ciftdemir M, Memişoğlu S. Functional results of patients treated with modular prosthetic replacement for bone tumors of the extremities. Acta Orthop Traumatol Turc. 2008;42(4):238–45.
13. de Visser E, Deckers JA, Veth RP, et al. Deterioration of balance control after limb-saving surgery. Am J Phys Med Rehabil. 2001;80(5):358–65.
14. Shehadeh A, El Dahleh M, et al. Standardization of rehabilitation after limb salvage surgery for sarcomas improves patients' outcome. Hematol Oncol Stem Cell Ther. 2013;6(3–4):105–11.
15. Brosseau L, Tousignant M, Budd J, Chartier N, Duciaume L, Plamondon S, O'Sullivan JP, O'Donoghue S, Balmer S. Intratester and intertester reliability and criterion validity of the parallelogram and universal goniometers for active knee flexion in healthy subjects. Physiother Res Int. 1997;2(3):150–66.
16. Medical Research Council. Aids to the investigation of peripheral nerve injuries. 2nd ed. London: Her Majesty's Stationery Office; 1943.
17. Davis AM, Wright JG, Williams JI, et al. Development of a measure of physical function for patients with bone and soft tissue sarcoma. Qual Life Res. 1996;5:508–16.
18. Podsiadlo D, Richardson S. The timed "up and go": a test of basic functional mobility for frail elderly persons. J Am Geriatr Soc. 1991;39(2):142–8.
19. Butland RJ, Pang J, Gross ER, Woodcock AA, Geddes DM. Two-, six-, and 12-minute walking tests in respiratory disease. Br Med J (Clin Res Ed). 1982; 284(6329):1607–8.
20. Ferrari S, Ruggieri P, Cefalo G, et al. Neoadjuvant chemotherapy with methotrexate, cisplatin, and doxorubicin with or without ifosfamide in nonmetastatic osteosarcoma of the extremity: an Italian sarcoma group trial ISG/OS-1. J Clin Oncol. 2012;30(17):2112–8.
21. Benedetti MG, Zati A, Mariani E, Ruggeri P. Neoplasie primitive dell'apparato muscolo scheletrico: LA RIABILITAZIONE. 2016.
22. Fung V, Ho A, Shaffer J, Chung E, Gomez M. Use of Nintendo Wii fit™ in the rehabilitation of outpatients following total knee replacement: a preliminary randomised controlled trial. Physiotherapy. 2012;98(3):183–8. https://doi.org/10.1016/j.physio.2012.04.001.
23. Benedetti MG, ErfeDelayon S, Colangeli M, et al. Rehabilitation needs in oncological patients: the on-rehab project results on patients operated for musculoskeletal tumors. Eur J Phys Rehabil Med. 2017;53(1):81–90.
24. Punzalan M, Hyden G. The role of physical therapy and occupational therapy in the rehabilitation of pediatric and adolescent patients with osteosarcoma. Cancer Treat Res. 2009;152:367–84. https://doi.org/10.1007/978-1-4419-0284-9_20.

21

Use of iliac crest allograft for Dega pelvic osteotomy in patients with cerebral palsy

Ki Hyuk Sung[1†], Soon-Sun Kwon[2†], Chin Youb Chung[1], Kyoung Min Lee[1], Jaeyoung Kim[3] and Moon Seok Park[1*] [iD]

Abstract

Background: Dega pelvic osteotomy is commonly performed procedure in patients with cerebral palsy (CP) undergoing hip reconstructive surgery for hip displacement. However, there has been no study investigating the outcomes after Dega pelvic osteotomy using allograft in patients with CP. This study investigated the outcomes of Dega pelvic osteotomy using iliac crest allograft in CP with hip displacement and the factors affecting allograft incorporation.

Methods: This study included 110 patients (150 hips; mean age 8y7mo; 68 males, 42 females) who underwent hip reconstructive surgeries including Dega pelvic osteotomy using iliac crest allograft. To evaluate the time of allograft incorporation, Goldberg score was evaluated according to the follow-up period on all postoperative hip radiographs. The acetabular index, migration percentage, and neck-shaft angle were also measured on the preoperative and postoperative follow-up radiographs.

Results: The mean estimated time for allograft incorporation (Goldberg score ≥ 6) was 1.1 years postoperatively. All hips showed radiographic union at the final follow-up and there was no case of graft-related complications. Patients with Gross Motor Function Classification System (GMFCS) level V had 6.9 times higher risk of radiographic delayed union than those with GMFCS level III and IV. Acetabular index did not increase during the follow-up period ($p = 0.316$).

Conclusions: Dega pelvic osteotomy using iliac crest allograft was effective in correcting acetabular dysplasia, without graft-related complications in patients with CP. Furthermore, the correction of acetabular dysplasia remained stable during the follow-up period.

Keywords: Dega osteotomy, Iliac crest allograft, Cerebral palsy, Goldberg score, Aceteabular dysplasia

Background

Cerebral palsy (CP) is defined as a group of permanent motor impairment disorders that are attributed to non-progressive disturbances in the brain of a developing fetus or infant. [1] Hip displacement (subluxation or dislocation) is common deformity in CP patients with severe impairment and is associated with acetabular dysplasia. [2] It can lead to pain and severe contractures, resulting in difficulties with perineal care, sitting balance, standing, and walking, as well as reduced quality of life. [3] Severely subluxated or dislocated hip can be corrected by hip reconstructive surgeries including proximal femoral varus osteotomy (FVO), either separately or in combination with several different types of pelvic osteotomy. [4] In patients with adequate sourcil and presence of a triradiate cartilage, reconstruction of the acetabulum using the Dega technique stabilizes the pelvis better than other techniques because it is a stable and incomplete osteotomy, and does not affect the medial cortex of the ilium. [5]

Most studies reported the use of iliac crest or femoral autograft as the interposition material for Dega osteotomy. The stability and the maintenance of osteotomy are dependent on the strength of the graft materials. [6] However, patients with CP have the osteoporotic features around the hip joint. [7] When an autogenous bone graft from the iliac crest is used, it may cause

---

* Correspondence: pmsmed@gmail.com
†Ki Hyuk Sung and Soon-Sun Kwon contributed equally to this work.
¹Department of Orthopaedic Surgery, Seoul National University Bundang Hospital, 82 Gumi-ro 173 Beon-gil, Bundang-Gu, Sungnam, Gyeonggi 13620, South Korea
Full list of author information is available at the end of the article

growth disturbances in the iliac bone due to splitting of the iliac apophysis, longer operation time, and increased blood loss. [8, 9] Therefore, our institution has been used iliac crest allograft as an interposition material for the Dega osteotomy in patients with CP.

Tricortical iliac allograft bone is widely available, has no donor site morbidity for harvesting, and has similar bone union rates as an autograft. [10, 11] Nevertheless, an allograft poses some concerns about the risk of transmission of infectious disease and graft rejection. [12, 13] However, a bone demineralization process can decrease the rates of disease transmission. [14] Several studies have reported allograft failure after operations on the spine, humerus, tibia and calcaneus. [15–19] However, to our knowledge, no study has investigated the outcomes after Dega pelvic osteotomy using allograft in patients with CP.

In the present study, we aimed to investigate the outcomes after Dega pelvic osteotomy, using iliac crest allograft in patients with CP. Furthermore, we also investigated the factors influencing allograft incorporation.

Methods

Participants

The inclusion criteria were (1) consecutive children with CP with hip displacement (2) patients who underwent hip reconstructive surgeries, including Dega pelvic osteotomy and FVO from 2003 to 2015, (2) patients with a minimum follow-up of 1 year, and (3) patients who had preoperative and at least two postoperative follow-up hip radiographs. Patients with a history of hip surgery and with inappropriate hip radiographs for assessment were excluded.

Surgical protocol

At our hospital, hip reconstructive surgeries, including Dega pelvic osteotomy and FVO, were performed in displaced hips by two pediatric orthopedic surgeons. Hip reconstructive surgery was indicated in patients with a migration percentage (MP) of more than 33%. For FVO, the osteotomy site at the intertrochanteric level was fixated using a blade plate (Stryker, Selzach, Switzerland) or a pediatric locking compression plate (Depuy Synthes, MA, USA). For Dega pelvic osteotomy, the osteotomy site was widened using a laminar spreader until sufficient coverage of the femoral head was achieved under C-arm fluoroscopy. A tricortical iliac crest allograft was trimmed and inserted into the osteotomy site. Internal fixation of the bone graft was not performed. After surgery, bilateral short leg cast with an abduction bar were applied to maintain hip abduction position for 6 weeks. [20] Thereafter, all patients returned to a local rehabilitation center to begin standing and weight-bearing exercises.

Consensus building

A consensus building session was conducted for the selection of the radiographic parameters; this session included 5 orthopedic surgeons. Previous studies regarding graft incorporation after bone grafting were reviewed, and the Goldberg scoring system was selected. [19, 21] In hip radiographs, graft appearance, bony union at the proximal end and bony union at the distal end, were defined and evaluated. For graft appearance, the score was 0 for resorbed, 1 for mostly resorbed, 2 for largely intact, and 3 for reorganizing. For bony union at the proximal and distal ends, the score was 0 for nonunion, 1 for possible union, and 2 for complete union. [19] The highest possible score was 7 points, which indicated excellent graft reorganization and radiographic union (Fig. 1). For our study, radiographic delayed union was defined as a Goldberg score < 6 by 6 months after the surgery.

Additionally, 3 radiographic parameters that were relevant to assessing hip displacement and acetabular dysplasia were selected from previous studies [3, 22–25]. These were the neck-shaft angle (NSA), MP, and acetabular index (AI) on hip radiographs (Fig. 2).

Reliability testing and radiographic measurements

To assess the inter-observer reliabilities of radiographic measurements, three orthopedic surgeons measured the radiographic indices including MP, NSA, AI, and the Goldberg score for 36 hips independently. Four weeks after the inter-observer reliability testing, one orthopedic surgeon (JYK) performed the measurements again for 36 hips to evaluate the intra-observer reliability. After the completion of reliability test, he performed the measurement for all preoperative and postoperative follow-up hip radiographs.

Statistical methods

Inter- and intra-observer reliabilities of radiographic measurements were assessed by the ICCs and their 95% CIs with the setting of a two-way mixed effects model, assuming a single measurement and absolute agreement. [26] Prior sample size estimation was performed for reliability testing with a target ICC value of 0.80 and a 95% CI width of 0.2 for 3 examiners. The minimum sample size was 36 hips, using Bonett's method. [27] An ICC value more than 0.8 represented excellent reliability. Repeated measures analysis of variance with a Bonferroni post hoc test was applied to compare the preoperative radiographic measurements to postoperative and final follow-up values.

Bilateral cases were included in this study, thus, a linear mixed model (LMM) and a generalized estimating equation (GEE) were used for statistical analysis. [28] The risk factors for radiographic delayed union were

Goldberg scoring system for pelvic bone graft

Graft appearance

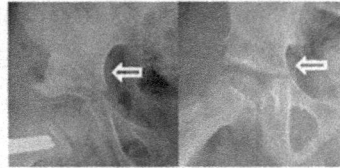

Index	Point	Check
1. Graft appeareance		
Resorbed	0	
Mostly resorbed	1	
Largely intact	2	
Reorganizing	3	
2. Bony union (Proximal)		
Nonunion	0	
Possible union	1	
Radiographic union	2	
3. Bony union (Distal)		
Nonunion	0	
Possible union	1	
Radiographic union	2	
Total		

Bone union (Proximal)

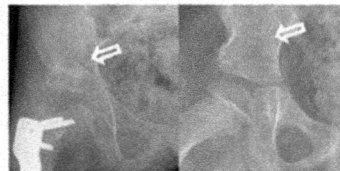

Bone union (Distal)

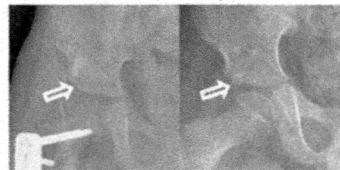

Fig. 1 Indices of the Goldberg scoring system are shown. A postoperative hip radiograph is used for the checklist. There was no case with scores 0 and 1 for graft appearance, and no case with score 0 for proximal and distal bony union. Modified from Goldberg VM, Powell A, Shaffer JW, Zika J, Bos GD, Heiple KG. Bone grafting: role of histocompatibility in transplantation. J Orthop Res. 1985;3:389–404.

evaluated by a GEE to calculate the adjusted odds ratios (ORs). The annual change in the MP, NSA, and AI was adjusted by multiple factors by using a LMM. R version 3.2.5 (R Foundation for Statistical Computing, Vienna, Austria) and SAS 9.4.2 (SAS Institute, Cary, NC, USA) were used for statistical analysis, and p-values less than 0.05 were considered to be significant.

Results

One hundred ten patients with 150 hips were enrolled in this study. The mean number of follow-up radiographs was 6 per patients (range, 2–15) (Table 1).

Inter- and intra-observer reliabilities of all radiographic measurements were excellent (ICC, 0.802 to 0.924) (Table 2). MP, NSA and AI were significantly improved after hip reconstructive surgery including the Dega osteotomy (all $p < 0.001$). AI was not changed at final follow-up ($p = 1.000$), but MP and NSA had significantly increased at final follow-up (both $p < 0.001$) (Table 3).

The mean estimated Goldberg score was 6 at 1.1 years after Dega osteotomy (Fig. 3). Twenty-four hips (16%, 4 hips with GMFCS level IV and 20 hips with GMFCS level V) were classified as radiographic delayed union (Goldberg score < 6) at 6 months after surgery. Nine hips (6%, all hips with GMFCS level V) had Goldberg score < 6 at 1 year after surgery. However, all hips showed radiographic union at the final

follow-ups and no hips underwent reoperation due to nonunion. There were no cases of bone graft resorption, nonunion, dislodgement, and graft-related infections (Fig. 4).

GMFCS level was significantly associated with radiographic delayed union ($p = 0.001$). Patients with GMFCS level V had 6.9 times higher risks for radiographic delayed union than those with GMFCS level III and IV. Other factors such as age, sex, anatomical type and body side were not associated with radiographic delayed union (Table 4).

AI was not increased by follow-up duration (0.2 degrees per year; $p = 0.316$). However, MP and NSA were significantly increased by follow-up duration (2.5%, $p < 0.001$ and 2.5 degrees, $p < 0.001$, respectively) (Table 5).

Discussion

To our knowledge, this is the largest study investigating outcomes after Dega osteotomy and the first study regarding the allograft behavior after Dega osteotomy in patients with CP. This study showed that a Dega pelvic osteotomy using an allograft could not only correct acetabular dysplasia, but also keep it stable over time. Therefore, an allograft can be a good option as the interposition material for Dega osteotomy if a femoral autograft is not available. Additionally, this study found that allograft incorporation in patients with GMFCS Level V

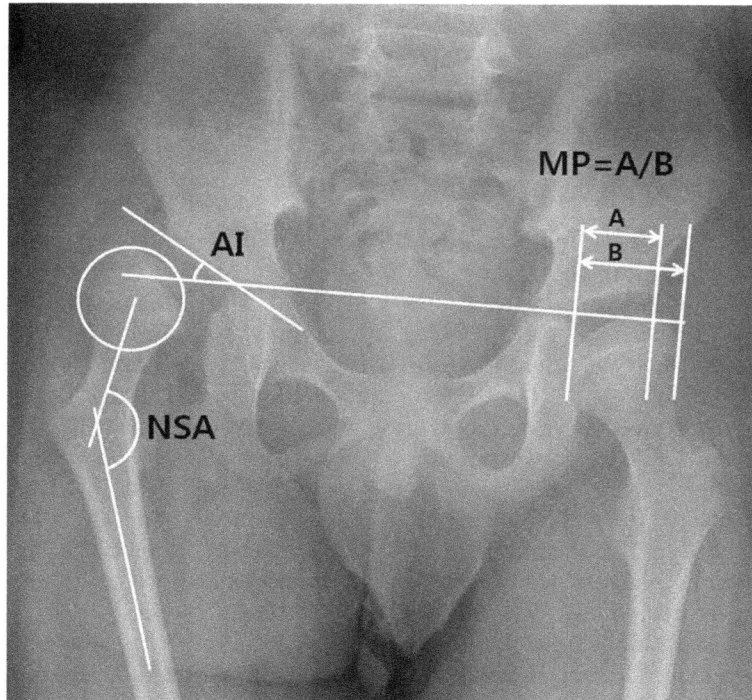

Fig. 2 Hip internal rotation view. For the right hip neck-shaft angle (NSA) was defined as the angle between a line passing through the center of the femoral shaft and another line connecting the center of the femoral head and the midpoint of the femoral neck. The center of the femoral head was the center of the largest best-fitting circle inside the femoral head. Acetabular index (AI) was defined as the angle between the acetabular roof and the Hilgenreiner's line. For the left hip, migration percentage (MP) was calculated by dividing the width of the femoral head lateral to Perkin's line (**a**) by the total width of the femoral head (**b**)

was significantly delayed compared to those with GMFCS level III and IV.

There were some limitations of this study. First, only retrospective review of medical records and radiographic assessments were used for evaluating surgical outcomes. However, we believe that allograft behavior can be reflected best by radiographic assessment. Second, all patients were not evaluated until skeletal maturity. However, all hips showed radiographic union at final follow-up without any allograft-related complication. Furthermore, our analysis showed that the correction of acetabular dysplasia remained stable throughout the follow-up duration. Therefore, we think that further

follow-up may not be necessary. Thirds, no comparison group that used autograft for Dega osteotomy was included. Therefore, further study comparing the outcomes of allografts and autografts as graft materials for Dega osteotomy is required.

Most of authors used the iliac crest autograft or femoral autograft obtained from femoral shortening osteotomy as a bone graft material for Dega osteotomy and showed good clinical and radiological outcomes in patients with CP and developmental dysplasia of the hip (DDH) (Table 6). [6, 29–45] Mallet et al. investigated the long-term results after one-stage hip reconstructive surgery in children with CP. [37] They found that correction of AI remained

Table 1 Summary of patient data

Parameters	Values
Male / Female	68 / 42
Anatomical type (diplegia / quadriplegia)	18 / 92
GMFCS level (III/IV/V)	17 / 39 / 54
Age at surgery (years)	8.7 ± 2.4 (2.8 to 13.8)
Follow-up duration (years)	2.9 ± 2.6 (1.0 to 12.0)
Age at final follow-up (years)	11.6 ± 3.8 (3.8 to 22.5)
Laterality (Right / Left)	80 / 70

GMFCS Gross Motor Function Classification System

Table 2 Intra- and inter-observer reliabilities of radiographic measurements

Measurements	Inter-observer reliability		Intra-observer reliability	
	ICC	95% CI	ICC	95% CI
Neck-shaft angle	0.808	0.655–0.894	0.802	0.645–0.894
Migration percentage	0.885	0.740–0.945	0.860	0.723–0.932
Acetabular index	0.817	0.709–0.895	0.833	0.732–0.904
Goldberg score	0.918	0.864–0.954	0.924	0.874–0.958

ICC intraclass correlation coefficient, CI confidence interval

Table 3 Summary of radiographic measurements

Radiographic index	Preoperative	Immediate postoperative	Final follow-up	p-value		
				Preop-postop	Preop-final	Postop-final
Acetabular index (degree)	32.2 ± 7.0	13.6 ± 5.5	13.8 ± 5.9	< 0.001	< 0.001	1.000
Neck-shaft angle (degree)	156.0 ± 9.8	119.9 ± 10.7	125.1 ± 13.6	< 0.001	< 0.001	< 0.001
Migration percentage (%)	75.2 ± 20.2	0.5 ± 2.3	11.7 ± 12.2	< 0.001	< 0.001	< 0.001

stable postoperatively for 9 years of follow-up. Joz-wiak et al. also reported that AI did not show any noticeable changes during the follow-up period after Dega pelvic osteotomy in patients with CP. [31] Our study also showed that AI did not increase during the follow-up period.

On the contrary, previous studies have found that both NSA and MP showed a tendency to worsen during the follow-up period after hip reconstruction, including Dega osteotomy, in CP . [31, 37] In addition, Bayusentono et al. showed that MP significantly increased by 2.0% per year in patients with GMFCS level IV and by 3.5% per year in those with GMFCS level V. [24] Our study also showed that MP and NSA were significantly increased during the follow-up period, as reported in previous studies.

Several studies showed good surgical outcome after pelvic osteotomy using allograft for DDH patients. Wade et al. investigated the radiologic results of 147 hips treated for DDH by Dega osteotomy with an iliac crest allograft. [6] They showed that

postoperative corrected AI had improved at 2 years of follow-up. McCarthy et al. compared the results of autograft and allograft in 36 hips after Pemberton osteotomy. [46] Almost all of the children with DDH had satisfactory results regardless of graft type, but allograft provided better results than iliac crest autograft in neuromuscular diseases. Kessler et al. also reported that allograft bone could be effectively used in Pemberton osteotomy in 26 hips with DDH or neuromuscular disorders. [47] The authors believed that the immediate stability, owing to the larger size and the mechanical properties of the graft, allowed for earlier rehabilitation.

Patients with CP have low BMD, which is highly correlated with GMFCS levels. Several factors, including physical disability, poor nutritional status, decreased calcium intake, low vitamin D level, prolonged immobilization, sarcopenia, and the use of anticonvulsant, were associated with the low BMD in patients with CP. [48–50] Moon et al. showed that bone attenuation of the acetabulum and femur neck was significantly

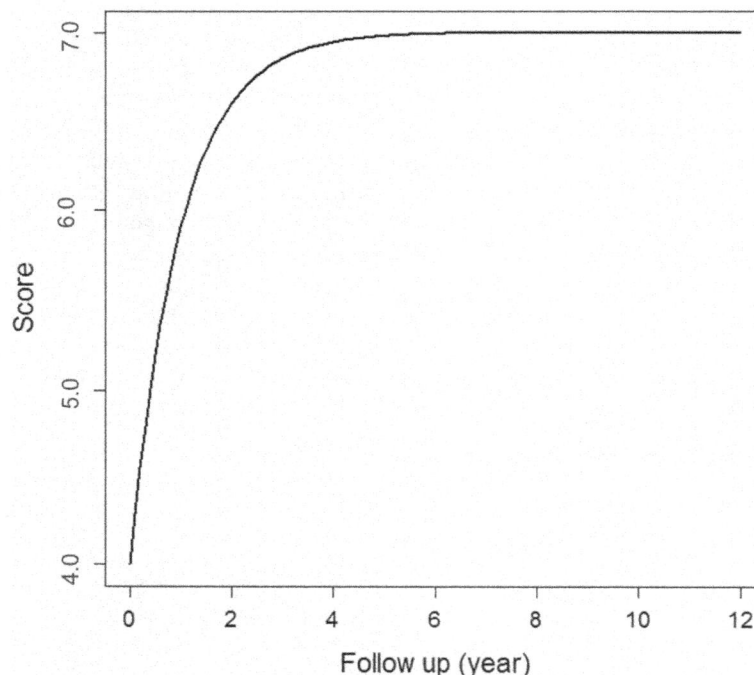

Fig. 3 Graph showing the mean Goldberg score according to the duration of follow-up after Dega osteotomy

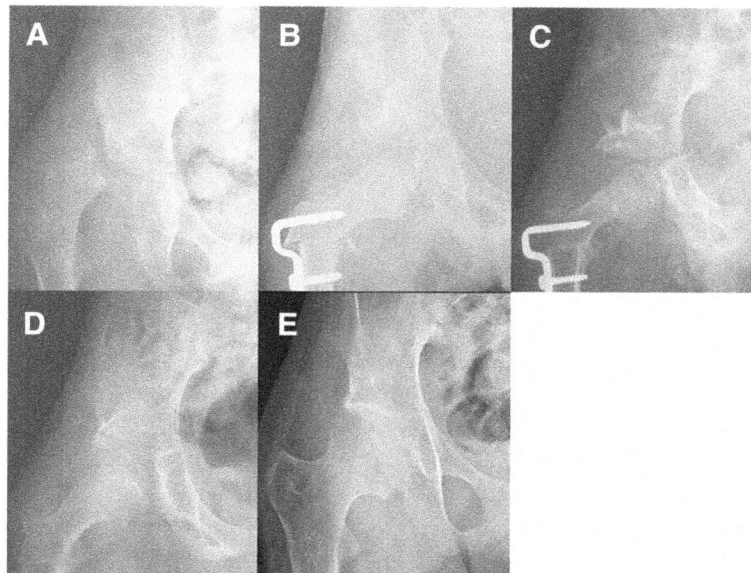

Fig. 4 a Preoperative hip radiograph of a 9-year-old body with cerebral palsy shows right hip dislocation and aceteabular dysplasia. **b** He underwent hip reconstructive surgery including Dega osteotomy using iliac crest allograft for right hip. **c** The osteotomy site was not incorporated yet at 6 months after the surgery (Goldberg score of 5), **d** It was completely incorporated at 1 year after the surgery (Goldberg score of 7). **e** Correction of acetabular dysplasia remained stable at 10 years after the surgery

affected by GMFCS levels and degree of hip displacement. [7] Because the osteoporotic features around hip joints in CP may not guarantee the initial mechanical stability of osteotomy site, we had used iliac crest allograft as the interposition material at the osteotomy site.

Allograft has been proven to be a good choice of graft in other pediatric orthopedic conditions. Wade et al. showed that all of the allografts were completely incorporated at 6 months after surgery with a mean incorporation time of 3 months in 147 hips treated for DDH by Dega osteotomy. [6] Lee et al. investigated the incidence and risk factors of allograft failure after lateral column lengthening for planovalgus foot deformity. [19] They reported that the mean estimated Goldberg score was 6 at 6 months after surgery and 4% of feet had Goldberg score < 6 at 6 months after surgery. Additionally, reoperation using an autogenous iliac bone graft bone was performed in four feet (1%). In our study, the mean

estimated Goldberg score was 6 at 1.1 years after Dega osteotomy and at 6 months after the surgeries, 16% of hips had a Goldberg score of < 6. Furthermore, allograft incorporation in patients with GMFCS Level V was significantly delayed than in those with GMFCS level III and IV. However, no hip underwent reoperation due to allograft failure. We think that the delayed allograft incorporation in our study, compared with previous studies, is due to the underlying CP in the included patients with GMFCS level III to V. On the other hand, Wade et al.'s study included patients with DDH, and Lee et al.'s study included patients with idiopathic planovalgus and ambulatory CP. We think that the delayed allograft incorporation in patients with GMFCS level V compared with those with GMFCS level III and IV is due to the severity of osteoporosis. Therefore, surgeons should remember that the degree of osteoporosis might affect the time to allograft incorporation and pay extra attention to the patients with GMFCS level V.

Table 4 Potential risk factors for radiographic delayed union

Factor	Adjusted OR (95% CI)	P-value
Age (per year)	0.9 (0.8 to 1.1)	0.443
Sex (male)	0.4 (0.2 to 1.0)	0.062
GMFCS level (V)	6.9 (2.2 to 22.2)	0.001
Anatomical type (quadriplegia)	2.3 (0.2 to 22.5)	0.476
Body side (right)	1.6 (0.6 to 4.0)	0.365

OR odds ratio, *CI* confidence interval, *GMFCS* Gross Motor Function Classification System; Multivariate analysis using generalized estimation equation is used to calculate the OR and CI

Conclusion

Dega pelvic osteotomy using iliac crest allograft was an effective procedure in the correction of acetabular dysplasia without graft-related complications in patients with CP. Additionally, the correction of acetabular dysplasia remained stable during the follow-up period. However, physicians should consider that allograft incorporation in patients with GMFCS level V can be delayed compared with those with GMFCS level III & IV.

Table 5 Factors affecting radiographic measurements after hip reconstructive surgery

	Acetabula index			Migration percentage			Neck-shaft angle		
	Estimate	SE	P-value	Estimate	SE	P-value	Estimate	SE	P-value
Follow-up duration (year)	0.2	0.2	0.316	2.5	0.2	< 0.001	2.5	0.3	< 0.001
Age at surgery	−0.0	0.2	0.919	0.2	0.2	0.349	−1.3	0.3	< 0.001
Sex	0.0	0.8	0.961	−2.3	1.1	0.036	2.5	1.7	0.127
GMFCS level									
V (reference)									
III	3.1	1.2	0.010	3.8	1.5	0.013	9.1	2.4	< 0.001
IV	1.2	0.9	0.198	0.6	1.2	0.600	3.1	1.8	0.086
Anatomical type	−0.2	1.2	0.873	−0.1	2.0	0.966	−2.2	2.8	0.445
Laterality	−1.1	0.8	0.001	−0.1	1.0	0.451	−1.2	1.6	0.835

A linear mixed model was used to estimate factors affecting AI, MP and NSA
SE standard error, *GMFCS* Gross Motor Function Classification System

Table 6 Previous studies on the outcome after Dega osteotomy

Author	Diagnosis	Graft material	No. of hips	Age at surgery (year)	Follow-up duration (year)	AI (°)			MP (%)			NSA (°)		
						Preop	Postop	final	Preop	Postop	final	Preop	Postop	final
Current study	CP	Iliac crest allograft	150	8.7	2.9	32.2	13.6	13.8	75.2	0.5	11.7	156	119.9	125.1
Mubarak [29]	CP	Iliac crest autograft	18	8.4	6.8	30		14	78		6.2	149		95
McNerney [30]	CP	Iliac crest autograft	104	8.1	6.9	26	13	11	66	5	14			
Jozwiak [31]	CP		30	7.0	12.0	32	22	23	65	11	20	152	133	140
Robb [32]	CP	Femoral autograft	52	14.0	4.0				70	10				
Kim [33]	CP	Iliac crest or femoral autograft	32	8.6	2.3	35.7	19		74.2	10.6				
Dhawale [34]	CP		22	7.5	11.7				79.4	4.3	7.9	151	112	120.6
Koch [35]	CP	Femoral autograft	115	9.0	5.5	30.7	21.3		98.3	16		142	119.6	119.3
Braatz [36]	CP	Femoral autograft		7.3	7.7				68	12	16			
Mallet [37]	CP	Femoral autograft	20	8.1	9.1	30.1	12.7	15.8	60.6	4.9	15.4	153	114.6	129.7
Reidy [38]	CP	Femoral autograft	57	8.9	5.4				63.6	2.7	9.7	152	132.6	137.2
Grudziak [39]	DDH	Iliac crest or femoral autograft or fibular allograft	24	5.8	4.6	33	12							
Karlen [40]	DDH	Iliac crest or femoral autograft	26	3.1	4.3	37	15	13						
	NM		24	6.3	4.7	36	16	14	84	8	14			
Wade [6]	DDH	Iliac crest allograft	147	2.9	2.0	43.2	24.3	16.9						
Al-Ghamdi [41]	DDH		21	4.6	7.3	37	17	19	38	−10	15			
Aksoy [42]	DDH	Iliac crest or femoral autograft	43	2.9	4.8	35	20	13						
Akgul [43]	DDH		26	3.2	3.5	39.4	18.3	15						
El-Sayed [44]	DDH	Iliac crest or femoral autograft	58	4.1	16.6	39	18	25				−21	19	
Issin [45]	DDH	Iliac crest autograft	10	2.1	5.6	46	23.4	15.9						

CP cerebral palsy, *DDH* developmental dislocation of hip, *NM* neuromuscular, *AI* acetabular index, *MP* migration percentage, *NSA* neck-shaft angle

Abbreviations

AI: Acetabular index; CP: Cerebral palsy; DDH: Developmental dysplasia of hip; FVO: Femoral varization osteotomy; GEE: Generalized estimating equation; GMFCS: Gross Motor Function Classification System; LMM: Linear mixed model; MP: Migration percentage; NSA: Neck-shaft angle

Acknowledgements

The authors thank Seung Joon Moon, MD and Arif Zulkarnain, MD for reliability measurements.

Funding

This research was supported by Korea Institute of Planning and Evaluation for Technology in Food, Agriculture, Forestry and Fisheries(IPET) throughHigh Value-added Food Technology Development Program, funded by Ministry of Agriculture, Food and Rural Affairs(MAFRA)(117051-3), by Ministry of SMEs and Startups (grant no. S2409723), and the SNUBH Research Fund (grant no. 03-2013-005).

Authors' contributions

All authors on this manuscript (KHS, SSK, CYC, KML, JK and MSP) made significant contributions to the study design. KHS, SSK, and JK were involved in acquisition of data. KHS, SSK, KML, JK and MSP were involved in the analysis and interpretation of data, as well as drafting the manuscript. All authors gave final approval of the version to be published.

Competing interests

The authors declare that they have no competing interests.

Author details

[1]Department of Orthopaedic Surgery, Seoul National University Bundang Hospital, 82 Gumi-ro 173 Beon-gil, Bundang-Gu, Sungnam, Gyeonggi 13620, South Korea. [2]Department of Mathematics, College of Natural Sciences, Ajou University, Suwon, Gyeonggi, South Korea. [3]Department of Orthopaedic Surgery, H Plus Yangji Hospital, Seoul, South Korea.

References

1. Bax M, Goldstein M, Rosenbaum P, Leviton A, Paneth N, Dan B, Jacobsson B, Damiano D. Executive Committee for the Definition of Cerebral P: Proposed definition and classification of cerebral palsy, April 2005. Dev Med Child Neurol. 2005;47:571–6.
2. Scrutton D, Baird G, Smeeton N. Hip dysplasia in bilateral cerebral palsy: incidence and natural history in children aged 18 months to 5 years. Dev Med Child Neurol. 2001;43:586–600.
3. Hagglund G, Lauge-Pedersen H, Wagner P. Characteristics of children with hip displacement in cerebral palsy. BMC Musculoskelet Disord. 2007;8:101.
4. Hoffer MM, Stein GA, Koffman M, Prietto M. Femoral varus-derotation osteotomy in spastic cerebral palsy. J Bone Joint Surg Am. 1985;67:1229–35.
5. Dega W. Transiliac osteotomy in the treatment of congenital hip dysplasia. Chir Narzadow Ruchu Ortop Pol. 1974;39:601–13.
6. Wade WJ, Alhussainan TS, Al Zayed Z, Hamdi N, Bubshait D. Contoured iliac crest allograft interposition for pericapsular acetabuloplasty in developmental dislocation of the hip: technique and short-term results. J Child Orthop. 2010;4:429–38.
7. Moon SY, Kwon SS, Cho BC, Chung CY, Lee KM, Sung KH, Chung MK, Zulkarnain A, Kim YS, Park MS. Osteopenic features of the hip joint in patients with cerebral palsy: a hospital-based study. Dev Med Child Neurol. 2016;58:1153–8.
8. Rossillon R, Desmette D, Rombouts JJ. Growth disturbance of the ilium after splitting the iliac apophysis and iliac crest bone harvesting in children: a retrospective study at the end of growth following unilateral Salter innominate osteotomy in 21 children. Acta Orthop Belg. 1999;65:295–301.
9. Goulet JA, Senunas LE, DeSilva GL, Greenfield ML. Autogenous iliac crest bone graft. Complications and functional assessment. Clin Orthop Relat Res. 1997;339:76–81.
10. Mahan KT, Hillstrom HJ. Bone grafting in foot and ankle surgery. A review of 300 cases. J Am Podiatr Med Assoc. 1998;88:109–18.
11. Dolan CM, Henning JA, Anderson JG, Bohay DR, Kornmesser MJ, Endres TJ. Randomized prospective study comparing tri-cortical iliac crest autograft to allograft in the lateral column lengthening component for operative correction of adult acquired flatfoot deformity. Foot Ankle Int. 2007;28:8–12.
12. Bauer TW, Muschler GF. Bone graft materials. An overview of the basic science. Clin Orthop Relat Res. 2000;371:10–27.
13. Cypher TJ, Grossman JP. Biological principles of bone graft healing. J Foot Ankle Surg. 1996;35:413–7.
14. Scarborough NL, White EM, Hughes JV, Manrique AJ, Poser JW. Allograft safety: viral inactivation with bone demineralization. Contemp Orthop. 1995;31:257–61.
15. Ehrler DM, Vaccaro AR. The use of allograft bone in lumbar spine surgery. Clin Orthop Relat Res. 2000;371:38–45.
16. Nugent PJ, Dawson EG. Intertransverse process lumbar arthrodesis with allogeneic fresh-frozen bone graft. Clin Orthop Relat Res. 1993;287:107–11.
17. Segur JM, Torner P, Garcia S, Combalia A, Suso S, Ramon R. Use of bone allograft in tibial plateu fractures. Arch Orthop Trauma Surg. 1998;117:357–9.
18. Tomford WW. Bone allografts: past, present and future. Cell Tissue Bank. 2000;1:105–9.
19. Lee IH, Chung CY, Lee KM, Kwon SS, Moon SY, Jung KJ, Chung MK, Park MS. Incidence and risk factors of allograft bone failure after calcaneal lengthening. Clin Orthop Relat Res. 2015;473:1765–74.
20. Sung KH, Kwon SS, Chung CY, Lee KM, Kim J, Lee SY, Park MS. Fate of stable hips after prophylactic femoral varization osteotomy in patients with cerebral palsy. BMC Musculoskelet Disord. 2018;19:130.
21. Goldberg VM, Powell A, Shaffer JW, Zika J, Bos GD, Heiple KG. Bone grafting: role of histocompatibility in transplantation. J Orthop Res. 1985;3:389–404.
22. Gordon GS, Simkiss DE. A systematic review of the evidence for hip surveillance in children with cerebral palsy. J Bone Joint Surg Br. 2006;88:1492–6.
23. Park JY, Choi Y, Cho BC, Moon SY, Chung CY, Lee KM, Sung KH, Kwon SS, Park MS. Progression of Hip Displacement during Radiographic Surveillance in Patients with Cerebral Palsy. J Korean Med Sci. 2016;31:1143–9.
24. Bayusentono S, Choi Y, Chung CY, Kwon SS, Lee KM, Park MS. Recurrence of hip instability after reconstructive surgery in patients with cerebral palsy. J Bone Joint Surg Am. 2014;96:1527–34.
25. Pidcock FS, Fish DE, Johnson-Greene D, Borras I, McGready J, Silberstein CE. Hip migration percentage in children with cerebral palsy treated with botulinum toxin type A. Arch Phys Med Rehabil. 2005;86:431–5.
26. Lee KM, Lee J, Chung CY, Ahn S, Sung KH, Kim TW, Lee HJ, Park MS. Pitfalls and important issues in testing reliability using intraclass correlation coefficients in orthopaedic research. Clin Orthop Surg. 2012;4:149–55.
27. Bonett DG. Sample size requirements for estimating intraclass correlations with desired precision. Stat Med. 2002;21:1331–5.
28. Park MS, Kim SJ, Chung CY, Choi IH, Lee SH, Lee KM. Statistical consideration for bilateral cases in orthopaedic research. J Bone Joint Surg Am. 2010;92:1732–7.
29. Mubarak SJ, Valencia FG, Wenger DR. One-stage correction of the spastic dislocated hip. Use of pericapsular acetabuloplasty to improve coverage. J Bone Joint Surg Am. 1992;74:1347–57.
30. McNerney NP, Mubarak SJ, Wenger DR. One-stage correction of the dysplastic hip in cerebral palsy with the San Diego acetabuloplasty: results and complications in 104 hips. J Pediatr Orthop. 2000;20:93–103.
31. Jozwiak M, Koch A. Two-stage surgery in the treatment of spastic hip dislocation–comparison between early and late results of open reduction and derotation-varus femoral osteotomy combined with Dega pelvic osteotomy preceded by soft tissue release. Ortop Traumatol Rehabil. 2011;13:144–54.
32. Robb JE, Brunner R. A Dega-type osteotomy after closure of the triradiate cartilage in non-walking patients with severe cerebral palsy. J Bone Joint Surg Br. 2006;88:933–7.
33. Kim HT, Jang JH, Ahn JM, Lee JS, Kang DJ. Early results of one-stage correction for hip instability in cerebral palsy. Clin Orthop Surg. 2012;4:139–48.
34. Dhawale AA, Karatas AF, Holmes L, Rogers KJ, Dabney KW, Miller F. Long-term outcome of reconstruction of the hip in young children with cerebral palsy. Bone Joint J. 2013;95-B:259–65.
35. Koch A, Jozwiak M, Idzior M, Molinska-Glura M, Szulc A. Avascular necrosis as a complication of the treatment of dislocation of the hip in children with cerebral palsy. Bone Joint J. 2015;97-B:270–6.
36. Braatz F, Staude D, Klotz MC, Wolf SI, Dreher T, Lakemeier S. Hip-joint congruity after Dega osteotomy in patients with cerebral palsy: long-term results. Int Orthop. 2016;40:1663–8.
37. Mallet C, Ilharreborde B, Presedo A, Khairouni A, Mazda K, Pennecot GF. One-stage hip reconstruction in children with cerebral palsy: long-term results at skeletal maturity. J Child Orthop. 2014;8:221–8.
38. Reidy K, Heidt C, Dierauer S, Huber H. A balanced approach for stable hips in children with cerebral palsy: a combination of moderate VDRO and pelvic osteotomy. J Child Orthop. 2016;10:281–8.

39. Grudziak JS, Ward WT. Dega osteotomy for the treatment of congenital dysplasia of the hip. J Bone Joint Surg Am. 2001;83-A:845–54.
40. Karlen JW, Skaggs DL, Ramachandran M, Kay RM. The Dega osteotomy: a versatile osteotomy in the treatment of developmental and neuromuscular hip pathology. J Pediatr Orthop. 2009;29:676–82.
41. Al-Ghamdi A, Rendon JS, Al-Faya F, Saran N, Benaroch T, Hamdy RC. Dega osteotomy for the correction of acetabular dysplasia of the hip: a radiographic review of 21 cases. J Pediatr Orthop. 2012;32:113–20.
42. Aksoy C, Yilgor C, Demirkiran G, Caglar O. Evaluation of acetabular development after Dega acetabuloplasty in developmental dysplasia of the hip. J Pediatr Orthop B. 2013;22:91–5.
43. Akgul T, Bora Goksan S, Bilgili F, Valiyev N, Hurmeydan OM. Radiological results of modified Dega osteotomy in Tonnis grade 3 and 4 developmental dysplasia of the hip. J Pediatr Orthop B. 2014;23:333–8.
44. El-Sayed MM, Hegazy M, Abdelatif NM, ElGebeily MA, ElSobky T, Nader S. Dega osteotomy for the management of developmental dysplasia of the hip in children aged 2-8 years: results of 58 consecutive osteotomies after 13-25 years of follow-up. J Child Orthop. 2015;9:191–8.
45. Issin A, Oner A, Kockara N, Camurcu Y. Comparison of open reduction alone and open reduction plus Dega osteotomy in developmental dysplasia of the hip. J Pediatr Orthop B. 2016;25:1–6.
46. McCarthy JJ, Palma DA, Betz RR. Comparison of autograft and allograft fixation in Pemberton osteotomy. Orthopedics. 2008;31:126.
47. Kessler JI, Stevens PM, Smith JT, Carroll KL. Use of allografts in Pemberton osteotomies. J Pediatr Orthop. 2001;21:468–73.
48. Henderson RC, Lark RK, Gurka MJ, Worley G, Fung EB, Conaway M, Stallings VA, Stevenson RD. Bone density and metabolism in children and adolescents with moderate to severe cerebral palsy. Pediatrics. 2002;110:e5.
49. Tatay Diaz A, Farrington DM, Downey Carmona FJ, Macias Moreno ME, Quintana del Olmo JJ. Bone mineral density in a population with severe infantile cerebral palsy. Rev Esp Cir Ortop Traumatol. 2012;56:306–12.
50. Houlihan CM, Stevenson RD. Bone density in cerebral palsy. Phys Med Rehabil Clin N Am. 2009;20:493–508.

22

The change of first metatarsal head articular surface position after Lapidus arthrodesis

Jan Klouda[1,2]* (iD), Rastislav Hromádka[2,3], Simona Šoffová[3], Stanislav Popelka Jr[2], Stanislav Popelka[2] and Ivan Landor[2]

Abstract

Background: The Lapidus procedure has been used for hallux valgus deformity correction since 1931. In some cases, the arthrodesis results in an unfavourable lateral inclination of first metatarsal head articular surface. The objective of our study was to evaluate the change of orientation of this articular surface in relation to the second metatarsal axis by comparing pre- and postoperative radiographs. The secondary target was to evaluate possible benefits of combination of Lapidus and Akin procedures in the reduction of hallux valgus deformity.

Methods: We evaluated 449 pre- and postoperative radiographs of 134 operations from 2010 to 2015. Routinely used angle measurements were performed on all X-rays. A sum of tangential angle to the second axis and distal articular set angle values was chosen as the best indicator for the deformity correction success.

Results: The mean value of these angles total was 5.2° ±9.3° before and 14.2° ±7.8° after the operation. In the group of patients, where the additional Akin osteotomy was used, the mean value was 5.3° ±8.4° before and 6.9° ±10.2° after the surgery. The mean difference in values between the two groups (with and without Akin procedure) was 7.3° of extra correction in favour of the group with the Akin osteotomy.

Conclusions: The mean worsening of the tangential angle after Lapidus operation was 6.1° ±6.9°, which counts for significant deterioration after a surgery. The Akin osteotomy was found to be a valuable addition to the Lapidus arthrodesis, which improves the position of articular surfaces in first metatarsophalangeal joint.

Keywords: Hallux valgus, Lapidus arthrodesis, Akin osteotomy, Tangential angle to the second axis, Proximal articular set angle, X-ray analysis

Background

Hallux valgus deformity has been attracting attention of orthopaedic surgeons from all over the world over the last 150 years. An abundance of reconstruction techniques has been described in the history and forefoot reconstruction surgery remains in the limelight even in the modern era of orthopaedics.

One of techniques routinely used for operative treatment of moderate to severe hallux valgus deformity with first metatarsocuneiform (MTC) joint hypermobility is the surgical procedure originally described by Albrecht

and popularized by Lapidus [1–3]. The procedure allows a very strong reduction of the deformity and a distinct change in position and rotation of the first metatarsal. Recent studies performed by Dayton et al. [4–7] and other authors [8–10] indicated that the rotational component of the deformity is key in its proper reduction.

The Lapidus procedure reduces first intermetatarsal angle (IMA) and changes the inclination and rotation of the first metatarsal head – that's how it indirectly changes the position of the distal articular surface of the first metatarsal. The proper alignment of the surface is important for the correction of the deformity. The position of the surface can be measured on weight-bearing radiographs pre- and postoperatively [11, 12].

The objective of our study was to evaluate the change of orientation of the distal articular surface of first

* Correspondence: jan.klouda@mail.com
[1]Department of Orthopaedics, Hospital Nemocnice České Budějovice, a.s., České Budějovice, Czech Republic
[2]Department of Orthopaedics, First Faculty of Medicine, Charles University and Motol University Hospital, Prague, Czech Republic
Full list of author information is available at the end of the article

metatarsal in relation to the second metatarsal axis by comparing pre- and postoperative radiographs. The study evaluates influence of the derotation of the first metatarsal during the Lapidus procedure. The tangential angle to the second metatarsal axis (TASA) was used as a tool for description of the change of first metatarsal articular surface position.

A secondary goal of our study was to find out, if TASA measurement is a useful tool in the preoperative setting.

The third target of our investigation was to evaluate the possible benefits of combination of Lapidus and Akin procedures in the reduction of hallux valgus deformity.

Methods

We retrospectively evaluated preoperative and postoperative radiographs of 134 feet (69 left, 65 right) of 110 patients (99 female, 11 male) who underwent the forefoot reconstruction surgery in Department of Orthopaedics, First Faculty of Medicine, Charles University in Prague at Motol University Hospital from 2010 to 2015. The mean age was 60.6 years (range 14 to 79). From the total of 110 patients, 19 patients (17%) had forefoot reconstruction surgery performed on both feet (not in one session). All patients were operated by 6 different surgeons.

The Lapidus procedure was performed from open medio-dorsal approach to the first MTC joint and the arthrodesis was fixed with 2–3 screws or 2 memory staples, in one case a plate was used for fixation during a revision surgery. The procedure was combined with other ones like Akin osteotomy or procedures on lesser toes. We used either open, miniinvasive or a combination of these approaches to the lesser toes and proximal phalanx of the hallux. The lateral release of first metatarsophalangeal (MTP) joint and medial eminence adjustment was done in all cases. The release was usually performed through longitudinal open approach in first web space or with McGlamry elevator through medial approach to the joint.

In every case, a preoperative weight-bearing X-ray (or X-rays) and a series of postoperative radiographs were obtained and separately evaluated by 2 investigators. The investigators measured totally 449 radiographs. An average set of radiographs for a case consisted of 3.3 X-ray pictures.

Two independent investigators assessed all X-rays using graphic analysis software (ImageJ). The first investigator (JK) was one of the surgeons, the other one (SS) was a clinical anatomist (Institute of Anatomy, First Faculty of Medicine, Charles University in Prague). They were blinded to each other's measurements. On each picture, they had drawn five lines that were used for measurements (Fig. 1a, b). Firstly, the axis of the first metatarsal was defined as axis of the bone shaft. Similarly, the axes of the second metatarsal and proximal phalanx of the hallux were drawn. Fourth line went

through medial and lateral margins of the articular surface of the first metatarsal head. Fifth line connected medial and lateral margins of proximal articular surface of the basal phalanx of the hallux.

Five angles were then measured on each radiograph: *hallux valgus angle* (HVA) – the angle between long axes of the first metatarsal and proximal phalanx, *intermetatarsal angle* (IMA) – the angle between long axes of the first and second metatarsal, *tangential angle to the second axis* (TASA) – the angle between the line connecting the medial and lateral margin of the articular surface of the first metatarsal head and a line drawn perpendicular to the long axis of the second metatarsal, *proximal articular set angle* (PASA) – the angle between long axis of the first metatarsal and a line drawn perpendicular to the articular surface of the first metatarsal head, *distal articular set angle* (DASA) – the angle between the long axis of proximal phalanx of the hallux and a line drawn perpendicular to its proximal articular surface (Fig. 1a, b).

After obtaining the data from selected patients' radiographs, a statistical analysis was performed. Data of all angle measurements were compared to evaluate interobserver reliability and the method of measurement. The standard protocol with Cohen's kappa coefficient for interrater reliability evaluation was used.

We evaluated the change of TASA, HVA, IMA and DASA caused by the surgery. The tangential angle to the second metatarsal axis (TASA) is one of angles, that can be assessed [13]. The angle is measured between the articular surface of the first metatarsal head and the long axis of the second metatarsal. It describes the inclination (even the rotation) of the articular surface in relation to the axis of the forefoot.

The TASA angle was chosen due to the type of surgery – Lapidus procedure does not include a distal metatarsal osteotomy, therefore a significant change of the first metatarsal articular surface position in relation to its axis (PASA) was not expected in the process.

The study was focused not only on differences between values of the TASA angle, but even on combination of angles. The group of patients was divided into two subgroups – one where only Lapidus procedure was performed and second group, where a complementary Akin operation was added. The DASA angle described the level of the closing wedge Akin osteotomy of the proximal phalanx. The sum of TASA and DASA values was chosen with intention to compare the subgroups to describe the alignment of first MTP joint after surgery.

Results

On the preoperative and postoperative radiographs, the hallux valgus angle (HVA), intermetatarsal angle (IMA), tangential angle to second axis (TASA) and distal

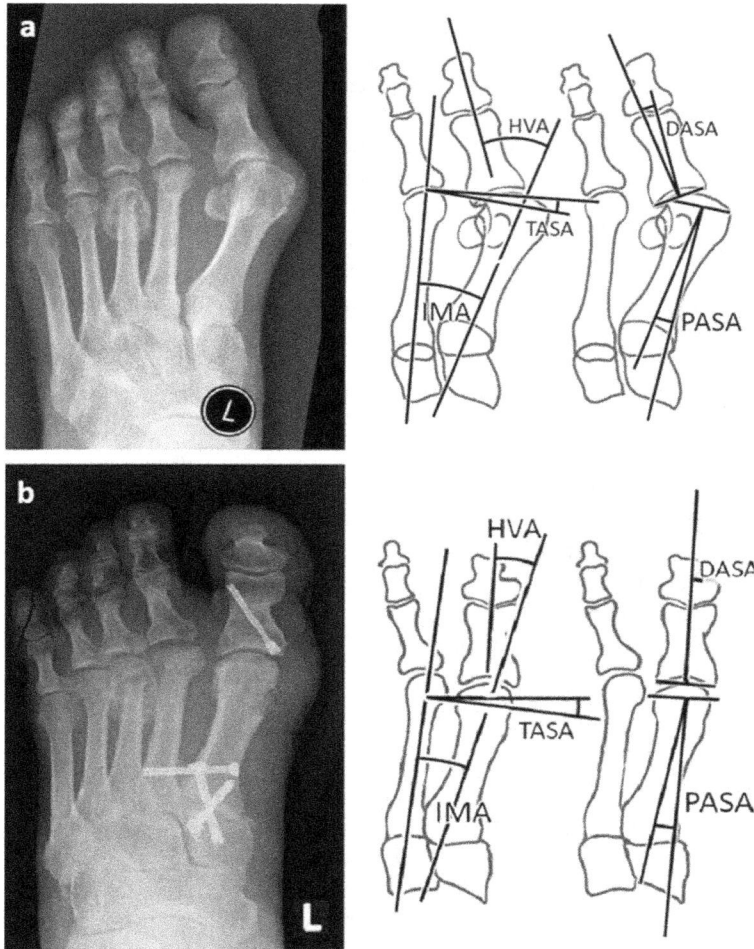

Fig. 1 a, b Pre- and postoperative dorsoplantar radiographs of a patient who underwent Lapidus and Akin procedure. *Measurements of the HVA, TASA, DASA, PASA, and IMA. HVA – hallux valgus angle; TASA – tangential angle to the second axis; DASA – distal articular set angle; PASA – proximal articular set angle; IMA – intermetatarsal angle*

articular set angle (DASA) were measured by two independent observers. There were no statistically significant differences found between the two observers' measurements ($p = 0.083$, $\eta^2 = 0.028$).

Evaluating our correction comparing preoperative to postoperative radiographs, these are the mean angle values for the whole group of 110 patients, not distinguishing the surgery type (both observers' measurements together):

Before the surgery: The mean HVA was 45.6° ± 20.5 (range 25.0° to 77.0°), the mean IMA was 16.9° ± 3,8° (range 8.5° to 28.5°), the mean TASA was 3.8° ± 8.5° (range – 17.0° to 26.0°), mean PASA was 20.5° ± 7.5° (range 3.3° to 40.0°) and the mean DASA was 1.5° ± 4.0° (range – 9.0° to 20.0°).

After the surgery: The mean HVA was 24.6° ± 14.4° (range 2.1° to 36.0°), mean IMA was 9.8° ± 5.3° (range – 2.0° to 27.8°), the mean TASA was 9.9° ± 6.9° (range

– 5.6° to 30.3°), mean PASA was 19.4° ± 6.9° (range 2.6° to 36.9°) and DASA 3.4° ± 5.2° (range – 13.5° to 15.0°). The summary of results is shown in Table 1.

We found out that there was a significant change of the TASA angle when comparing preoperative to postoperative radiographs ($p < 0.001$, $\eta^2 = 0.361$). The average change was 6.1° ± 6.9°. The distribution of TASA angle values recorded by two observers is displayed in Fig. 2.

We also compared two subgroups of patients according to the surgical procedure used. The first group underwent Lapidus arthrodesis only and the second one had Lapidus procedure combined with Akin osteotomy. Results of HVA and TASA measurements in both groups before and after surgery are displayed in Table 2. The distribution of HVA angle values recorded for Akin +/Akin- groups of patients is shown in Fig. 3.

The Fig. 4 shows distribution of TASA and DASA sums. The mean value of these angles total for a Lapidus

Table 1 Angles of interest measured on X-rays before and after the Lapidus operation

Angle	Preoperatively	Postoperatively
HVA	45.6° ± 20.5 (range 25.0° to 77.0°)	24.6° ± 14.4° (range 2.1° to 36.0°)
IMA	16.9° ± 3.8° (range 8.5° to 28.5°)	9.8° ± 5.3° (range – 2.0° to 27.8°)
TASA	3.8° ± 8.5° (range – 17.0° to 26.0°)	9.9° ± 6.9° (range – 5.6° to 30.3°)
PASA	20.5° ± 7.5° (range 3.3° to 40.0°)	19.4° ± 6.9° (range 2.6° to 36.9°)
DASA	1.5° ± 4.0° (range – 9.0° to 20.0°)	3.4° ± 5.2° (range – 13.5° to 15.0°)

HVA – hallux valgus angle, IMA – intermetatarsal angle, TASA – tangential angle to the second axis, DASA – distal articular set angle; values mean ± standard deviation (range)

only procedure was 5.2° ± 9.3° before and 14.2° ± 7.8° after the operation. In the group of patients, where the additional Akin osteotomy was used, the mean value was 5.3° ± 8.4° before the operation and 6.9° ± 10.2° after the two procedures. A significant difference, comparing these two groups, was found ($p = 0.005$, $\eta^2 = 0.075$). The mean difference in values (TASA+DASA) between the two groups was 7.3° of extra correction in favour of the group with an additional Akin osteotomy.

Discussion

Bunion surgery is a common part of the orthopaedic practice. The reduction of hallux valgus angle (HVA) using various types of osteotomies is one of the main purposes of the surgery. The proper alignment of the hallux is achievable only by a combination of soft tissue

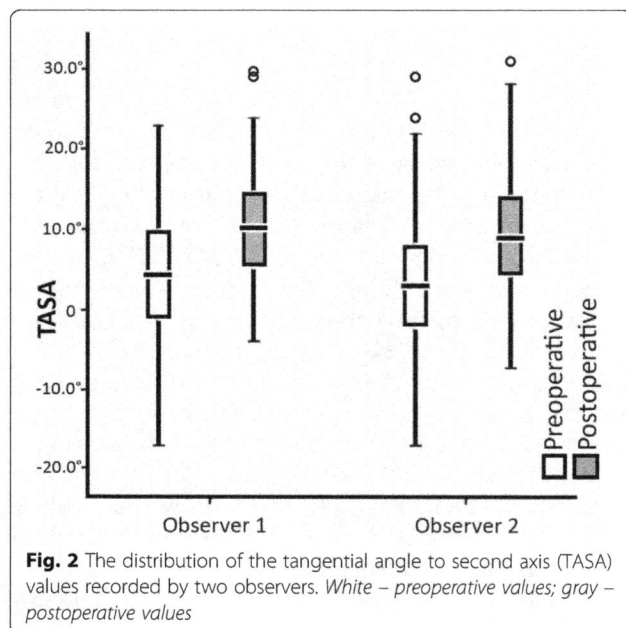

Fig. 2 The distribution of the tangential angle to second axis (TASA) values recorded by two observers. *White – preoperative values; gray – postoperative values*

and bony procedures changing position of articular surfaces.

The Lapidus procedure is an effective operation that can reduce deformity of the forefoot and improve position of the hallux. The surgery allows not only a reduction of the first intermetatarsal angle, but, more importantly, it can change the rotation and length of the first metatarsal [4–10]. The procedure has even disadvantages. The operative technique is demanding for the skill of the surgeon, since the position of the arthrodesis must address the deformity in all 3 dimensions. Especially important is the rotational part of the deformity. That leads to a lower reproducibility of the surgery results when comparing the work of more surgeons, as the personal experience with the arthrodesis positioning is crucial and the learning curve is longer. Beside that, there is an insufficient control over the first metatarsal's distal articular surface position, if fluoroscopy imaging is not used peroperatively.

The reduction of IMA, which is also usually pursued by any type of reconstruction surgery, may lead to an increase in TASA value as well. Theoretically, in normal conditions the formula TASA = PASA-IMA is valid [14]. The PASA angle describes the orientation of the distal articular surface in relation to the first metatarsal shaft axis. The angle is not changed by the Lapidus type arthrodesis. In our study, the mean TASA value increase was 6.1 ± 6.9°, while there was a mean decrease of 7.1° in IMA values. The average difference was 1° and the median was 0°. The TASA angle will increase equally to the decrease of IMA after the Lapidus procedure. Surgeons should expect it especially when the TASA is positive before the operation.

The outcome of the operation depends not only on IMA reduction, but also on the rotation of the first metatarsal. The pronation of the metatarsal is an integral and logical by-product of every hallux valgus deformity and its precise correction (derotation) is an essential part of the correction process. [4, 5]. Originally, we thought that the derotation of the first metatarsal would strongly influence the TASA angle. Our anticipation was, that correction of the pronation would lead to an improvement in TASA values. Contrary to that, our results showed that the derotation generally does not influence the TASA angle at all. Since there is not enough evidence in the literature about the use of TASA in the planning of surgery, our aim was to assess its usefulness in this field. We found out that there were enormous individual differences in TASA values among various patients´ cases (ranging from – 20° to 26°). We do not recommend using this method in precise preoperative measurements.

The DASA and PASA compile a set of angles. The set of these angles i.e. articular surfaces position is

Table 2 Angles of interest measured on X-rays before and after Lapidus procedure

Angle	Preoperatively		Postoperatively	
	without Akin	with Akin	without Akin	with Akin
HVA	45.6° ± 20.5° (range 25.0° to 77.0°)	42.7° ± 20.7° (range 28.0° to 56.0°)	26.2° ± 15.1° (range 2.1° to 36.0°)	17.3° ± 11.9° (range 6.6° to 26.6°)
TASA	3.7° ± 8.5° (range − 17.0° to 23.4°)	4.7° ± 8.0° (range − 6.0° to 23.5°)	9.7° ± 6.5° (range − 5.6° to 27.8°)	10.9° ± 8.5° (range − 2.5° to 30.1°)
DASA	1.5° ± 4.1° (range − 9.0° to 20.0°)	1.1° ± 3.8° (range − 5.8° to 7.5°)	4.6° ± 4.1° (range − 8.3° to 15.0°)	-4.3° ± 4.8° (range − 13.5° to 5.9°)

HVA – hallux valgus angle, TASA – tangential angle to second axis, DASA – distal articular set angle
values: mean ± standard deviation (range)

important for correction of the hallux valgus deformity. The size of DASA angle influences not only the mechanical axis of the toe, but even takes an effect in the action of extrinsic muscles as well [15]. The lower the DASA value is after surgery, the better deformity correction was achieved [16]. The DASA should not be influenced by Lapidus operation. Nevertheless, we recorded a change in DASA values before and after surgical procedure. The average change was 2.5° without Akin procedure and 7.0° using the procedure. The significant change in cases without using a phalangeal osteotomy was due to an initial pronation of the toe (as a part of the hallux valgus deformity). The change was a consequence of restoring the physiological position of first metatarsal in coronal plane.

In our study, we evaluated the influence of an additional Akin procedure on the forefoot reconstruction using Lapidus procedure. Not many current studies have assessed the hallux valgus correction results depending on the use of Akin osteotomy [17]. The sum of TASA and DASA angles was evaluated for a foot operated only with Lapidus arthrodesis or both Lapidus and Akin procedures. The Fig. 3 shows distribution and average values of the set of angles. The study demonstrates, beside other things, that if Lapidus procedure increases the TASA angle, a reduction of the DASA can improve position of the set of articular surfaces. The mean statistical difference in the correction of articular surfaces position with and without Akin osteotomy is 7.3° (TASA +DASA sums), the reduction of DASA achieved by an additional Akin procedure was an extra 8.9° (4.6° postoperatively in the Akin- group vs. − 4.3° in the Akin+ group, see Table 2). We recommend performing an additional Akin procedure in every case, where the first MTP joint soft tissue release cannot ensure a sufficient correction of hallux valgus deformity.

In our opinion, the unfavourable change of TASA by Lapidus arthrodesis can't be influenced by any osteotomy at the level of first MTC joint or proximal part of

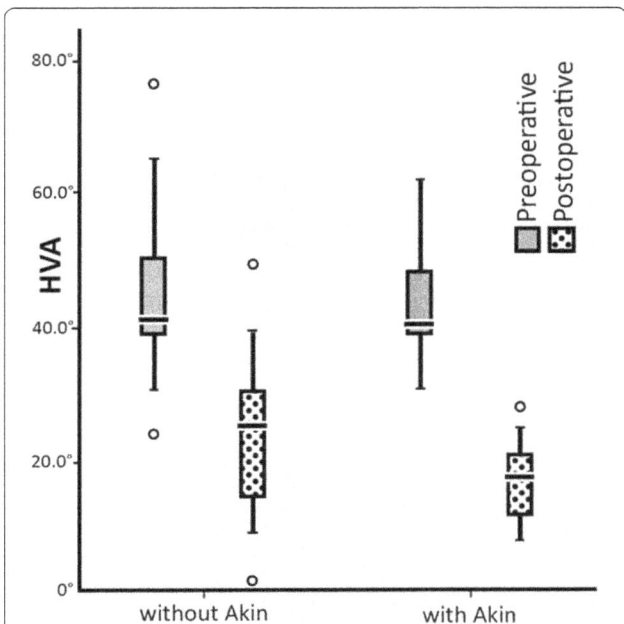

Fig. 3 The distribution of HVA values before and after surgery. *Patients who had the Lapidus procedure only are shown on the left side. Patients who had a combination of the Lapidus and Akin procedures are shown on the right side. Gray area denotes preoperative values; dotted area denotes postoperative values*

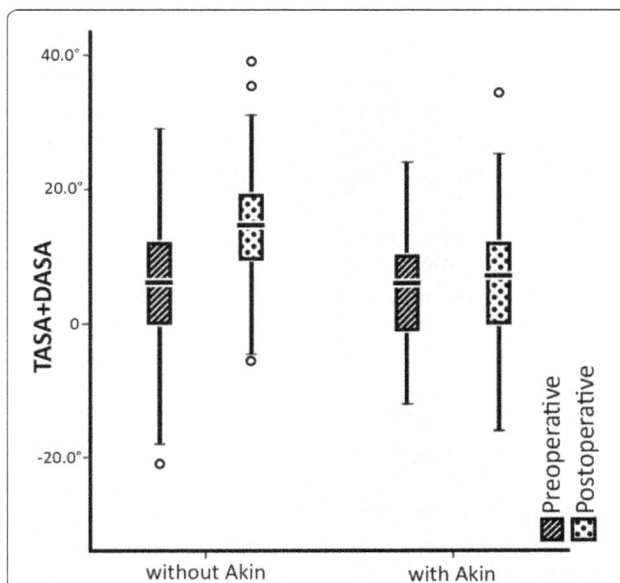

Fig. 4 The distribution and comparison of sums of TASA and DASA angles. *Patients who had the Lapidus procedure only are shown on the left side. Patients who had a combination of the Lapidus and Akin procedures are shown on the right side. Striped area denotes preoperative values; dotted area denotes postoperative values*

the first metatarsal. Another possible solution than Akin operation would be adding of a distal metatarsal osteotomy (e.g. Reverdin-Isham osteotomy [18]) to the first MTC joint fusion. However, this could possibly lead to the stiffness of first MTP joint.

Our radiographic study didn't evaluate the soft tissue balance. The soft tissue balance and different amount of weight-bearing changes position of the toe and hallux valgus angle. The soft tissue procedures such as lateral release of first MTP joint to restore physiological position of the sesamoids or release of long extensor hallucis tendon were used as a complementary procedure.

An example of the use of our measurements can be seen in above mentioned illustrations. The TASA angle value (Fig. 1a) is negative (– 10°). After the reduction of IMA, it switches to positive values (2°). Equation TASA = PASA-IMA is valid and PASA value wasn't changed by surgery. The IMA was reduced by 12°. The PASA and DASA angles preoperatively are approx. 30° (Fig. 1a). The PASA value is more or less the same after the arthrodesis (Fig. 1b). The DASA is reduced nearly to 0° by an Akin osteotomy. If only a lateral release was used as a complementary procedure to Lapidus arthrodesis, the final position of the hallux under full weight-bearing would be unsatisfactory. Therefore, an additional Akin osteotomy was used to improve the axis of the hallux. Surgeons should be careful especially in a case where TASA angle is positive before the operation.

There are several limitations of our study – we have not evaluated tibial sesamoid position (TSP) on pre- and postoperative radiographs. This variable is important for the clinical outcome of any reconstruction surgery. The present study was aimed predominantly on the articular surface position before and after the surgery and on the role of TASA angle in hallux valgus surgery assessment and planning, not on the correction success rate. On the other hand, we admit, that the inclusion of TSP measurement would bring even deeper insight into the surgery impact.

Another possible limitation of the study is the variety of fixation techniques used – the arthrodesis of first MTC joint was done mostly with memory staples but in some cases also using 2 or 3 screws or a plate. Additionally, the peroperative fluoroscopic control of the desis position was not available in all cases. These facts decrease the homogeneity of the studied group of patients and the reproducibility of the surgery results.

Further research is also needed to compare the Lapidus osteotomy with Akin procedure before and after surgery using subjective outcome scoring systems (AOFAS Forefoot score etc.).

Conclusions

The results of our X-ray analysis confirm the hypothesis of an unfavourable lateral inclination of the articular surface of first metatarsal head after the Lapidus procedure. The mean worsening of TASA angle after performing of Lapidus operation is $6.1° \pm 6.9°$. The significant deterioration after the operation corresponds with reduction of IMA and it is not caused by the derotation of the first metatarsal. The Akin osteotomy of the proximal phalanx is a suitable complement to the Lapidus arthrodesis and improves the articular set (position of the articular surfaces) of the first MTP joint.

Abbreviations
AOFAS: American Orthopaedic Foot & Ankle Society; DASA: Distal articular set angle; HVA: Hallux valgus angle; IMA: Intermetatarsal angle; MTC: Metatarsocuneiform; MTP: Metatarsophalangeal; PASA: Proximal articular set angle; TASA: Tangential angle to the second metatarsal axis; TSP: Tibial sesamoid position

Acknowledgements
The results of our study were previously published in the poster section of the 6th Triennial IFFAS Scientific Meeting 2017, Lisbon. The abstract was subsequently published in Foot and Ankle Surgery Journal (*Hromadka R, Klouda J, Soffova S. The change of first metatarsal head articular surface position after Lapidus procedure. Foot Ankle Surg. 2017;23:42.*)

Funding
Supported by Ministry of Health, Czech Republic - conceptual development of research organization, Motol University Hospital, Prague, Czech Republic 00064203.

Author's contributions
JK, SPJ and RH conceived the study, participated in its design and coordination, and helped draft the manuscript. JK and SS performed the X-ray analysis, RH, as a consultant for statistical analysis, performed the statistical analysis. JK, SPJ and RH analyzed and interpreted the data. JK was a major contributor in writing the manuscript. SP and IL were a part of the surgical team and participated in the study design and coordination. They also gave assessment guidance during this study, reviewed the first version of the text and helped draft the manuscript. All authors have read and approved the final manuscript.

Competing interests
The authors declare that they have no competing interests.

Author details
Department of Orthopaedics, Hospital Nemocnice České Budějovice, a.s., České Budějovice, Czech Republic. [2]Department of Orthopaedics, First Faculty of Medicine, Charles University and Motol University Hospital, Prague, Czech Republic. [3]Institute of Anatomy, First Faculty of Medicine, Charles University, Prague, Czech Republic.

References
1. Lapidus PW. The author's bunion operation from 1931 to 1959. Clin Orthop. 1960;16:119.
2. Lapidus PW. A quarter of a century of experience with the operative correction of the metatarsus varus primus in hallux valgus. Bull Hosp Joint Dis. 1956;17:404.
3. Lapidus PW. Operative correction of the metatarsus varus primus in hallux valgus. Surg Gynecol Obstet. 1934;58:183.
4. Dayton P, Feilmeier M, Hirschi J, Kauwe M, Kauwe JS. Observed changes in radiographic measurements of the first ray after frontal plane rotation of the first metatarsal in a cadaveric foot model. J Foot Ankle Surg. 2014;53:274.
5. Dayton P, Feilmeier M, Kauwe M, Hirschi J. Relationship of frontal plane rotation of first metatarsal to proximal articular set angle and hallux alignment in patients undergoing tarsometatarsal arthrodesis for hallux abducto valgus: a case series and critical review of the literature. J Foot Ankle Surg. 2013;52:348.

6. Dayton P, Feilmeier M, Kauwe M, Holmes C, McArdle A, Coleman N. Observed changes in radiographic measurements of the first ray after frontal and transverse plane rotation of the hallux: does the hallux drive the metatarsal in a bunion deformity? J Foot Ankle Surg. 2014;53:584.

7. Dayton P, Kauwe M, Feilmeier M. Is our current paradigm for evaluation and management of the bunion deformity flawed? A discussion of procedure philosophy relative to anatomy. J Foot Ankle Surg. 2015;54:102.

8. Mortier JP, Bernard JL, Maestro M. Axial rotation of the first metatarsal head in a normal population and hallux valgus patients. Orthop Traumatol Surg Res. 2012;98:677.

9. DiDomenico LA, Fahim R, Rollandini J, Thomas ZM. Correction of frontal plane rotation of sesamoid apparatus during the Lapidus procedure: a novel approach. J Foot Ankle Surg. 2014;53:248.

10. Klemola T, Leppilahti J, Kalinainen S, Ohtonen P, Ojala R, Savola O. First tarsometatarsal joint derotational arthrodesis--a new operative technique for flexible hallux valgus without touching the first metatarsophalangeal joint. J Foot Ankle Surg. 2014;53:22.

11. Lee KM, Ahn S, Chung CY, Sung KH, Park MS. Reliability and relationship of radiographic measurements in hallux Valgus. Clin Orthop Relat Res. 2012; 470:2613.

12. Coughlin MJ, Jones CP. Hallux valgus: demographics, etiology, and radiographic assessment. Foot Ankle Int. 2007;28:759.

13. Shechter DZ, Doll PJ. Tangential angle to the second axis. A new angle with implications for bunion surgery. J Am Podiatr Med Assoc. 1985;75:505.

14. Bettazzoni F, Leardini A, Parenti-Castelli V, Giannini S. Mathematical model for pre-operative planning of linear and closing-wedge metatarsal osteotomies for the correction of hallux valgus. Med Biol Eng Comput. 2004;42:209.

15. Coughlin MJ, Mann RA, Saltzman CL. Surgery of the foot and ankle. 8th ed. Amsterdam, The Netherlands: Elsevier Health Sciences; 2006.

16. Balding M, Jr LS. Distal articular set angle. Etiology and x-ray evaluation. J Am Podiatr Med Assoc. 1985;75:648.

17. Shibuya N, Thorud JC, Martin LR, Plemmons BS, Jupiter DC. Evaluation of hallux Valgus correction with versus without akin proximal phalanx osteotomy. J Foot Ankle Surg. 2016;55:910.

18. Isham SA. The Reverdin-Isham procedure for the correction of hallux abducto valgus. A distal metatarsal osteotomy procedure. Clin Podiatr Med Surg. 1991;8:81.

23

Treatment of osteoarthritis of the elbow with open or arthroscopic debridement: a narrative review

Keshav Poonit[1], Xijie Zhou[1], Bin Zhao[1], Chao Sun[1], Chenglun Yao[1], Feng Zhang[2], Jingwei Zheng[3] and Hede Yan[1*]

Abstract

Background: Elbow osteoarthritis (OA) is a common disabling condition because of pain and loss of motion. Open and arthroscopic debridement are the preferred treatment, however there is no consensus on which treatment modality is suited to which category of patient or stage of disease. The objective of this study was to narratively review the literature for a more comprehensive understanding of its treatment options and associated outcomes, trying to provide a better treatment plan.

Methods: The PubMed database, EMBASE, Cochrane Library, and Google Scholar were searched, using the keywords (elbow [title/abstract] and osteoarthritis [title/abstract] and (surgery or open or arthroscop* or debridement or ulnohumeral arthroplasty) including all possible studies with a set of inclusion and exclusion criteria.

Results: A total of 229 studies were identified. Twenty-one articles published between 1994 and 2016 satisfied the inclusion and exclusion criteria including 651 elbows in 639 patients. After comparison, mean postoperative improvement in (ROM) was 28.6° and 23.3°,Mayo elbow performance score/index(MEPS/MEPI) 31 and 26.8 and the total complication rate was 37(11.5%), and 18(5.5%) for open and arthroscopic procedure.

Conclusions: This narrative review could not provide an insight on which surgical procedure is superior to the other due to the poor orthopedics literature. However, from the data we obtained the open and arthroscopic debridement procedures seem to be safe and effective in the treatment of elbow OA. The optimal surgical intervention for the treatment of symptomatic elbow OA should be determined depending on patients' conditions.

Keywords: Elbow, Osteoarthritis, Elbow stiffness, Open, Arthroscopy, Surgery, Debridement

Background

Arthritis of the elbow is characterized mainly by chronic musculoskeletal pain, stiffness, reduction in the ROM and most importantly a decrease in the quality of life of the patient. Elbow OA has had less focus than lower extremity joints but it can cause severe disability in patients involving their daily living activities [1]. Although the normal range of flexion to extension of the elbow is from 0 degrees to 145 degrees, most daily activities can be accomplished without discomfort within the functional range of 100 degrees (range, 30 degrees-130 degrees) elbow flexion [2]. Nonetheless the elbow provides power for lifting and stability for precision tasks. Consequently, restoration of the normal ROM in a stiff elbow is a major concern [3]. OA is a chronic disorder of synovial joints where there is a progressive disintegration and softening of articular cartilage followed by regeneration of new cartilage and bone at the joint margins (osteophytes), cyst formation and sclerosis in the subchondral bone, mild synovitis and capsular fibrosis contributing to swelling, elbow stiffness and chronic pain. Most patients can go along well with the limitation of ROM, but can't stand the pain, which severely affects the quality of patients' life [4].

Numerous procedures have been described in the literature in order to address these symptoms, including arthroscopic soft tissue release, debridement, interposition

* Correspondence: yanhede@hotmail.com
[1]Department of Orthopedics (Division of Plastic and Hand Surgery), The Second Affiliated Hospital and Yuying Children's Hospital of Wenzhou Medical University, Key Laboratory of Orthopedics of Zhejiang Province Wenzhou, China, 109 West Xueyuan Road, Lucheng District, Wenzhou 325027, Zhejiang Province, China
Full list of author information is available at the end of the article

arthroplasty and total elbow arthroplasty [5–11]. In the recent years, total elbow arthroplasty has shown promising results, but in comparison with hip and knee arthroplasties, a lot more is desired. Due to this reason, procedures like open and arthroscopic debridement have gained popularity and became the mainstay of treatments [12]. In literature, there has been an increased focus on arthroscopic debridement; however there is no consensus on which treatment modality is suited to which category of patient or stage of disease,also there is no objective evidence of clear superiority of any one technique. Each one of the different surgical approaches for elbow OA has its own advantages and disadvantages (see Table 1). The objective of this study was to narratively review the literature for a more comprehensive understanding of its treatment options and associated outcomes, trying to provide a better treatment plan.

Methods

The PubMed database, EMBASE, Cochrane Library, and Google Scholar were searched for related articles, using the following keywords (elbow [title/abstract] and osteoarthritis[title/abstract] and (surgery or open or arthroscop* or debridement or ulnohumeral arthroplasty) to ensure the inclusion of all possible studies. The search was restricted to articles written in English. In addition, references regarding elbow OA were hand-searched for potential studies. Figure 1 shows the methodology of the review.

Inclusion and exclusion criteria

To be eligible for inclusion, the studies had to: (1) be published clinical trials; (2) meet the diagnostic criteria for primary elbow OA; (3) report operative treatment of open or arthroscopic and outcomes of elbow OA in humans (4) Articles published in English (5) outcome

Table 1 Advantages and disadvantages of Open and Arthroscopic Debridement

Surgery	Advantages	Disadvantages
Open	-Good visualization of joint	-Soft tissue damage
	-Extensive debridement possible	-Larger scars
	-Larger working space	-Risk of soft tissue contraction
	-Most pathologies can be addressed	-Longer rehabilitation
		-Greater risk of infection and hematoma
Arthroscopic	-Minimally invasive	-Tight working space
	-Smaller scars on the skin	-Risk of injury to nerves
	-Less soft tissue damage	-Mainly dependent on surgeon skills
	-Quicker Rehabilitation	-Cannot be used in advanced cases of osteoarthritis due to nerve adhesion

reported should include at least one of the patient important outcomes (pain, ROM, and functional recovery).

Exclusion criteria were: studies involving Total elbow arthroplasty, elbow replacement, tendon disorders, Fracture of the elbow, interposition arthroplasty, osteochondritis dissicans were excluded.

Each article was thoroughly read and data regarding pre-operative/post-operative flexion, extension, gain in range of motion, complications were retrieved and an average was performed to obtain the gain in range of motion in both groups. Many different scoring methods were used to measure the outcomes of the elbow debridement including (ROM), (MEPS), (MEPI), Andrew and Carson Score, Hospital for Special Surgery (HSS) elbow scoring system, Disabilities of Arm Shoulder and Hand (DASH), Japanese orthopedic association score, Visual Analogue Scale for pain (VAS), Oxford Elbow Score (OES), American Shoulder and Elbow Score (ASES), Quick DASH [12–23]. The most popular scoring system was the ROM and the MEPS which was used in most of the 23 articles. We compared both groups using average gain in range of motion and MEPS but unfortunately the uses of quantitative quality appraisals, quantitative meta-analysis or statistical analysis were not possible because of the limited data available in the literature.. The studies found could not provide solid evidences to aid clinical practice and also the data retrieved were not uniform among all the papers as it was reported by different authors all around the world. We used a narrative literature synthesis approach to summarize the literature, and quantitatively analyzed longitudinal trends across studies where possible.

Results

A total of 229 studies were identified in the initial search. After a careful review of the lists, full texts were retrieved for 16 articles. The rest of articles that did not meet the inclusion criteria were excluded. A search of the reference lists of selected articles identified 5 more relevant articles; the search was updated with no more relevant articles, leaving a total of 21 articles for the final inclusion. Of the 21 articles 11 were on open joint debridement; 10 were on arthroscopic joint debridement, one study included both open and arthroscopic debridement. These 21 studies included the results of 651 elbows in 639 patients. Of the elbows, 328 were treated arthroscopically, 323 with the open debridement method. Mean improvement in ROM after surgery was 28.6° for Open, 23.3°for Arthroscopic group,mean improvement in MEPS/MEPI after surgery was 31 for Open and 26.8 for Arthroscopic group as shown in Table 2. The difference between the two groups was not significant. All the studies reported good to excellent pain relief after both open and arthroscopic debridement (see Table 3 and Table 4). On the other hand, the

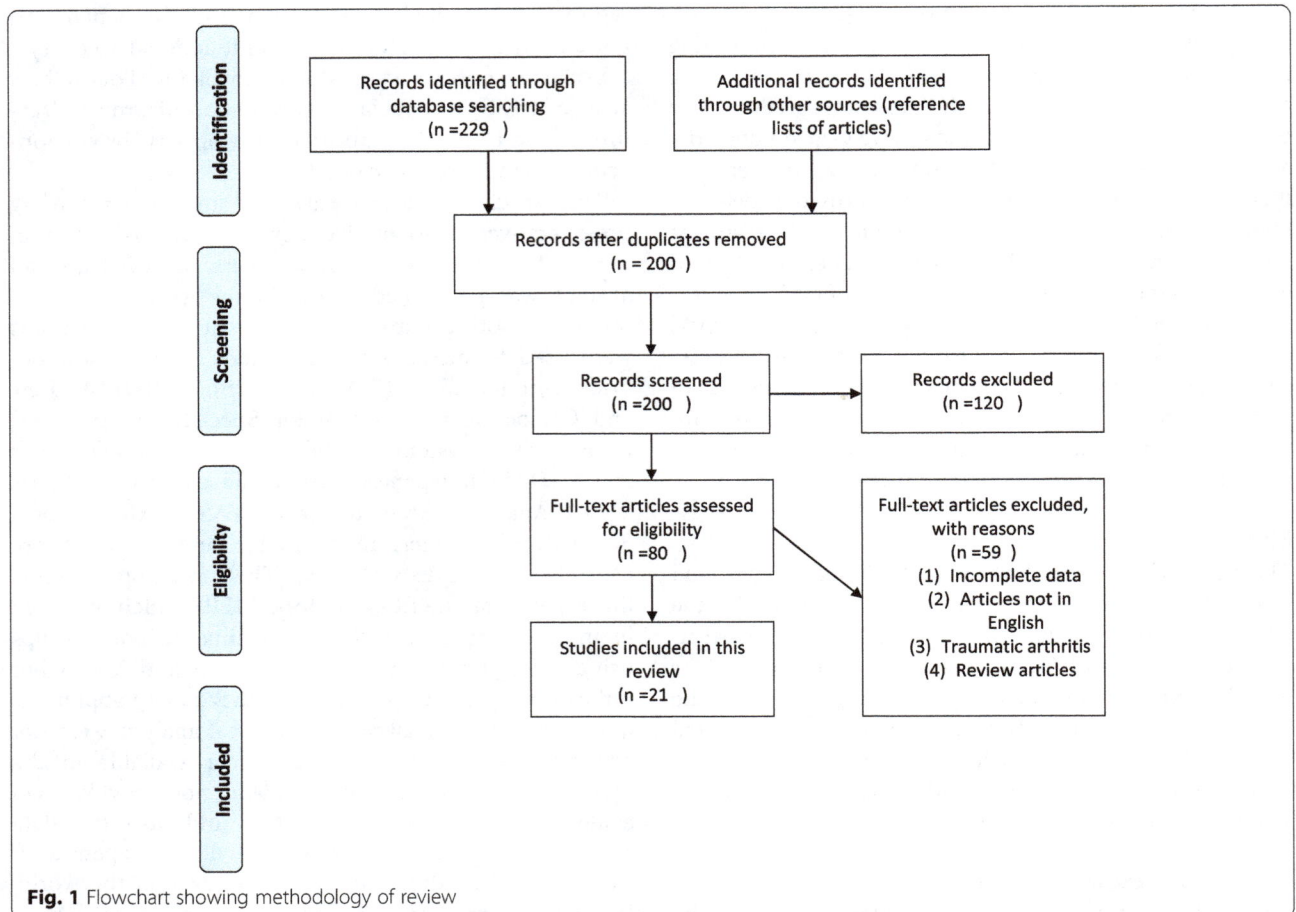

Fig. 1 Flowchart showing methodology of review

pre-operative ROM in the arthroscopic group with an average ROM of 97.2 (87.5–105.3) was much better than that of the open group with an average ROM of 73.3(66.5–77.4). In addition, a significant difference in pre-operative ROM between the two groups was noted in the summary plot, indicating that open procedure is better suited for advanced cases with more limitation of elbow motion (Fig. 2). The total complication rate for the Open procedure was 37(11.5%), and 18(5.5%) for the Arthroscopic procedure as summarized in Table 5. The most

Table 2 Comparison of open and arthroscopic procedures

	Open	Arthroscopic
ROM (Mean Arc) articles	12	10
Patients	323	328
Improvement	28.6°	23.3°
MEPS/MEPI articles	2	6
Patients	76	203
Pre-Operative Score	57.5	60.74
Post-Operative score	88.5	87.6
Improvement	31	26.8

Abbreviations: Range Of Motion (ROM), Mayo Elbow Performance Score(MEPS)

common complications for both procedures were ulnar nerve symptoms and hematoma.

Discussion

The etiology of primary OA of the elbow has not been fully elucidated. Several studies have proposed environmental factors as the primary etiology. No known morphologic features of the elbow have been identified as a predisposition to the development of primary OA of the elbow [24].The cardinal features of OA are (1) progressive cartilage destruction, (2) subarticular cyst formation, (3) sclerosis of surrounding bone (4) osteophyte formation (5) capsular fibrosis. Patients complain of pain and stiffness at the extremes of movements. This can be caused by degenerative changes at the radio-capitellar, ulnohumeral joint or due to ulnar nerve symptoms [5].

Non-operative management which includes elbow sleeves, non-steroidal anti-inflammatory medications, and intra-articular corticosteroid injections remains the mainstay of initial treatment for both primary OA of the elbow and posttraumatic arthritis of the elbow [3, 25, 26]. In the management of primary OA of the elbow, surgical interventions are used when conservative measures like

Table 3 Summary of Open Procedures

First Author	Year	Patient Mean Age (year)	Patient Symptoms	Number of patients and elbow (n=)	Type of treatment	Follow Up (Months) Range/mean	Evaluation Methods	Pain scale	Treatment Outcomes (Mean ROM)
Tsuge K et al [19]	1994	59	Pain and loss of range of motion	28 patients, 29 elbows	Open joint debridement	64	System of Japanese Orthopedic association	Good pain relief. No measure reported	Improvement of 33.2°
Minami et al[27]	1996	48.6	Pain on terminal motion, loss of range of motion	44 patients, 44 elbows	Outerbridge Kashiwagi procedure	127	(ROM)	27 out of 44 reported good pain relief. No measure reported	Improvement by 17°
Y.Oka[28]	1998	32	Severe pain at terminal flexion and extension, loss of range of motion	26 patients, 26 elbows	Open procedure (lateral and medial approach) and Outerbridge Kashiwagi procedure	46	ROM	0-2 grading scale (before 2 to after 0.24)	Improvement of 24°
Cohen et al[14]	2000	55	Pain, Stiffness, Locking	16 Patients, 18 Elbows	O-K Procedure	35.3	ROM and pain score	0-6 Likert scale from MEPI (after 2 points)	Improvement of 15°
Forster et al[20]	2001	55	Pain, decrease in range of motion, locking	35 patients, 36 elbows	Outerbridge Kashiwagi prOcedure	39	ROM, pain score	Morrey's system (0-3 Likert scale). (1.8 before to 1.1 after)	(PRE OP39°-108°) (POST OP27°-121°)
Antuna et al[21]	2002	48	Pain with terminal elbow extension	45patients, 46 elbows	Open ulnohumeral arthroplasty	80	MEPS	76% had complete pain relief. No measure reported	Improvement of 22°
Philips et al[29]	2003	51.4	Pain and loss of flexion/ extension	19 patients, 20 elbows	O-K procedure	75	(DASH) and (MEPS)	All patients reported pain relief. No measure reported.	Improvement of 20°
Sarris et al[30]	2004	52	patients was pain in terminal flexion and extension	17 patients, 17 elbows	Outerbridge Kashiwagi procedure	36	Pain scale, ROM	Morrey's system (0-3 Likert scale). All patient 0 post operatively.	PRE OP(26° to 98°) POST OP(14° to 118°)
Wada et al[32]	2005	50	Loss of range of motion,pain	32 patients 33 elbows	Debridement arthroplasty	121	ROM	Improved from 13 to 27	Improvement of 24°
Ugurlu et al[22]	2009	47	Pain and loss of range of motion	10 patients 10 elbows	Ulnohumeral arthroplasty	25 to 46	Andrews and Carson score	VAS (before 8; after 3.1)	flexion-extension arc improved from 63.4° to 120°
Hattori et al[23]	2011	59	Pain at the end points of motion	31 patients 31 elbows	Debridement arthroplasty combined with capsulectomy	19±7	(MEPS)	23 painful, 8 mildly painful post operatively. No measure reported.	mean arc of elbow motion Increased by 40° +/_ 13°.
Raval et al[12]	2015	54	Pain and stiffness at the extremes of movements	13 Patients 13 elbows	Ulnohumeral arthroplasty	48	(Quick DASH), (VAS)	VAS (before 8 after 2)	Improvement of 27 degrees in the flexion extension arc

Abbreviations: Range Of Motion(ROM), Mayo Elbow Performance Score(MEPS), Disabilities of Arm Shoulder and Hand(DASH), American Shoulder and Elbow Score(ASES), Visual Analogue Scale(VAS), Oxford Elbow Score(OES), Mayo Elbow Performance Index(MEPI), Hospital for Special Surgery (HSS) elbow scoring system。

Table 4 Summary of Arthroscopic Procedures

Author	Year	Patient Mean Age (years)	Patient Symptoms	Number of patients and elbow (n=)	Type of treatment	Follow Up (Months) Range/mean	Evaluation Methods	Pain scale	Treatment Outcomes (average Flexion/extension arc)
Cohen et al. [14]	2000	46	Pain, Stiffness, Locking	26 Patients, 26Elbows	Arthroscopic debridement	35.3	ROM and pain score	0–6 Likert scale from MEPI (after 2.9 points)	Improvement of 18°
Kelly et al. [33]	2007	51	Pain and loss of range of motion	24 patients 25 elbows	Arthroscopic debridement	24 to 123	Andrews and Carson score	Decreased from 7 to 2	Improved by 21°
Krishnan et al. [15]	2007	36	Pain and loss of range of motion	11 patients 11 elbows	Arthroscopic ulnohumeral arthroplasty	24–29	(VAS),(MEPS)	Decreased from 9.2 to 1.7	improvement of 73°
Adams et al. [37]	2008	52.8	Pain and loss of range of motion	50 patients 52 elbows	Arthroscopic debridement	26–68	ROM,MEPI	Subjective pain(0–5) Decreased 2.86 to 1.44	Improvement of 26.23°
Yan Hui et al. [16]	2011	23 ± 5	Pain, Locking, Loss of Range of motion	35 Patients 36 elbows	Arthroscopic debridement	16–98	(HSS), ROM,pain scale	All atheletes reported pain improvement.	Improved by 16°
MacLean et al. [17]	2013	42	Pain and locking	20 patients 21 elbows	arthroscopic debridement	66	(DASH), Mayo, and ROM	Measure not reported.	unchanged
Lim et al.(8)	2014	51.4	Terminal pain at flexion and extension with limitation of motion	43 patients 43 elbows	Arthroscopic d ebridement	38	(VAS),(MEPI)	Decreased from 4.5 to 2.2	mean flexion improved from 103° to 116°
Miyake et al. [34]	2014	38	Pain at the endpoints of movement and stiffness, catching or locking	20 patients 20 elbows	Arthroscopic debridement	24 to 29	Mayo Elbow Performance Score, Range of motion	No measure reported, pain disappeared or decreased post operatively.	Flexion PRE OP from 121° to to 130° POST OP
Merolla et al. [35]	2015	48	Pain, limited range of motion	48 patients 48 elbows	Arthroscopic joint debridement	44	(ROM), pain score, (OES), and (MEPS)	Decreased from 7.2 ± 1.6 to 4.3 ± 1.1	Flexion PRE OP from 115.73° ± 16.53° to128.75° ± 12.35° POST OP
Galle et al. [36]	2016	48	Loss of elbow motion, Pain	46 patients 46 elbows	Arthroscopic osteo-capsular arthroplasty	40.8	(VAS), (MEPS), (DASH), (ASES)	ASES pain Score post op 40 +/–12	flexion (PRE OP from 126° to 135° POST OP

Abbreviations: Range Of Motion(ROM), Mayo Elbow Performance Score(MEPS), Disabilities of Arm Shoulder and Hand(DASH), American Shoulder and Elbow Score(ASES), Visual Analogue Scale(VAS), Oxford Elbow Score(OES), Mayo Elbow Performance Index(MEPI), Hospital for Special Surgery (HSS) elbow scoring system

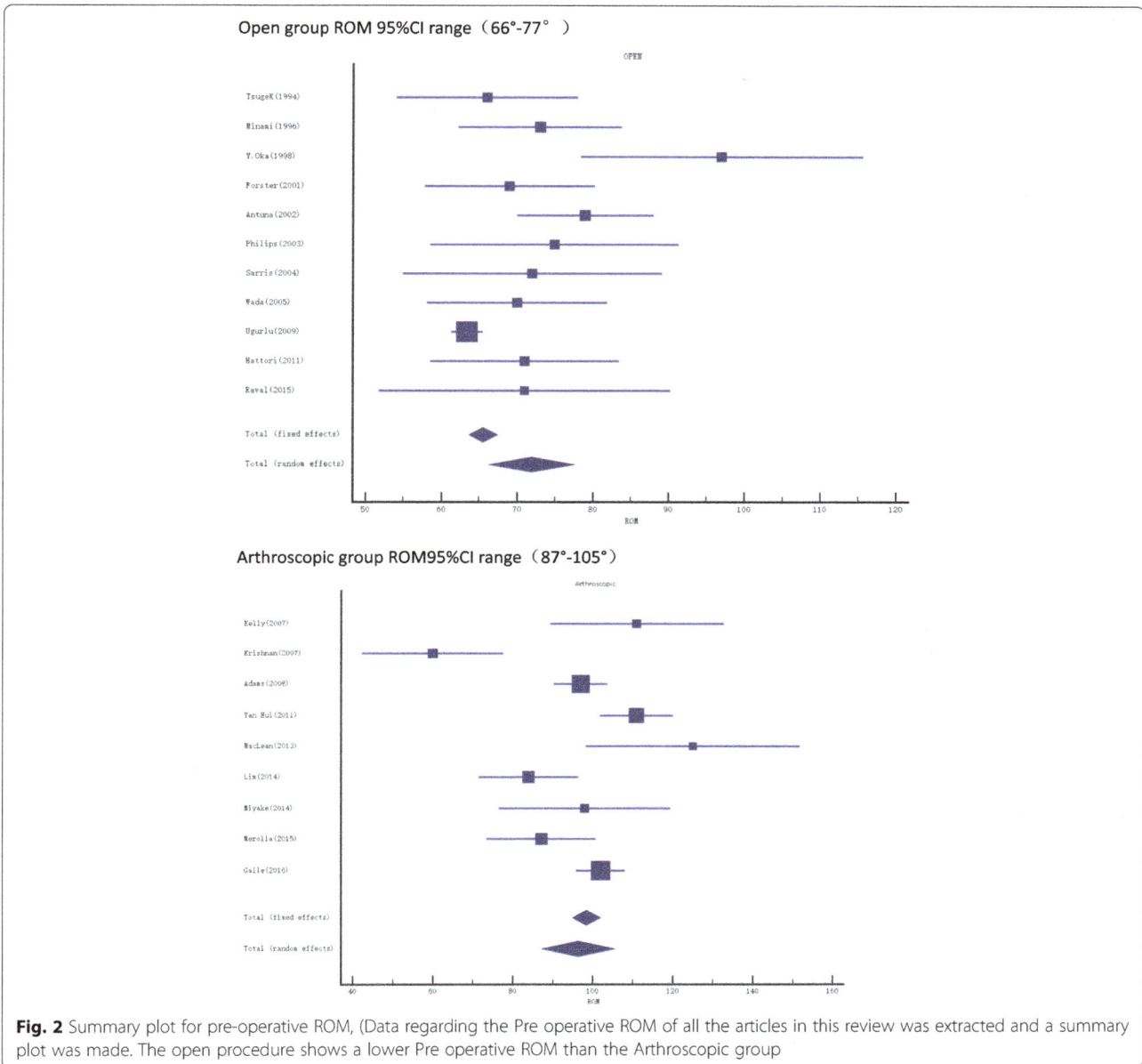

Fig. 2 Summary plot for pre-operative ROM, (Data regarding the Pre operative ROM of all the articles in this review was extracted and a summary plot was made. The open procedure shows a lower Pre operative ROM than the Arthroscopic group

physiotherapy and medical management fail. The most common indications for surgery are end range pain, stiffness, loose bodies, and locking of the elbow joint. Open and arhroscopic debridement are the preferred surgical management. In terms of these two procedures nearly all the studies in this review reported excellent reduction of pain, substantial increase in ROM, and functional recovery, however, a lack of trials limits the ability to directly compare different treatment options. All the studies included did not use the same scoring system and as a result direct comparison was not always possible. However, ROM and MEPS were used in some studies and therefore a direct comparison was made possible and the results of were as follows: Mean improvement in ROM after surgery

was 28.6° for Open, 23.3°for Arthroscopic group,mean improvement in MEPS/MEPI after surgery was 31 for Open and 26.8 for Arthroscopic group. Both groups had similar outcomes in terms of improvement therefore it shows that both open and arthroscopic procedures still have its role in the treatment of osteoarthritis.

In this study we found that by comparing the open [12, 14, 19–23, 27–32] and the arthroscopic [13–18, 33–37] procedures, both procedures have comparable outcomes concerning ROM and MEPS. This proves that both open and arthroscopic procedure can improve function, ROM and relieve pain in patients with elbow OA. Pain is the major complaint for patients resorting to surgery. In this review most studies reported good to

Table 5 Complications of open and arthroscopic debridement (n = number of elbows)

Complications	Open (n=)	Arthroscopic (n=)
	323	328
superficial wound infection	3	2
shoulder-hand syndrome	1	–
deep wound infection	1	1
ulnar nerve symptoms	27	6
Radial nerve palsy	1	–
residual loose bodies	–	2
hematoma	4	5
Recurrent effusions	–	2
Total	37(11.5%)	18(5.5%)

excellent pain relief after open joint debridement. However, to evaluate pain different scores were used, including (VAS) [3, 25], Morrey's 0–3 Likert scale pain grading system [6, 26], but other studies [8, 14] despite achieving satisfactory relief in pain did not mention the outcome measure they used. Similarly after arthroscopic debridement, every author reported excellent pain relief. The VAS was adopted in five studies and significant changes in pain levels were reported [15–19]. Krishnan et al. [15] followed 11 elbows and mentioned a change in the mean VAS scores from 9.2 Pre-surgery to 1.43 after final follow up at 26 months. A Likert scale from 0 to 5 was used in one study [11]. Others studies used Morrey's scoring system, elbow scoring systems like MEPI and good amelioration in pain levels were reported. In terms of complications the open group had a higher rate (11.5%) than the arthroscopic group (5.5%). Some of the complications reported were superficial wound infection, shoulder-hand syndrome, deep wound infection, ulnar nerve symptoms, Radial nerve palsy, residual loose bodies, hematoma and recurrent effusions. The two most common complications in both groups were ulnar nerve symptoms and hematoma formation. Open debridement requires an extensive soft tissue dissection, division of collateral ligament whereas arthroscopic debridement requires small stab incision and is minimally invasive; it requires expertise and specialized equipment's. This may explain why open group had a higher complication rate than the arthroscopic group but there is also the fact that open group had lower preoperative ROM which means that the patients were in a much advanced stage of osteoarthritis than the arthroscopic group, this might also contribute to a higher complication rate in the open group.

Cohen et al. [14] compared open joint debridement (18 elbows) to arthroscopic debridement (26 elbows) in 44 elbows. After a total follow up of 3 years they found a greater mean increase in flexion-extension arc of 21 degrees in the open debridement group, and a mean increase of 7 degrees in the arthroscopic debridement group. Although the authors reported superior pain relief with the arthroscopic procedure, a greater improvement in flexion was noted with the standard open procedure. This finding is not surprising as anterior capsular contractures are much more amenable to arthroscopic release than are contractures involving the posterior structures. Because the posterior bundle of the medial collateral ligament contracts and prevents flexion in patients with a long-standing lack of flexion, gains in extension are greater after arthroscopic release [4]. Therefore, more studies comparing different treatment options are needed to be able to gain insight on which procedure is superior to the other.

Open and Arthroscopic Procedure also proved to be safe in athletes, and a younger generation of patients. Two studies performed debridement in professional athletes' with one using open procedure and the other using the arthroscopic procedure. Oka et al. [28] treated twenty-six elbows in 26 patients using open debridement, preoperatively all patients complained of pain level around grade 2 or grade 3. There was limited ROM with a mean lack of extension of 16° (range 0°–30°), and a mean flexion range of 113° (range 80°–140°). In all cases severe pain occurred at the end of flexion or extension. As a result, anxiety and a decrease in performance while performing physical activities were noted. The concerned sports included baseball and Judo each affecting (9 cases), aikido (3 cases), apparatus gymnastics (2 cases), and karate, volleyball and bodybuilding (one case each). The mean sport participation time was 12 (3–30) years. Surgery resulted in improved pain relief and ROM. However, there was one case that suffered residual pain rated as grade 2. Each and every athlete returned to their prior activities and first class accomplishments was achieved by a few. Despite a minor recurrence of osteophytes, long-term results also indicated that the improvement in pain and ROM was maintained over a prolonged period.

Yan et al. [16] used the arthroscopic procedure to treat 35 professional athletes. The concerned sports included wrestling affecting 8 elbows in 7 athletes, weightlifting and judo both affecting 5 cases each, shooting, boxing, diving, ping-pong, and rowing (one case each), and badminton (3 cases), gymnastics, javelin, softball, basketball and baseball (2 cases each). All the 35 patients complained of pain. Before surgery, mean total arc of motion was (111 ± 28) ° (range 50°–150°), mean loss of extension was (14 ± 12) ° (range 0° – 40°), and mean flexion was (125 ± 20) ° (range 75°–150°). The mean sport participation time was (8 ± 6) years (range 2–20 years). Before surgery all patients reported difficulties performing physical activity: slightly affected in 2 (6%) elbows, severely affected in 24 (67%) and unable to participate in 10 (28%). Postoperatively as per the HSS scoring system, the outcome was as follows: poor for 6, good for 14 and excellent for 16 elbows. Pain improvements were reported by all athletes. After debridement, mean total arc of motion was $127° ± 26°$ (range $80°$–$150°$), mean extension loss was $7° ± 12°$ ($0°$–$30°$), and mean flexion was $134° ± 17°$ ($95°$–$150°$). Post-surgery total arc of motion increased $16°$, extension increased $7°$ and flexion increased $9°$.

A basic treatment strategy was proposed according to our findings from studies selected in this narrative review as shown in Fig. 3. We have detailed the treatment of osteoarthritis and classified it into early stage, mild to moderate stage, severe stage and further explained which treatment is more appropriate for each stage and the severity/type of pain for each stage has been described. This treatment strategy will benefit the surgeon to identity the stage of osteoarthritis and have a general idea about the treatment needed for that stage, furthermore open treatment seems to have its place mostly in rural institutions where there are less facilities available and the surgeons doesn't require much expertise to perform the operation, whereas arthroscopic treatment is becoming popular in urban institutions but it requires a greater learning curve and is more challenging than open technique. People in urban areas want a smaller scar and a quicker recovery and tend to be able to afford the high cost of the operation. The orthopedic literature is poor and the studies used in this narrative review are case series which prevent us to draw a valid conclusion, this calls for more Randomized controlled trials comparing different surgical options either in terms of short- or long-term follow-up that will enable us to better compare these two procedures.

Recently, arthroscopy has gained popularity in clinical practice and we found that similar outcomes were achieved by both open and arthroscopic procedures, but the complication rate was lower in the arthroscopic group. However differences in pre-operative ROM was significantly different, the results of the summary plot showed a better pre-operative ROM in the arthroscopic group compared to the open group, indicating that open procedure is better suited for advanced cases and the arthroscopic procedure may be more acceptable for mild to moderate cases.

This narrative review had limitations as there is a scarcity of data on comparative outcomes and a lack of prospective studies that directly compare the two surgical techniques. The most noticeable finding was a lack of Randomized controlled trials that bear comparison with short- or long-term benefit among different debridement procedures. However, reviews that analyze and summarize these procedures could boost our confidence about joint debridement procedures being safe and efficacious. The uses of quantitative quality appraisals, quantitative meta-analysis or statistical analysis were not possible because of the limited data available in the literature. Furthermore, there were many scoring methods used to measure the outcomes of the elbow debridement. Researchers used more than 1 score, but direct comparison of all results was not possible because of this heterogeneity. The vast variety of scores calls for a widely acceptable questionnaire that will give us the possibility to measure the wide range of patients. As a matter of fact, we also noticed that patients in the open

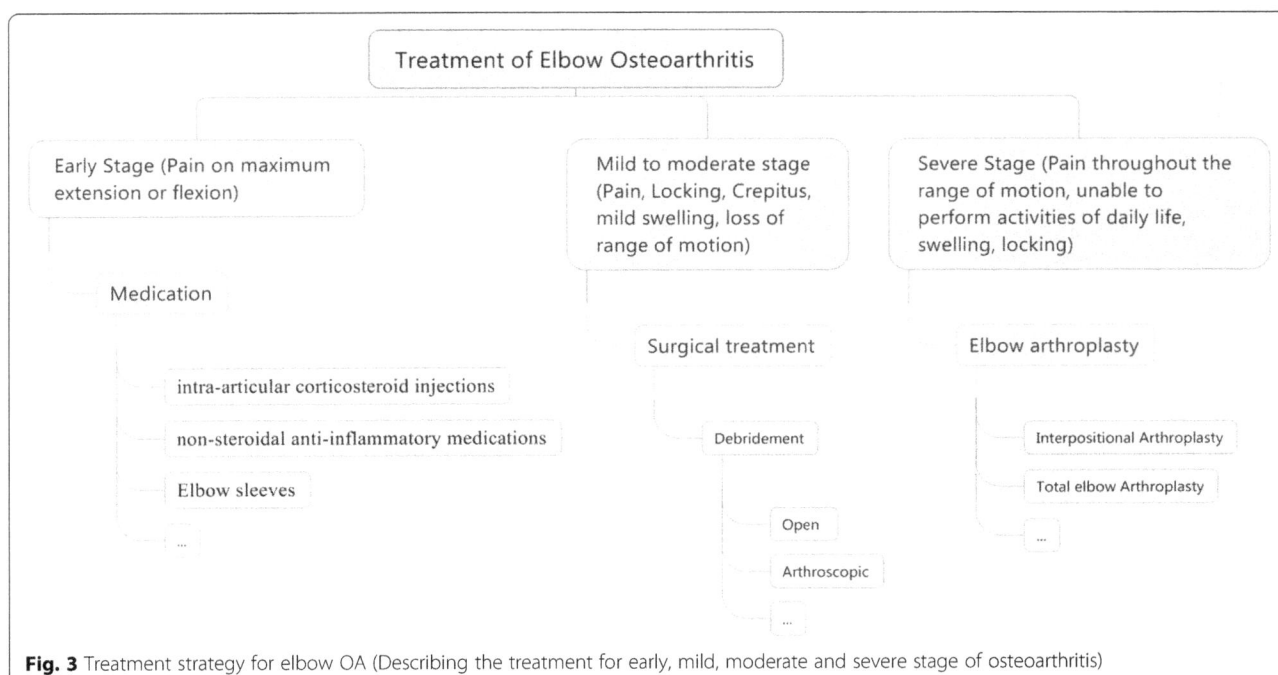

Fig. 3 Treatment strategy for elbow OA (Describing the treatment for early, mild, moderate and severe stage of osteoarthritis)

surgery group seemed to suffer from a more severe OA with low pre-operative ROM than those in the arthroscopic group, which may definitely cause selection bias for analysis. To our knowledge this is the first review that compares results across the two most common debridement procedures and this can help the general audience to better understand the outcomes, benefits and complications of these two procedures.

Conclusion

The optimal surgical procedure for the treatment of OA of the elbow is controversial. This narrative review could provide an insight on which surgical procedure is superior to the other due scarcity of data from the literature. However, from the data we obtained the open and arthroscopic debridement procedures seem to be safe and effective in the treatment of elbow OA. The optimal surgical intervention for the treatment of symptomatic elbow OA should be determined depending on patients' conditions. A clear understanding and knowledge of each approach will help the surgeon to evaluate the most appropriate approach for any given surgery. Reviews and case series directly comparing the two approaches and longer-term follow-up are the key to clearly elucidate the respective roles of these two surgical approaches.

Abbreviation
ASES: American Shoulder and Elbow Score; DASH: Disabilities of Arm Shoulder and Hand; HSS: Andrew and Carson Score, Hospital for Special Surgery elbow scoring system; MEPS/MEPI: Mayo elbow performance score/index; OA: Osteoarthritis; OES : Oxford Elbow Score; ROM: Range of motion; VAS: Visual Analogue Scale for pain,

Acknowledgements
The authors thank Miss Yulia Pidhorna for English revision.

Funding
This study was funded by the National Natural Science Foundation of China (81571185) for collection and interpretation of the data.

Author's contributions
KP and HY conducted the conception and design of the study, acquisitioned interpretation of data, drafting the article; XZ, BZ, CY, CS,FZ conducted final drafting, English editing and JZ performed statistical analysis and took part in drafting of the article. All authors have reviewed, read and approved the manuscript.

Competing interests
The authors declare that they have no competing interests.

Author details
[1]Department of Orthopedics (Division of Plastic and Hand Surgery), The Second Affiliated Hospital and Yuying Children's Hospital of Wenzhou Medical University, Key Laboratory of Orthopedics of Zhejiang Province Wenzhou, China, 109 West Xueyuan Road, Lucheng District, Wenzhou 325027, Zhejiang Province, China. [2]Joseph M. Still Burn and Reconstructive Center, 346 Crossgates Blvd, Suite, Brandon, MS 202, USA. [3]Department of Clinical Research Center, The Affiliated Eye Hospital of Wenzhou Medical University, Wenzhou, China.

References
1. Vincent JI, Vandervoort AA, Macdermid JC. A literature synthesis indicates very low quality, but consistent evidence of improvements in function after surgical interventions for primary osteoarthritis of the elbow. Arthritis. 2013; 8340:487–615. https://doi.org/10.1155/2013/487615.
2. Morrey BF. Primary degenerative arthritis of the elbow. Treatment by ulnohumeral arthroplasty. Journal of Bone & Joint Surgery-british Volume. 1992;74(3):409–13.
3. Biswas D, Wysocki RW, Cohen MS. Primary and posttraumatic arthritis of the elbow. Arthritis. 2013;27:131–7. https://doi.org/10.1016/j.hcl.2011.02.001.
4. Gramstad GD, Galatz LM. Management of elbow osteoarthritis. J Bone Joint Surg Am. 2006;88:421–30. https://doi.org/10.2106/JBJS.E.00568.
5. Gallo RA, Payatakes A, Sotereanos DG. Surgical options for the arthritic elbow. J Hand Surg [Am]. 2008;33:746–59. https://doi.org/10.1016/j.jhsa.2007.12.022.
6. Katolik LI. Osteocapsular debridement for elbow arthritis. Hand Clin. 2011;27: 165–70. https://doi.org/10.1016/j.hcl.2011.03.001.
7. Blonna D, Lee GC, O'Driscoll SW. Arthroscopic restoration of terminal elbow extension in high-level athletes. Am J Sports Med. 2010;38:2509–15. https://doi.org/10.1177/0363546510376727.
8. McAuliffe JA. Surgical alternatives for elbow arthritis in the young adult. Hand Clin. 2002;18:99–111.
9. Sanchez-Sotelo J. Total elbow arthroplasty. Open Orthop J. 2011;5:115–23. https://doi.org/10.2174/1874325001105010115.
10. DeGreef I, Samorjai N, De Smet L. The Outerbridge-Kashiwaghi procedure in elbow arthroscopy. Acta Orthop Belg. 2010;76:468–71.
11. Wright TW, Wong AM, Jaffe R. Functional outcome comparison of semiconstrained and unconstrained total elbow arthroplasties. J Shoulder Elbow Surg. 2000;9:524–31. https://doi.org/10.1067/mse.2000.109408.
12. Raval P, Ellanti P, Harrington P. Ulnohumeral debridement arthroplasty: a retrospective study and midterm outcome results. Eur J Orthop Surg Tr. 2015;25:847–50. https://doi.org/10.1007/s00590-015-1593-6.
13. Savoie FH 3rd, Nunley PD, Field LD. Arthroscopic management of the arthritic elbow: indications, technique, and results. J Shoulder Elbow Surg. 1999;8:214–9.
14. Cohen AP, Redden JF, Stanley D. Treatment of osteoarthritis of the elbow. Arthroscopy. 2000;16:701–6.
15. Krishnan SG, Harkins DC, Pennington SD, et al. Arthroscopic ulnohumeral arthroplasty for degenerative arthritis of the elbow in patients under fifty years of age. J Shoulder Elbow Surg. 2007;16:443–8. https://doi.org/10.1016/j.jse.2006.09.001.
16. Yan H, Cui GQ, Wang JQ, et al. Arthroscopic debridement of osteoarthritic elbow in professional athletes. Chin Med J. 2011;124:4223–8.
17. MacLean SB, Oni T, Crawford LA, et al. Medium-term results of arthroscopic debridement and capsulectomy for the treatment of elbow osteoarthritis. J Shoulder Elbow Surg. 2013;22:653–7. https://doi.org/10.1016/j.jse.2013.01.030.
18. Miyake J, Shimada K, Oka K, et al. Arthroscopic debridement in the treatment of patients with osteoarthritis of the elbow, based on computer simulation. Bone Joint J. 2014;96:237–41. https://doi.org/10.1302/0301-620X.96B2.30714.
19. Tsuge K, Mizuseki T, Debridement arthroplasty for advanced primary osteoarthritis of the elbow. Results of a new technique used for 29 elbows. J Bone Joint Surg Br. 1994;76:641–6. https://doi.org/10.2106/JBJS.D.02684.
20. Forster MC, Clark DI, Lunn PG. Elbow osteoarthritis: prognostic indicators in ulnohumeral debridement--the Outerbridge-Kashiwagi procedure. J Shoulder Elb Surg. 2001;10:557–60. https://doi.org/10.1067/mse.2001.118416.
21. Antuna SA, Morrey BF, Adams RA, et al. Ulnohumeral Arthroplasty for Primary Degenerative Arthritis of the Elbow. J Bone Joint Surg Am. 2002;84: 2168–73. https://doi.org/10.1007/s00590-015-1593-6.

22. Ugurlu M, Senkoylu A, Ozsoy H, et al. Outcome of ulnohumeral arthroplasty in osteoarthritis of the elbow. Acta Orthopaedica Belgica. 2009;75:606–10.
23. Hattori Y, Doi K, Sakamoto S, et al. Capsulectomy and debridement for primary osteoarthritis of the elbow through a medial trans-flexor approach. J Hand Surg Am. 2011;36:1652–8. https://doi.org/10.1016/j.jhsa.2011.07.018.
24. Rettig LA, Hastings H 2nd, Feinberg JR. Primary osteoarthritis of the elbow: lack of radiographic evidence for morphologic predisposition, results of operative debridement at intermediate follow-up, and basis for a new radiographic classification system. J Shoulder Elb Surg. 2008;17:97–105. https://doi.org/10.1016/j.jse.2007.03.014.
25. van Brakel RW, Eygendaal D. Intra-articular injection of hyaluronic acid is not effective for the treatment of post-traumatic osteoarthritis of the elbow. Arthroscopy. 2006;22:1199–203. https://doi.org/10.1016/j.arthro.2006.07.023.
26. Kokkalis ZT, Schmidt CC, Sotereanos DG. Elbow arthritis: current concepts. J Hand Surg Am. 2009;34:761–8. https://doi.org/10.1016/j.jhsa.2009.02.019.
27. Minami M, Kato S, Kashiwagi D. Outerbridge-Kashiwagi's method for arthroplasty of osteoarthritis of the elbow — 44 elbows followed for 8–16 years. J Orthop Sci. 1996;1:11–5. https://doi.org/10.1007/BF01234111.
28. Oka Y, Ohta K, Saitoh I. Debridement Arthroplasty for Osteoarthritis of the Elbow. Clin Orthop Relat Res. 1998;351:127–34.
29. Phillips NJ, Ali A, Stanley D. Treatment of primary degenerative arthritis of the elbow by ulnohumeral arthroplasty. A long-term follow-up. J Bone Joint Surg Br. 2003;85:347.
30. Sarris I, Riano FA, Goebel F, et al. Ulnohumeral arthroplasty: results in primary degenerative arthritis of the elbow. Clin Orthop Relat Res. 2004;420:190–3.
31. Vingerhoeds B, Degreef I, De Smet L. Debridement arthroplasty for osteoarthritis of the elbow (Outerbridge-Kashiwagi procedure). Acta Orthop Belg. 2004;70:306–10.
32. Wada T, Isogai S, Ishii S, et al. Debridement arthroplasty for primary osteoarthritis of the elbow. Surgical technique. J Bone Joint Surg Am. 2005; 87:95–105. https://doi.org/10.2106/JBJS.D.02684.
33. Kelly EW, Bryce R, Coghlan J, et al. Arthroscopic debridement without radial head excision of the osteoarthritic elbow. Arthroscopy. 2007;23:151–6. https://doi.org/10.1016/j.arthro.2006.10.008.
34. Lim TK, Koh KH, Lee HI, et al. Arthroscopic debridement for primary osteoarthritis of the elbow: analysis of preoperative factors affecting outcome. J Shoulder Elbow Surg. 2014;23:1381–7. https://doi.org/10.1016/j.jse.2014.01.009.
35. Merolla G, Buononato C, Chillemi C, et al. Arthroscopic joint debridement and capsular release in primary and post-traumatic elbow osteoarthritis: a retrospective blinded cohort study with minimum 24-month follow-up. Musculoskelet Surg. 2015;99:83–90. https://doi.org/10.1007/s12306-015-0365-0.
36. Galle SE, Beck JD, Burchette RJ, et al. Outcomes of Elbow Arthroscopic Osteocapsular Arthroplasty. J Hand Surg Am. 2016;41:184–91. https://doi.org/10.1016/j.jhsa.2015.11.018.
37. Adams JE, Wolff LH 3rd, Merten SM, et al. Osteoarthritis of the elbow: results of arthroscopic osteophyte resection and capsulectomy. J Shoulder Elbow Surg. 2008;17:126–31. https://doi.org/10.1016/j.jse.2007.04.005.

24

Re-infection rates and clinical outcomes following arthrodesis with intramedullary nail and external fixator for infected knee prosthesis

Giovanni Balato[1*], Maria Rizzo[1], Tiziana Ascione[2], Francesco Smeraglia[1] and Massimo Mariconda[1]

Abstract

Background: Knee arthrodesis with intramedullary (IM) nail or external fixator (EF) is the most reliable therapeutic option to achieve definitive infection control in patients with septic failure of total knee arthroplasty (TKA). The first aim of this study was to compare re-infection rates following knee arthrodesis for periprosthetic joint infection (PJI) with IM nail or EF. The second aim was to compare rates of radiographic union, complication, and re-operation as well as clinical outcomes.

Methods: A systematic search was performed in electronic databases for longitudinal studies of PJIs (minimum ten patients; minimum follow-up = 1 year) treated by knee arthrodesis with IM nail or EF. Studies were also required to report the rate of re-infection as an outcome measure. Eligible studies were meta-analyzed using random-effect models.

Results: The rate (95% confidence intervals) of re-infection was 10.6% (95% CI 7.3 to 14.0) in IM nail arthrodesis studies. The corresponding re-infection rate for EF was 5.4% (95% CI 1.7 to 9.1). This difference was significant ($p = 0.009$). The use of IM nail resulted in more advantages than EF for frequency of major complications and limb shortening. Other postoperative clinical and radiographic outcomes were similar for both surgical strategies.

Conclusions: The available evidence from the aggregate published data suggests that knee arthrodesis with EF in the specific context of PJI has a reduced risk of re-infection in comparison with the IM nail strategy. The use of IM nail is more effective for the complication rate and shortening of the affected limb.

Keywords: Periprosthetic joint infection, Intramedullary nail, External fixator, Knee arthrodesis, Knee arthroplasty, Re-infection

Background

Periprosthetic joint infection (PJI) is one of the most serious complications of total knee arthroplasty (TKA). Two-stage revision is considered as the most effective surgical technique for treating chronic PJI of the knee [1], but the one-stage revision has been recently gaining popularity [2]. These revision strategies have a re-infection rate of 8.8% and 7.6%, respectively [1]. Risk factors for the development of recurrent infection after revision surgery include isolation of difficult micro-organisms [3, 4], co-morbidities [3], and previous surgeries [4]. Once any measures to salvage a functional TKA through multiple revision procedures have been exhausted, knee arthrodesis or the above-knee amputation represent the only options to eradicate the infection. Amputation should only be performed in conditions of severe and irreversible damage of the bone and soft-tissues [2, 5] because of its unsatisfactory functional results [6, 7]. Conversely, knee arthrodesis

* Correspondence: giovannibalato@gmail.com
[1]Department of Public Health, Section of Orthopaedic Surgery, "Federico II" University, Via S. Pansini 5, Building 12, 80131 Naples, Italy
Full list of author information is available at the end of the article

can provide acceptable quality of life and functionality of the knee when there is sufficient residual bone stock [8]. Currently, the external fixator (EF) and intramedullary (IM) nail represent preferred methods to achieve knee arthrodesis in the context of septic failure of TKA [9]. Published results of these two surgical strategies have been variable [9–13]. Ideally, to compare EF and IM nail for knee arthrodesis would require evidence from carefully designed randomized clinical trials that are unlikely to occur given the low PJI event rates recorded after TKA [1]. The lack of robust evidence from randomized clinical trials results in uncertainty on the effectiveness of these surgical options. Hence, there is a need for further work to compare these strategies for arthrodesis. Using a meta-analytic approach, our first aim was precisely to evaluate the effectiveness of IM nail and EF knee arthrodesis adopting re-infection rate as the primary endpoint. Other relevant outcomes including the rate of radiographic union, complication, and re-operation as well as the postoperative limb length discrepancy (LLD), pain, and functional status were also investigated. Moreover, we aimed to compare and describe the differences in these outcomes between the two surgical options.

Methods

Data sources and search strategy

We searched for studies investigating different outcomes following knee arthrodesis performed with IM nail and/or EF in MEDLINE, Scopus, EMBASE, Web of Science, and Cochrane databases from inception up to September 2017. The Preferred Reporting Items for Systematic Review and Meta-Analyses (PRISMA) [14] methodology guidance was employed. The search strategy used a combination of the following key words: Knee arthroplasty OR Knee replacement OR Knee prosthesis AND Infection OR Septic AND Nail OR Fixator AND Arthrodesis OR Fusion. No language restrictions were employed. The reference lists of selected articles were also examined for any additional articles not identified from the database search.

Eligibility criteria

We included longitudinal studies comprising of consecutive unselected patients affected by PJI who were treated by knee arthrodesis using an IM nail or EF. We excluded: (i) studies that reported on these surgical methods in selected group of patients (such as patients with a specific infection or single preoperative diagnosis); (ii) studies with less than 1 year of minimum follow-up; (iii) studies with less than 10 participants; and (iiii) studies including patients with knee arthrodesis for causes of TKA failure different from infection where the outcome in septic patients could not be specifically assessed.

Study assessment and data extraction

Initial screening of titles and abstracts was performed by two pairs of independent reviewers (GB and MR, FS and TA). Full text was obtained for all abstracts that appeared to meet the inclusion criteria or where there was any uncertainty. Each article was assessed by two independent reviewers (GB, FS) using the inclusion criteria and any discrepancies regarding the eligibility of an article were solved with a third author (MM). Thereafter, relevant data were extracted from each included study. Two authors (MR, TA) performed quality assessment of eligible articles using the Methodological Index for Non-Randomized Studies (MINORS) criteria [15]. MINORS is a valid instrument designed to assess the methodological quality of non-randomized surgical studies. It yields a maximum score of 16 and 24, respectively, for non-comparative and comparative studies.

Statistical analysis

The rate of re-infection (i.e. number of re-infections at follow-up/total number of participants) with 95% confidence interval (CI) represented the primary outcome. Secondary outcomes were the rate of radiographic union, surgical complication, and re-operation as well as several clinical findings recorded at follow-up including the quality of life (SF-36 or SF-12 Questionnaire), functionality of knee (Oxford Knee score, Knee Society score etc.), severity of pain (Visual analog scale), and LLD. Subgroup analysis was undertaken, based on the effect of different types of IM nail and EF on different outcomes (re-infection rate, fusion rate, and time to fusion). Two broad types of IM nail (i.e. long and short) were identified. For EF arthrodesis, the subgroup analysis compared the effect of unilateral vs biplanar/circular and pins vs wires EF. Heterogeneity between studies was tested using the I^2 statistic (0% to 40% = not relevant; 30% to 60% = moderate; 50% to 90% = substantial; 75% to 100% = considerable) [14]. The primary and secondary outcomes were pooled using random effects models to account for the effect of between-study heterogeneity. Due to the unsuitability of pooling data for LLD, knee functional scales, the pain severity, and quality of life questionnaires, these outcomes were assessed using a comparison of means. A two-sample t test and chi-square test were used to test the significance of cross-sectional differences between the IM nail and EF knee arthrodesis and between different subgroups of surgical implant. We utilized Open Meta Analyst (Center for Evidence Synthesis, RI, USA) and SPSS version 23 (SPSS, Chicago, IL, USA) for all statistical analyses. $P \leq 0.05$ was considered significant.

Results

The flow diagram of our search strategy is reported in Fig. 1. The computer search and manual screening of reference lists of relevant studies identified 803 potentially relevant citations. After initial screening based of titles and abstracts, 74 articles remained for full text evaluation. After detailed assessment, we excluded 48 references. The remaining 26 articles [5, 10, 12, 13, 16–37] were included in the meta-analysis. Two of these [10, 22] were retrospective studies comparing outcomes of nail and EF arthrodesis. Hence, data from 18 and 10 studies were used for the assessment of surgical results of knee arthrodesis with IM nail and EF, respectively (Table 1).

Re-infection

Studies reporting on re-infection outcome after IM nail arthrodesis included 422 participants with 66 re-infections at follow-up. The pooled random-effects re-infection rate was 13.3% (95% CI 8.7 to 17.8, $p < 0.001$). There was moderate heterogeneity between the contributing studies ($I^2 = 54\%$; $p = 0.004$). On the exclusion of one single outlier study [12], the pooled re-infection rate decreased to 10.6% (95% CI 7.3 to 14.0, p < 0.001) and the heterogeneity was not significant (Fig. 2). There was evidence of publication bias (Egger's $p = 0.006$). Ten studies including 152 participants reported the re-infection rate in patients who had undergone EF arthrodesis. There were 15 re-infections and the corresponding pooled re-infection rate was 7.2%

(95% CI 2.3 to 12.1, $p = 0.004$). The heterogeneity between studies ($I^2 = 41\%$; $p = 0.086$) was lower in comparison with IM nail studies. When 1 single outlier was excluded [21], there was no more heterogeneity between studies and the pooled re-infection rate decreased to 5.4% (95% CI 1.7 to 9.1, p = 0.004) (Fig. 3). There was evidence of publication bias (Egger's $p = 0.001$). The difference in re-infection rate between IM nail and EF once heterogeneity between studies was removed was significant in favour of EF arthrodesis ($p = 0.009$). When the effect of different surgical implants was analyzed using a subgroup analysis, the pooled re-infection rate of arthrodesis with short and long IM nail was 13.1% (95% CI 7.6 to 18.6) and 14.4% (95% CI 6.7 to 22.2), respectively, with no significant difference (Table 2). The heterogeneity of the model was moderate to substantial ($I^2 = 54\%$, $P = 0.004$). The subgroup analysis did not show any differences in re-infection rate between unilateral (7.5%; 95% CI 1.3 to 13.7) and biplanar/circular (8.5%; 95% CI 0.8 to 16.1) EF arthrodesis. The heterogeneity for this model was not significant ($I^2 = 27\%$, $p = 0.179$). The re-infection rate between EF with pins (5.4%; 95 CI 1.3 to 9.5) or wires (5.4%; 95% CI 3.1 to 14.0) was identical, once the heterogeneity between studies was eliminated ($I^2 = 0\%$; $p = 0.990$) by removing 1 outlier study [21] from the model. Details of the subgroups analysis for EF arthrodesis are provided in Table 3.

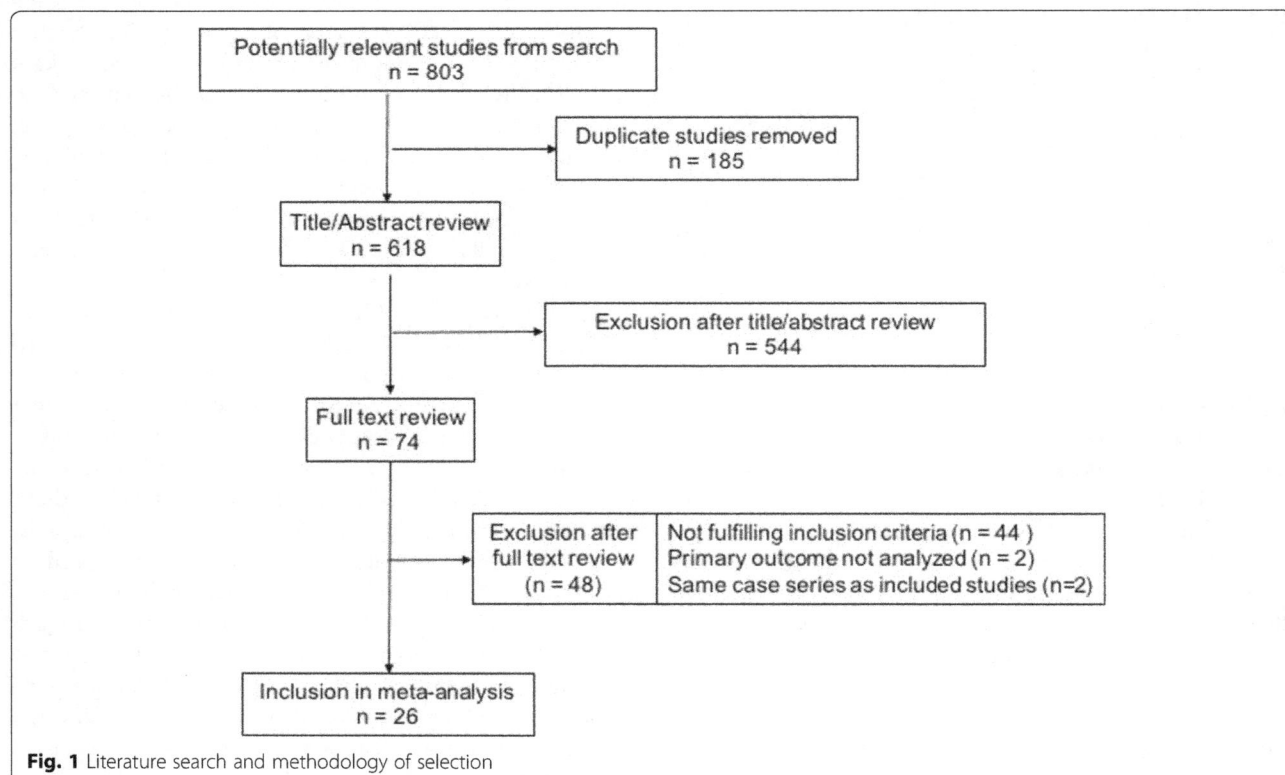

Fig. 1 Literature search and methodology of selection

Table 1 Characteristics of the studies included in the systematic review and meta-analysis

Lead Author, Publication Date	Location	Year of study	Mean age (years)	% male	Mean follow up (months)	Participants n	Two-stage/ one-stage	Surgical implant	Re-infections/ persisting infections n (%)	Fusion rate % (time to fusion - months)	Major complications n	Reoperations n	Postoperative limb length discrepancy (mm)	Quality score
Intramedullary nail														
Hungerer et al., 2017 [26]	Germany	2003–2012	68.6	43	53 (12–119)	55	NS	Short modular nail	12 (21.8%)	NS	13	20	18	9/16
Friedrich et al., 2017 [23]	Germany	2008–2014	70.2	NS	31 (12–74)	37	37/0	Short modular nail	5 (13.5%)	NS	2	7	22	10/16
Hawi et al., 2015 [5]	Germany	2002–2012	68.8	63	67 (24–143)	27	0/27	Short modular cemented nail	4 (14.8%)	NS	0	3	NS	11/16
Röhner et al., 2015 [12]	Germany	1997–2013	68	31	71 (12–204)	26	26/0	Short modular cemented nail	13 (50%)	NS	0	13	NS	10/16
Miralles-Muñoz et al., 2014 [29]	Spain	2001–2010	74.6	14	50 (36–60)	29	29/0	Short modular cemented nail	2 (6.9%)	NS	4	3	8	12/16
Scarponi et al., 2014 [33]	Italy	2000–2011	65	47	62 (24–105)	38	38/0	Short modular cementless nail	4 (10.5%)	NS	5	5	13	9/16
Iacono et al., 2013 [10]	Italy	2004–2009	69.3	NS	34(13–72)	21	21/0	Short modular cementless nail	3 (14.3%)	NS	0	3	8	9/16
Putman et al., 2013 [31]	France	2005–2008	67	NS	50 (28–90)	31	25/6	Short modular cementless nail	6 (19.4%)	68 (NS)	10	3	10	10/16
Barton et al., 2008 [17]	UK	1993–2004	NS	NS	53	10	9/1	Short modular nail	1 (10%)	100 (8)	2	2	NS	8/16
Talmo et al., 2007 [34]	USA	NS	67	41	48 (13–114)	29	25/4	Long modular cementless nail	4 (13.8%)	83 (6)	2	5	30	11/16
Bargiotas et al., 2006 [16]	USA	1999–2003	68	42	49 (18–72)	12	12/0	Long locked cementless nail	2 (16.6%)	83 (5.5)	2	2	55	10/16
Crockarell and Mihalko, 2005 [19]	USA	1991–2000	70.5	40	68 (24–96)	10	9/1	Long locked cementless nail	1 (10%)	100 (NS)	NS	NS	37	9/16
Domingo et al., 2004 [22]	Spain	1990–2001	67.8	50	Minimum 1 year	10	10/0	Short locked cementless nail	1 (10%)	90 (5)	2	1	NS	8/16
Volpi et al., 2004 [35]	France	1997–2001	68.6	43	19	12	12/0	Short modular cementless nail	2 (16.6%)	100 (3.6)	1	1	NS	7/16

Table 1 Characteristics of the studies included in the systematic review and meta-analysis (Continued)

Lead Author, Publication Date	Location	Year of study	Mean age (years)	% male	Mean follow up (months)	Participants n	Two-stage/ one-stage	Surgical implant	Re-infections/ persisting infections n (%)	Fusion rate % (time to fusion - months)	Major complications n	Reoperations n	Postoperative limb length discrepancy (mm)	Quality score
Gore and Gassner, 2003 [24]	USA	1977–2001	71.5	56	54 (12–288)	16	14/2	Long Kuntscher or modular nail	2 (12.5%)	87.5 (NS)	3	4	NS	8/16
Waldman et al., 1999 [36]	USA	NS	64	38	29 (24–90)	21	21/0	Short modular cementless nail	0 (0%)	95 (6.3)	2	2	NS	8/16
Lai et al, 1998 [28]	Taiwan	1988–1994	68.2	43	47 (18–94)	28	8/20	Short locked cementless nail	1 (3.6%)	93 (5.2)	2	1	25	9/16
Wilde and Stearns, 1989 [37]	USA	1983–1988	65	33	Minimum 24	10	10/0	Long Kuntscher nail	3 (30%)	60 (6.6)	6	6	36	8/16
External fixator														
Balci, 2016 [13]	Turkey	1999–2012	67	18	51	17	17/0	Unilateral EF	1 (6%)	94 (7.6)	4	6	29	11/16
Corona et al., 2013 [18]	Spain	2004–2009	81	48	50 (12–81)	21	0/21	Unilateral EF	3 (14%)	81 (10.3)	NS	NS	47	9/16
Iacono et al., 2013 [10]	Italy	2001–2004	68.5	NS	93 (82–110)	10	10/0	Semi circular Hoffmann EF	0 (0%)	90 (6.7)	1	2	45	9/16
Reddy et al., 2011 [32]	India	2003–2010	62.2	63	46 (12–84)	16	3/16	Ilizarov frame	1 (6%)	94 (6.6)	6	6	44	9/16
Parratten et al., 2007 [30]	France	1990–2003	64.8	43	88 (12–162)	14	6/8	2 unilateral EF	0 (0%)	93 (7.3)	2	2	45	9/16
Klinger et al., 2006 [27]	Germany	1990–2002	66.2	61	56 (24–132)	18	11/7	Unilateral EF	1 (6%)	83 (6.3)	3	2	36	9/16
Domingo et al., 2004 [22]	Spain	1990–2001	69.1	45	Minimum 1 year	11	11/0	Unilateral EF (3) Biplanar EF (8)	0 (0%)	100 (6.7) 100 (6.1)	1	0	NS	8/16
David et al., 2001 [20]	Israel	1988–	65.9	39	41 (18–60)	10	NS	Ilizarov frame	0 (0%)	100 (6.4)	1	0	37	8/16
Hak et al., 1995 [25]	USA	1973–1990	58.5	45	43 (12–186)	20	NS	Unilateral EF (7) Biplanar EF (13)	1 (5%)	57 (7.1) 62 (7.1)	13	4	NS	8/16
De Cloedt et al, 1994 [21]	Belgium	1984–1992	67.7	40	68 (14–108)	15	NS	2 unilateral EF	8 (53%)	67 (7.3)	NS	8	NS	8/16

NS Not stated, *EF* External fixator

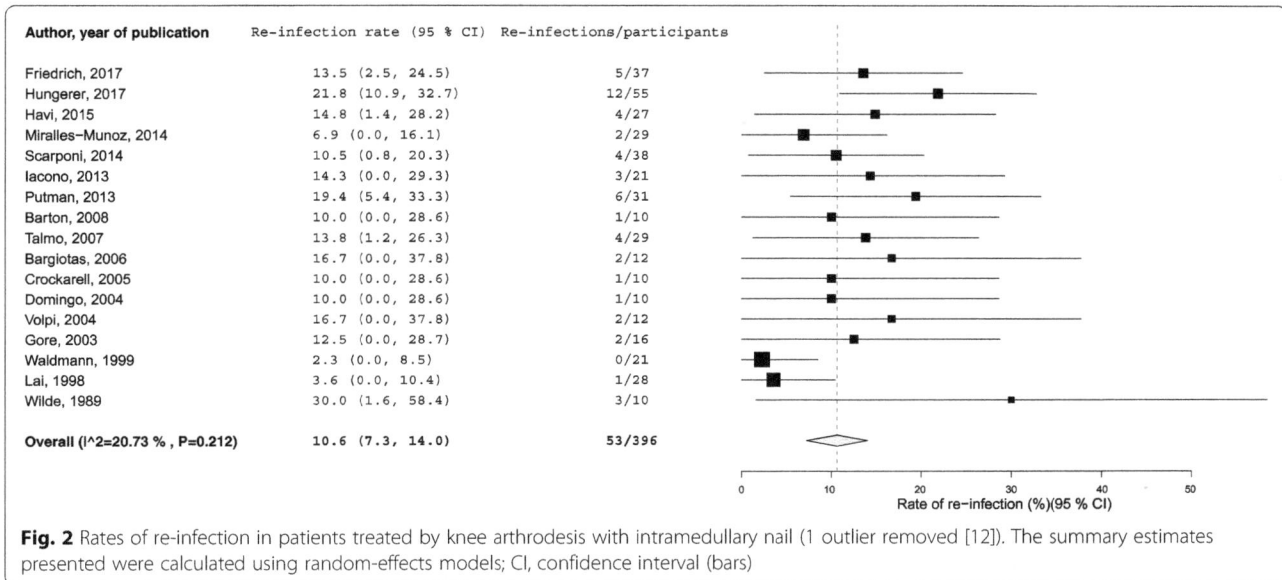

Fig. 2 Rates of re-infection in patients treated by knee arthrodesis with intramedullary nail (1 outlier removed [12]). The summary estimates presented were calculated using random-effects models; CI, confidence interval (bars)

Major complications and re-operations

Data for major complications (excluding re-infection) were pooled across 17 and 8 studies, respectively, for IM nail and EF arthrodesis. The most frequent major complication for IM nail and EF were implant failure and non-union, respectively. Pin track infection was reported with high frequency in all series of EFs but was not regarded as a major complication. The pooled random effects complication rate was 11.0% (95% CI 6.5 to 15.5, $p < 0.001$) for IM nail and 22.3% (95% CI 9.6 to 34.9, p < 0.001) for EF. Analysis of data revealed significant difference for treatment effect in favour of IM nail (p < 0.001). Heterogeneity between studies was substantial for both treatment strategies (IM nail – $I^2 = 66\%$; EF – $I^2 = 72\%$). Seventeen and 9 studies reported data regarding re-operations for arthrodesis with IM nail and EF, with a pooled random effects rate of 17.2% (95% CI 11.4 to 23.1, p < 0.001; $I^2 = 66\%$) and 19.3% (95% CI 9.4 to 29.3; p < 0.001; $I^2 = 66\%$), respectively. This difference was not significant ($p = 0.447$).

Radiographic union

Overall, the rate of radiographic union was not significantly different between IM nail and EF arthrodesis but the mean time to fusion was shorter with IM nail (5.78 range 3.6–8.0 months vs. 7.19 range 6.3–10.3 months; $p = 0.031$). In detail, data on the radiographic union rate following arthrodesis with IM nail were obtained from 11 of 18 studies. No such data were available in more recent articles (i.e. after 2013). The pooled random effects union rate for IM nail arthrodesis was 89.4% (95% CI 84.1 to 94.8, p < 0.001), with non-relevant heterogeneity between studies ($I^2 = 40\%$; $P = 0.082$). The subgroup analysis did not show significant differences in rate of bone union following knee arthrodesis with short periarticular (91.2%; 95% CI 84.4 to 98.1) or long IM nail (86.1%; 95% CI 77.4 to 94.7) (Table 2). All 10 studies on EF investigated radiographic union as an outcome. The pooled random effects union rate for this surgical option was 87.9% (95% CI 81.0 to 94.9, p < 0.001), with moderate

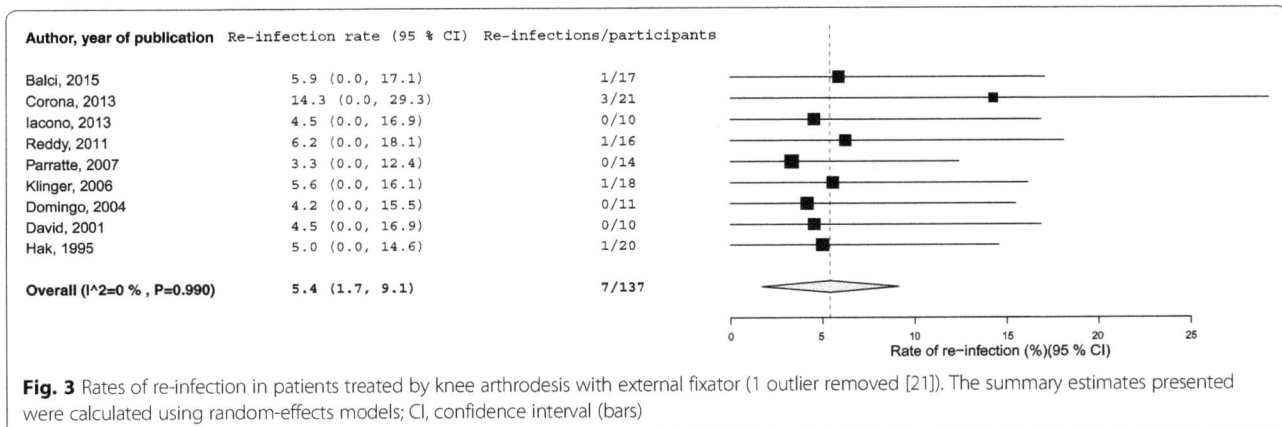

Fig. 3 Rates of re-infection in patients treated by knee arthrodesis with external fixator (1 outlier removed [21]). The summary estimates presented were calculated using random-effects models; CI, confidence interval (bars)

Table 2 Subgroup analysis of intramedullary nail arthrodesis studies

Outcome	Publications (n)	Cases	Long nail	Short nail	P
Re-infection	18	Total	77	345	
		No	65	291	0.998
		Yes	12	54	
Bone fusion	11	Total	77	112	
		No	13	14	0.397
		Yes	64	98	
Time to fusion (months ± SD)	8		5.62 ± 1.6	6.03 ± 0.6	0.626

SD Standard deviation

heterogeneity between studies ($I^2 = 57\%$; $p = 0.013$). On the exclusion of the two oldest studies,[21,25] the pooled union rate for EF increased to 92.0% (95% CI 87.5 to 96.4, p < 0.001) and no heterogeneity was present ($I^2 = 0\%$; $p = 0.484$). Uniplanar and biplanar/circular EF had similar rate of bone fusion (Unilateral = 86.1%; 95% CI 77.1 to 95.1; biplanar/circular = 89.1%; 95% CI 81.4 to 96.8), but a nearly significant difference in this outcome was detected when EF with pins (85.8%; 95% CI 77.9 to 93.7) was compared to EF with wires (94.6 95% CI 86.0 to 103.1). The mean time to bone fusion also was shorter for the wire EF than for pin EF. Details of the subgroup analysis for EF arthrodesis are given in Table 3.

Clinical outcomes

The comparison of clinical outcomes following IM nail and EF knee arthrodesis is reported in Table 4. With the numbers available, the only significant difference between these two surgical options was a bigger LLD in patients who had undergone arthrodesis with EF in comparison with those treated with IM nail. The extreme variability in assessment tools prevented us to perform any comparative analyses of knee functionality.

Discussion

Knee arthrodesis with IM nail or EF is the most reliable therapeutic option to achieve definitive infection control in patients with septic failure of TKA [8, 9]. Deficient

bone stock, impaired quality of bony surfaces, and shortened limbs may compromise the success of the procedure and lead to poor functional results [38]. To the best of our knowledge, this is the first review that compares IM nail and EF to achieve knee arthrodesis in the specific context of PJI. Indeed, two previous systematic reviews [11, 38] were not limited to studies of septic patients only. The most recent meta-analysis on the same topic [11] is different from our study for eligibility criteria and the primary endpoint. Indeed, White et al. [11] evaluated comparative studies that included also patients who had undergone knee arthrodesis for aseptic failure of TKA. The rate of radiographic union was assessed as a primary outcome. The inclusion criteria led these authors to select 12 comparative studies for the analysis, none of which was a randomized trial. Only two of these studies [10, 22] were used in our meta-analysis in that remaining studies did not fulfilled our stringent exclusion criteria because of methodological issues (e.g. mixed diagnosis and surgical strategy, small sample size, short follow-up period etc.). Conversely, we performed the meta-analysis by selecting studies that reported results of knee arthrodesis with EF or IM nail only in the specific context of septic failure of TKA. This approach has already be used in one previous meta-analysis that specifically dealt with the surgical revision of infected TKA [1]. Following previous studies [1], our primary outcome was the re-infection rate. Actually, infection control is the main goal of treatment when salvage surgery is performed for septic failure of TKA. Differently from the meta-analysis of White et al. [11], we assessed bone fusion as a secondary outcome. Indeed, achieving bone fusion may not be necessary in knee arthrodesis with the use of modular locking IM nails [33]. The eligibility criteria and selection of outcomes in the current analysis also enabled us to include studies on knee arthrodesis performed with the most recent modular IM nails that were completely excluded from the study of White et al. [11].

The present analysis showed that IM nail or EF arthrodesis have similar re-infection rates. However, most studies in the current meta-analysis only provided data on one of these two treatment strategies, which made

Table 3 Subgroup analysis of external fixator arthrodesis studies

Outcome	Publications (n)		Unilateral n = 66	Bipl/Circ n = 86	p	Pins n = 126	Wires n = 26	P
Re-infection	10	No	61	76	0.410	105[a]	25	0.745
		Yes	5	10		6[a]	1	
Bone fusion	10	No	11	13	0.795	23	1	0.066
		Yes	55	73		103	25	
Time to fusion (months ± SD)	10		7.60 ± 1.6	6.77 ± 0.5	0.314	7.38 ± 1.3	6.45 ± 0.2	0.086

Bipl/Circ Biplanar/Circular, *SD* Standard deviation
[a]1 outlier study removed

Table 4 Clinical Outcomes

		Intramedullary nail				External Fixator				P value
		Studies (n)	Patients (n)	Mean	SD	Studies (n)	Patients (n)	Mean	SD	
SF-36 or SF-12 questionnaire	PCS	3	94	35.0	8.7	2	38	41.1	2.5	0.357
	MCS	3	94	48.3	4.7	2	38	49.0	14.6	0.941
	PF	3	63	25.5	15.3	1	18	32.1		
	BP	3	63	43.8	17.8	1	18	47.4		
	RP	3	63	31.6	15.3	1	18	30.8		
	GH	3	63	45.9	10.3	1	18	46.9		
	SF	3	63	56.1	12.6	1	18	56.4		
	RE	3	63	45.4	24.7	1	18	46.7		
	VT	3	63	43.6	9.8	1	18	43.1		
	MH	3	63	63.5	11.8	1	18	58.3		
VAS pain		7	180	2.5	1.7	3	49	2.9	0.8	0.627
LLD (mm)		11	300	23.8	14.8	7	108	40.4	6.6	0.005

SD Standard deviation, *SF-36* Short form-36, *SF-12* Short form-12, *PCS* Physical component summary, *MCS* Mental component summary, *PF* Physical functioning, *BP* Bodily pain, *RP* Role-physical, *GH* General health, *SF* Social functioning, *RE* Role-emotional, *VT* Vitality, *MH* Mental health, *VAS* Visual analogue scale, *LLD* Limb length discrepancy

internal matching of studied samples missing. This makes more important to remove outliers and reduce heterogeneity, so that fair comparisons between the two groups could be made. Actually, an excess rate of re-infection after IM nail arthrodesis became evident once outlier studies were dropped off from the meta-analysis. Increased risk of recurrent infection with IM nailing as compared to EF arthrodesis has been previously reported [9, 10], even though this finding is not supported by one recent meta-analysis [11]. Overall, these results suggest caution if the use of IM nailing is planned in difficult-to-treat PJIs (i.e. isolation of multi-resistant micro-organisms, multiple comorbidities etc).

The present meta-analysis has shown that patients who had undergone arthrodesis with IM nail have lower rate of major complications in comparison with those treated with EF, but the pooled rate of re-operation is similar. Besides major complications, the need for daily pin site care to prevent local complications represents a drawback when using the EF [9].

The rate of radiographic union in the studies included in this review was similar between IM nail and EF, differently from one recent meta-analysis [11] that found better results with IM nailing. With the numbers available, no differences in fusion rate emerged between long and short periarticular nails. Several recent studies reporting results of modular IM implants disregarded bony union as an endpoint since it was not considered essential to obtain successful outcome [5, 10, 12, 23, 26, 29, 33]. Conversely, bony union is of outmost importance for EF arthrodesis. Indeed, Corona et al. [18] showed that 82% of patients treated with EF who achieve fusion is satisfied with the result. Among those who do not achieve fusion, 75% is dissatisfied. No significant difference in the rate and time of bone fusion was detected when unilateral or biplanar/circular EF was used to obtain knee arthrodesis. However, there was a tendency toward better results using circular fixators and wires. Despite numerous disadvantages (frame maintenance, cosmetic discomfort, risk of neurovascular damage during wire insertion), circular external fixation offers possible progressive adjustment to stimulate the bony fusion while keeping maximum triplanar stability at the arthrodesis site [32]. The severe bone defect represents a specific problem following multiple revisions for PJI and direct bony union in these circumstances will result in marked LLD. The shortening of limb has detrimental effect on functional outcome [8], with a breakpoint of 2 to 3 cm [39]. Friedrich et al. [23] set a minus two centimeters to allow walking without circumduction of the leg after IM nailing. The mean LLD following IM nailing in the present analysis was about 2 cm and was significantly smaller than that recorded after EF arthrodesis, confirming previous positive results of modular nail without bone fusion [5]. No significant differences in the quality of life and severity of pain between the two surgical strategies were detected in this study, but these findings should be interpreted with caution in the context of the limited available data. Moreover, the paucity of literature data prevented us to perform a subgroup analysis that related the bone union to clinical outcomes. Previous studies reported moderate physical disability and mild mental disability after knee arthrodesis independent of the surgical strategy [17, 19]. Literature data for postoperative pain are inconclusive. Significant postoperative improvement in pain has been reported following IM nail arthrodesis [10, 16, 40], but other authors [12] obtained much worse results. Ramazzini-Castro et al. [41] found better result for pain in patients who had undergone arthrodesis with EF when compared to other surgical strategies.

The limitations of this study deserve attention. First, this meta-analysis was performed on cohort studies, because of the lack of randomized controlled trials on the outcome of knee arthrodesis with EF and IM nail. Hence, there was low quality of evidence for each outcome. Moreover, variable design and the different way to assess results may have contributed to the heterogeneity between studies that emerged for some outcomes assessed in the present meta-analysis. Nevertheless, once few outliers were excluded the heterogeneity disappeared. We also acknowledge the limited number of studies on EF arthrodesis. This limitation prevented us to perform a robust comparison between the two procedures, especially for secondary clinical endpoints, and to carry out a subgroup analysis to assess the influence of different factors (i.e. number of surgical stages, number of previous surgeries, bone fusion etc.) on the outcomes. Lastly, significant publication bias was identified in both treatment groups, which might undermine the conclusion of the study.

This study also shows different strengths. First, we adopted stringent eligibility criteria that led to the exclusion of studies that assessed results of knee arthrodesis for causes different from the septic failure of TKA. Actually, knee arthrodesis for PJI compels the surgeon to deal with specific clinical and microbiologic problems. Furthermore, unlike one recent meta-analysis [11], we included only studies with adequate sample size and follow-up interval. Indeed, studies with less than 10 participants are more likely to be case series which do not include consecutive patients [1]. Similarly, a follow-up time of less than 1 year is not suitable to compare decision-making outcomes in a meta-analysis [14]. Another strength of this study is the use of a validated instrument for non-randomized surgical studies to assess the methodological quality of studies included. Finally, we compared post-operative clinical outcomes that have not been considered in previous reviews [11, 38].

Conclusions

The available evidence suggests that knee arthrodesis with EF in the specific context of PJI has a reduced risk of re-infection in comparison with the IM nail strategy. Hence, caution should be exercised particularly when the use of IM nail is planned in difficult-to-treat PJIs. The use of IM nail is more advantageous than EF with respect to important clinical outcomes such as the frequency of major complications and postoperative LLD.

Abbreviations
CI: Confidence interval; EF: External fixator; IM: Intramedullary; LLD: Limb length discrepancy; MINORS: Methodological Index for Non-Randomized Studies; PJI: Periprosthetic joint infection; PRISMA: Preferred Reporting Items for Systematic Review and Meta-Analyses; SF-12: 12-item short form health survey; SF-36: 36-item short form health survey; TKA: Total knee arthroplasty

Authors' contributions
GB, MR, TA, FS and MM were involved in the conceptual discussion and design of the review, in the critical appraisal of the content and have given final approval to the version to be published.

Competing interests
The authors declare that they have no competing interests.

Author details
[1]Department of Public Health, Section of Orthopaedic Surgery, "Federico II" University, Via S. Pansini 5, Building 12, 80131 Naples, Italy. [2]Department of Infectious Diseases, D. Cotugno Hospital - AORN dei Colli, Naples, Italy.

References
1. Kunutsor SK, Whitehouse MR, Lenguerrand E, Blom AW, Beswick AD, INFORM Team. Re-infection outcomes following one- and two-stage surgical revision of infected knee prosthesis: a systematic review and meta-analysis. PLoS One. 2016;11:e0151537.
2. Gehrke T, Alijanipour P, Parvizi J. The management of an infected total knee arthroplasty. Bone Joint J. 2015;97-B(10 Suppl A):20–9.
3. Ascione T, Pagliano P, Balato G, Mariconda M, Rotondo R, Esposito S. Oral therapy, microbiological findings, and comorbidity influence the outcome of prosthetic joint infections undergoing 2-stage exchange. J Arthroplast. 2017;32:2239–43.
4. Schwarzkopf R, Oh D, Wright E, Estok DM, Katz JN. Treatment failure among infected periprosthetic patients at a highly specialized revision TKA referral practice. Open Orthop J. 2013;7:264–71.
5. Hawi N, Kendoff D, Citak M, Gehrke T, Haasper C. Septic single-stage knee arthrodesis after failed total knee arthroplasty using a cemented coupled nail. Bone Joint J. 2015;97-B:649–53.
6. Chen AF, Kinback NC, Heyl AE, McClain EJ, Klatt BA. Betterfunction for fusions versus above-the-knee amputations for recurrent periprosthetic knee infection. Clin Orthop Relat Res. 2012;470:2737–45.
7. Conway JD, Mont MA, Bezwada HP. Arthrodesis of the knee. J Bone Joint Surg Am. 2004;86-A:835–48.
8. Wu CH, Gray CF, Lee GC. Arthrodesis should be strongly considered after failed two-stage reimplantation TKA. Clin Orthop Relat Res. 2014;472:3295–304.
9. Mabry TM, Jacofsky DJ, Haidukewych GJ, Hanssen AD. Comparison of intramedullary nailing and external fixation knee arthrodesis for the infected knee replacement. Clin Orthop Relat Res. 2007;464:11–5.
10. Iacono F, Raspugli GF, Bruni D, et al. Arthrodesis after infected revision TKA: retrospective comparison ofintramedullary nailing and external fixation. HSS J. 2013;9:229–35.
11. White CJ, Palmer AJR, Rodriguez-Merchan EC. External fixation vs intramedullary nailing for knee arthrodesis after failed infected total knee arthroplasty: a systematic review and meta-analysis. J Arthroplasty. 2017;33:1288-95.
12. Röhner E, Windisch C, Nuetzmann K, Rau M, Arnhold M, Matziolis G. Unsatisfactory outcome of arthrodesis performed after septic failure of revision total knee arthroplasty. J Bone Joint Surg Am. 2015;97-A:298–301.
13. Balci HI, Saglam Y, Pehlivanoglu T, Sen C, Eralp L, Kocaoglu M. Knee arthrodesis in persistently infected total knee arthroplasty. J Knee Surg. 2016;29:580–8.
14. Shamseer L, Moher D, Clarke M, et al. Preferred reporting items for systematic review and meta-analysis protocols (PRISMA-P) 2015: elaboration and explanation. BMJ. 2015;350:g7647.
15. Slim K, Nini E, Forestier D, Kwiatkowski F, Panis Y, Chipponi J. Methodological index for non-randomized studies (MINORS): development and validation of a new instrument. ANZ J Surg. 2003;73:712–6.
16. Bargiotas K, Wohlrab D, Sewecke JJ, Lavinge G, Demeo PJ, Sotereanos NG. Arthrodesis of the knee with a long intramedullary nail following the failure of a total knee arthroplasty as the result of infection. J Bone Joint Surg Am. 2006;88:553–8.

17. Barton TM, White SP, Mintowt-Czyz W, Porteous AJ, Newman JH. A comparison of patient based outcome following knee arthrodesis for failed total knee arthroplasty and revision knee arthroplasty. Knee. 2008;15:98–100.
18. Corona PS, Hernandez A, Reverte-Vinaixa MM, Amat C, Flores X. Outcome after knee arthrodesis for failed septic total knee replacement using a monolateral external fixator. J Orthop Surg (Hong Kong). 2013;21:275–80.
19. Crockarell JR Jr, Mihalko MJ. Knee arthrodesis using an intramedullary nail. J Arthroplast. 2005;20:703–8.
20. David R, Shtarker H, Horesh Z, Tsur A, Soudry M. Arthrodesis with the Ilizarov device after failed knee arthroplasty. Orthopedics. 2001;24:33–6.
21. De Cloedt P, Emery R, Legaye J, Lokietek W. Infected total knee prosthesis. Guidance for therapeutic choice. Rev Chir Orthop Reparatrice Appar Mot. 1994;80:626–33.
22. Domingo LJ, Caballero MJ, Cuenca J, Herrera A, Sola A, Herrero L. Knee arthrodesis with the Wichita fusion nail. Int Orthop 2004;28:25–27.
23. Friedrich MJ, Schmolders J, Wimmer MD, et al. Two-stage knee arthrodesis with a modular intramedullary nail due to septic failure of revision total knee arthroplasty with extensor mechanism deficiency. Knee. 2017;24:1240–46.
24. Gore DR, Gassner K. Use of an intramedullary rod in knee arthrodesis following failed total knee arthroplasty. J Knee Surg. 2003;16:165–7.
25. Hak DJ, Lieberman JR, Finerman GA. Single plane and biplane external fixators for knee arthrodesis. Clin Orthop Relat Res. 1995;316:134–44.
26. Hungerer S, Kiechle M, von Rüden C, Militz M, Beitzel K, Morgenstern M. Knee arthrodesis versus above-the-knee amputation after septic failure of revision total knee arthroplasty: comparison of functional outcome and complication rates. BMC Musculoskelet Disord. 2017;18:443.
27. Klinger HM, Spahn G, Schultz W, Baums MH. Arthrodesis of the knee after failed infected total knee arthroplasty. Knee Surg Sports Traumatol Arthrosc. 2006;14:447–53.
28. Lai KA, Shen WJ, Yang CY. Arthrodesis with a short Huckstep nail as a salvage procedure for failed total knee arthroplasty. J Bone Joint Surg Am. 1998;80-A:380–8.
29. Miralles-Muñoz FA, Lizaur-Utrilla A, Manrique-Lipa C, López-Prats FA. Arthrodesis without bone fusion with an intramedullary modular nail for revision of infected total knee arthroplasty. Rev Esp Cir Ortop Traumatol. 2014;58:217–22.
30. Parratte S, Madougou S, Villaba M, Stein A, Rochwerger A, Curvale G. Knee arthrodesis with a double mono-bar external fixators to salvage infected knee arthroplasty: retrospective analysis of 18 knees with mean seven-year follow-up. Rev Chir Orthop Reparatrice Appar Mot. 2007;93:373–80.
31. Putman S, Kern G, Senneville E, Beltrand E, Migaud H. Knee arthrodesis using customised modular intramedullary nail in failed infected total knee arthroplasty. Orthop Traumatol Surg Res. 2013;99:391–8.
32. Reddy VG, Kumar RV, Mootha AK, Thayi C, Kantesaria P, Reddy D. Salvage of infected total knee arthroplasty with Ilizarov external fixator. Indian J Orthop. 2011;45:541–7.
33. Scarponi S, Drago L, Romanò D, et al. Cementless modular intramedullary nail without bone-on-bone fusion as a salvage procedure in chronically infected total knee prosthesis: long-term results. Int Orthop. 2014;38:413–8.
34. Talmo CT, Bono JV, Figgie MP, Sculco TP, Laskin RS, Windsor RE. Intramedullary arthrodesis of the knee in the treatment of sepsis after TKR. HSS J. 2007;3:83–8.
35. Volpi R, Dehoux E, Touchard P, Mensa C, Segal P. Knee arthrodesis using a customized intramedullary nail: 14 cases. Rev Chir Orthop Reparatrice Appar Mot. 2004;90:58–64.
36. Waldman BJ, Mont MA, Payman KR, et al. Infected total knee arthroplasty treated with arthrodesis using a modular nail. Clin Orthop Relat Res. 1999; 367:230–7.
37. Wilde AH, Stearns KL. Intramedullary fixation for arthrodesis of the knee after infected total knee arthroplasty. Clin Orthop Relat Res. 1989;248:87–92.
38. Damron TA, McBeath AA. Arthrodesis following failed total knee arthroplasty: comprehensive review and meta-analysis of recent literature. Orthopedics. 1995;18:361–8.
39. Gurney B, Mermier C, Robergs R, Gibson A, Rivero D. Effects of limb-length discrepancy on gait economy and lower-extremity muscle activity in older adults. J Bone Joint Surg Am. 2001;83-A:907–15.
40. Wilding CP, Cooper GA, Freeman AK, Parry MC, Jeys L. Can a silver-coated arthrodesis implant provide a viable alternative to above knee amputation in the unsalvageable, infected total knee arthroplasty? J Arthroplast. 2016;31: 2542–7.
41. Ramazzini-Castro R, Pons-Cabrafiga M. Knee arthrodesis in rescue surgery: a study of 18 cases. Rev Esp Cir Ortop Traumatol. 2013;57:45–52.

25

Clinical implications of fracture-associated vascular damage in extremity and pelvic trauma

F. Gilbert[1,7]* ⓘD, C. Schneemann[2], C. J. Scholz[3], R. Kickuth[4], R. H. Meffert[1], R. Wildenauer[2], U. Lorenz[2], R. Kellersmann[5]* and A. Busch[2,6]*

Abstract

Background: Vascular damage in polytrauma patients is associated with high mortality and morbidity. Therefore, specific clinical implications of vascular damage with fractures in major trauma patients are reassessed.

Methods: This comprehensive nine-year retrospective single center cohort study analyzed demography, laboratory, treatment and outcome data from 3689 patients, 64 patients with fracture-associated vascular injuries were identified and were compared to a control group.

Results: Vascular damage occurred in 7% of patients with upper and lower limb and pelvic fractures admitted to the trauma room. Overall survival was 80% in pelvic fracture and 97% in extremity fracture patients and comparable to non-vascular trauma patients. Additional arterial damage required substantial fluid administration and was visible as significantly anemia and disturbed coagulation tests upon admission. Open procedures were done in over 80% of peripheral extremity vascular damage. Endovascular procedures were predominant (87%) in pelvic injury.

Conclusion: Vascular damage is associated with high mortality rates especially in combination with pelvic fractures. Initial anemia, disturbed coagulation tests and the need for extensive pre-clinical fluid substitution were observed in the cohort with vascular damage. Therefore, fast diagnosis and early interventional and surgical procedures are necessary to optimize patient-specific outcome.

Keywords: Fracture-associated vascular damage, Surgical trauma room, Extremity trauma, Pelvic trauma, Endovascular repair, Level of evidence: IV

Background

Trauma is one of the leading causes of death in western countries, and the most frequent one in people below forty [1]. Whenever the body's integrity is compromised by contusion, concussion or fracture, surgical trauma care is necessary for rapid damage control and specific individualized treatment. This remains, a major challenge for clinicians due to varying patterns of injuries and occasional major traumas, requiring urgent, yet highly specialized therapy [2, 3]. Fast, conclusive and complete injury assessment by examination of head and neck, thorax, abdomen, pelvis and the extremities is further supported by computed tomography (CT) and CT-angiography (CTA) [4, 5].

Head and thoracic injuries are found in approximately 50% of all trauma patients and extremity or pelvic fractures in roughly 30% [6]. Additional vascular damage, especially of arteries or venous plexus is acutely life threatening and further reduces time for decision-making and treatment [7]. Vascular damage in combination with fractures is associated with higher mortality and inferior outcome, especially due to rapid and voluminous blood loss into pelvic or femoral soft tissue compartments. Correct diagnosis may be difficult due to low body temperature and masking effects of other injuries [8–10].

* Correspondence: gilbert_f@ukw.de; kellersman_r@ukw.de; Albert.Busch@mri.tum.de
[1]Department of Orthopaedic Trauma, Hand, Plastic and Reconstructive Surgery, University Hospital Würzburg, Würzburg, Germany
[5]Department of Vascular Surgery, Klinikum Fulda, Fulda, Germany
[2]Department for General Visceral, Vascular & Paediatric Surgery, University Hospital Würzburg, Würzburg, Germany
Full list of author information is available at the end of the article

Doppler ultrasound and CTA increase the detection rate, yet incorrect diagnosis remains frequent thus requiring re-examination after initial stabilization [11, 12]. Depending on type and extent of trauma, presentations may be acute bleeding, hemodynamic instability, pulsating tumors, massive hematoma or ischemic and pulseless extremities [13]. Additionally, vasospasm or complete vascular disruption both may mimic ischemia [14].

Despite recognized difficulties in detecting vascular injury in extremity trauma as well as an increased mortality rate in combination with pelvic trauma, limited data about the immediate clinical implications of vascular damage associated with fractures is available. We therefore analyzed thoroughly demography, initial laboratory results, treatment and outcome of extremity and pelvic fracture-associated vascular injuries in a trauma cohort of 64 patients versus a comparable cohort of patients with isolated osseous damage in a nine-year retrospective single-center study was carried out.

Aim of the study:

The aim of this retrospective cohort study was to recognize patterns of injury where vascular damage and fracture occur and also identification of surrogate parameters which may suspect a vascular involvement in major trauma patients. In addition, the influences of concomitant vascular damage to patient's management and outcome were analyzed.

Methods
Facility
A university hospital and level-one trauma center, embedded in the regional trauma network (Traumanetzwerk Nordbayern-Würzburg) was analyzed. A multidisciplinary team provides twenty-four-seven trauma care; following standard operating procedures according to guidelines of the German National Society for Trauma Surgery (DGU) are implemented. Ultrasound, X-ray and multi-slice computed tomography (CT) are available on site in the trauma room. A board-certified vascular surgeon and an interventional radiologist are part of the trauma team.

Patient identification.

A retrospective analysis of all admissions to the surgical trauma room from December 2005 until December 2013 identified 3689 cases, including primary trauma admissions and secondary transfers from other centers.

The initial analysis included trauma mechanism and pattern of injuries, specifically identifying all vascular damages. Additional examination included fractures, immediate vascular, visceral, urologic or pediatric surgery or invasive vascular diagnostics and interventions. Every case with vascular involvement and extremity or pelvic fracture was then analyzed for age, sex, blunt or penetrating trauma, hospital stay, intensive care unit (ICU) stay, number of operations, method of treatment,

amputation, death, trauma scores (Glasgow coma scale, GCS; injury severity index, ISS; Revised Injury Severity Classification Score, RISC I), preclinical fluid management and initial laboratory results. Data were available for 100% of patients, except for preclinical fluid management (36.7 and 49.3% for vascular injury group and fracture only group, respectively).

This cohort (vascular injury group) was then subdivided in regard to localization of the fracture, upper/lower extremity or pelvis, and the corresponding vascular damage. Patients with vascular involvement of the head and neck ($N = 36$), i.e. carotid artery dissection, were excluded in this study.

Control group
In order to compare outcome and laboratory results, a control group consisting of 60 major trauma patients with limb/pelvic fractures only and no additional vascular damage, based on CTA, clinical assessment and clinical course, was selected. Inclusion criteria were surgical trauma room admission and fractures without further vascular, visceral, thoracic, spinal or cranial damage.

Statistics
Group comparisons of count data were performed with $\chi 2$ tests when the smallest value in the contingency table was 5 or more, otherwise Fisher's exact test was performed. Normally distributed measurement values (Shapiro-Wilk $p \geq 0.05$) were examined with the Welch two sample t-test, in cases where the normality assumption did not hold (Shapiro-Wilk $p < 0.05$) the Wilcoxon rank sum test was applied. Dependencies between measurement values were examined with linear regression. Endpoint (survival) analyses were performed with Cox regression. P-values < 0.05 were considered significant.

Results
Demographic data
Within the nine-year study period, 3689 patients were admitted to the trauma room. Fractures of the extremities, the pelvis or the shoulder girdle (i.e. clavicula, scapula) were found in 904 patients. A third presented with multiple (≥ 2) fractures (Additional file 1: Table S1).

Vascular damage associated with a corresponding fracture of the extremities or the pelvis, requiring specific vascular repair, was identified in 64 cases (Fig. 1). Vessel injuries were confined to the arterial system in lower and upper limb, while arterial damage was the reason to treat in 66% in pelvic fractures and venous damage requiring treatment was seen in 34%. The mean age of this cohort was 49 ± 17 years, 78% were male and 94% sustained blunt trauma

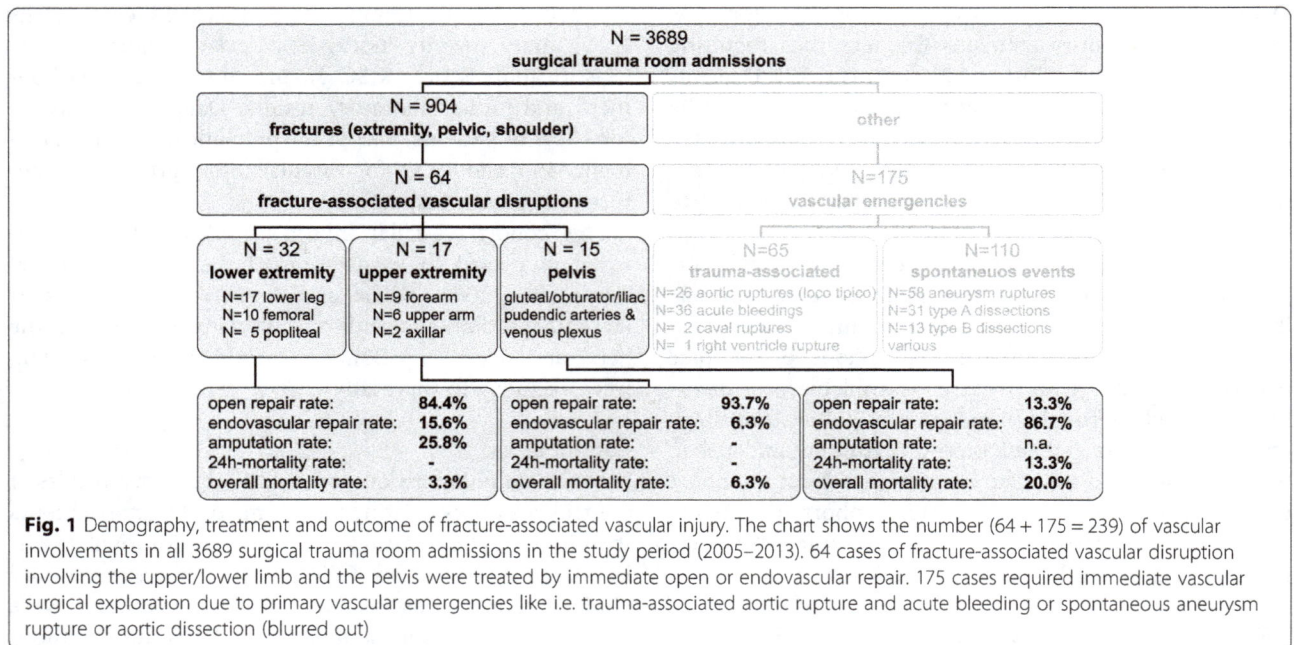

Fig. 1 Demography, treatment and outcome of fracture-associated vascular injury. The chart shows the number (64 + 175 = 239) of vascular involvements in all 3689 surgical trauma room admissions in the study period (2005–2013). 64 cases of fracture-associated vascular disruption involving the upper/lower limb and the pelvis were treated by immediate open or endovascular repair. 175 cases required immediate vascular surgical exploration due to primary vascular emergencies like i.e. trauma-associated aortic rupture and acute bleeding or spontaneous aneurysm rupture or aortic dissection (blurred out)

(79.4% traffic accident; 12.6% fall; 7.9% work-related accident) (Additional file 1: Table S1). The lower limb and its vessels were involved twice as often as upper limb and pelvis, however facture-associated vascular injury occurred at almost same rates in either localization (4.2, 6.2, 6.1% for upper limb, pelvis and lower limb, respectively) (Figs. 2 and 3). All patients had a CTA of the clinically suspected trauma area after exclusion of cerebral hemorrhage by native CT in cases of suspected head trauma. Depending on the treatment strategy, patients were then immediately transferred to the operating room or the angiography suite. A specific trauma mechanism could not be linked to vascular damage.

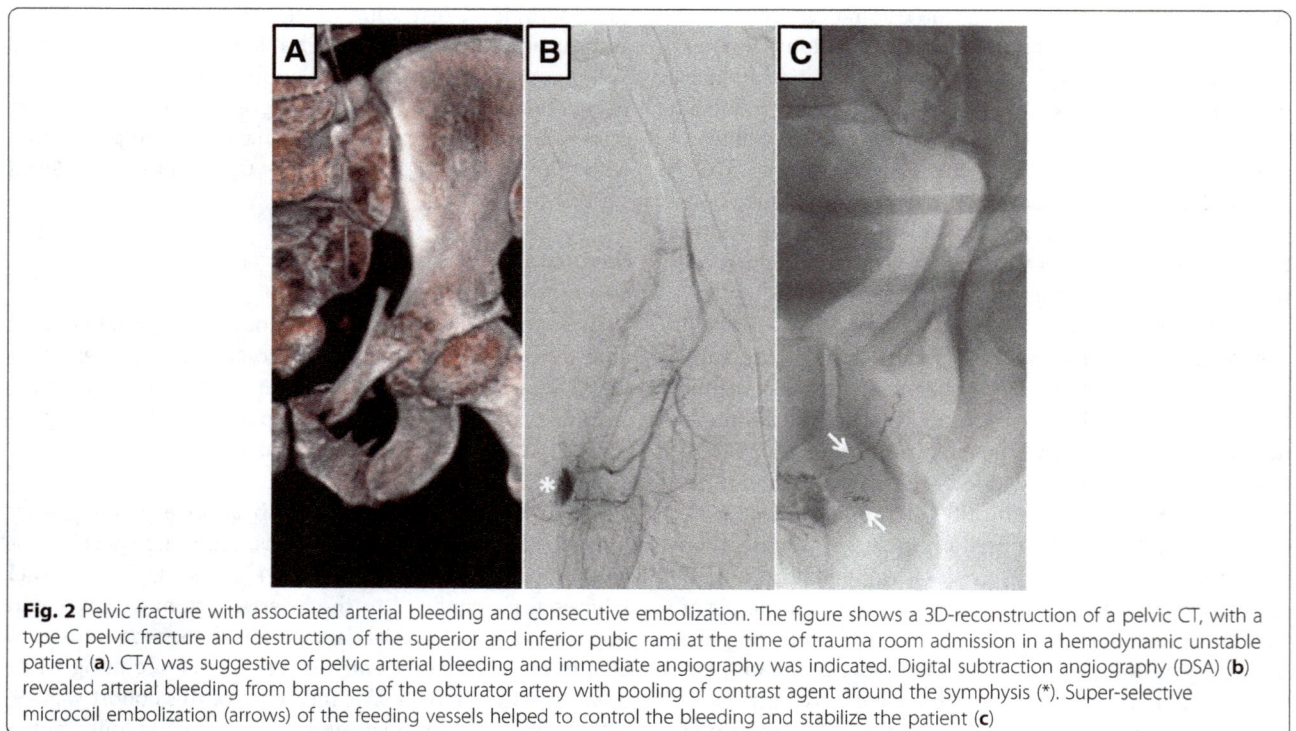

Fig. 2 Pelvic fracture with associated arterial bleeding and consecutive embolization. The figure shows a 3D-reconstruction of a pelvic CT, with a type C pelvic fracture and destruction of the superior and inferior pubic rami at the time of trauma room admission in a hemodynamic unstable patient (a). CTA was suggestive of pelvic arterial bleeding and immediate angiography was indicated. Digital subtraction angiography (DSA) (b) revealed arterial bleeding from branches of the obturator artery with pooling of contrast agent around the symphysis (*). Super-selective microcoil embolization (arrows) of the feeding vessels helped to control the bleeding and stabilize the patient (c)

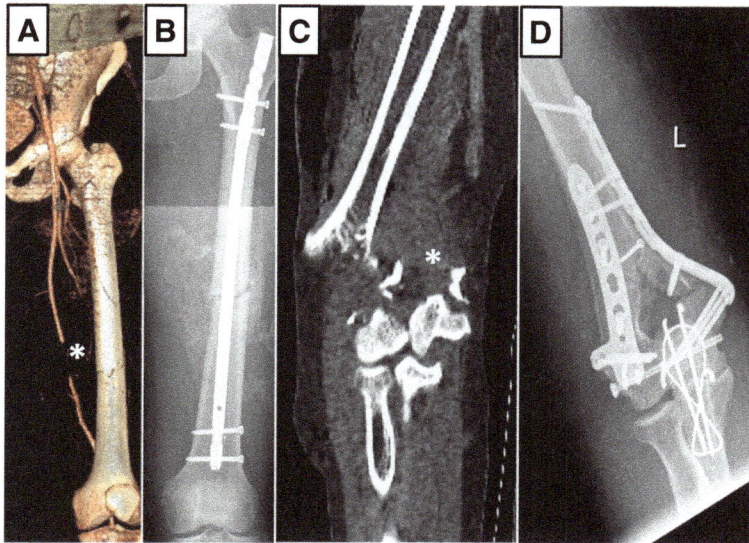

Fig. 3 Extremity fractures with associated vascular damage. 3D-reconstruction (**a**) of the initial CT of a patient after motorcycle accident with closed femoral shaft fracture and disruption of the superficial femoral artery (★) with active bleeding palpable as pulsatile femoral mass (signal loss of soft tissue contrast agent pooling due to 3D-reconstruction sequence). Of note, fracture lines (**a**) indicate medial translocation of the osseous fragment towards the artery, probably causative of arterial rupture. Initial treatment included immediate open arterial reconstruction with vein graft interposition and external stabilization and after 12 days intramedullary nail repair (**b**). CTA with active pooling of contrast agent (*) from the brachial artery in a patient after fall with a grade IIIb open fracture of the humeral shaft (**c**). Initial treatment included patch plasty of the brachial artery, external fixation and fasciotomy of the forearm compartments. After 10 days the elbow joint was reconstructed with open reduction and plate fixation, an olecranon osteotomy was performed for better joint visualization

In total, 239 (6.5%) cases of all trauma room admissions had vascular implications that required immediate vascular repair (Fig. 1).

Laboratory results

Comparing this group with a similar non-vascular trauma group, no differences in baseline characteristics were seen (Additional file 1: Table S1). However, fracture-associated arterial damage and consecutive blood loss into the surrounding soft tissues seriously aggravated the initial clinical presentation. Hemoglobin levels, a surrogate marker of blood loss, and prothrombin time (Quick) as well as activated partial thromboplastin time (PTT) were significantly lower in the vascular trauma group. Concordantly fibrinogen was at the lower limit (Table 1). These effects were pronounced in the pelvis and the lower extremity (Additional file 2: Table S2). Markers of cellular stress and disintegration, lactate, myoglobin and creatine kinase were elevated in both groups, yet showed no statistically significant difference (Table 1).

Subsequent analysis of the pre-clinical fluid administration revealed a significantly higher need of total volume to secure safe transport (Table 1). As expected, the total volume correlated inversely with the initial hemoglobin measurement at admission ($p < 0.001$). Regression analysis revealed lowering of the hemoglobin-value by 1 mg/dl with every 200 ml of fluids administered. This effect was four times stronger in the vascular trauma group (Additional file 3: Table S3). Unfortunately, initial blood pressure measurements and reports about tourniquet or pelvic clamp usage were not available. A drop in fibrinogen by 1 g/L was associated with roughly 700 ml of fluid administration. No significant values were detected in both groups, yet the observed trends suggest a stronger effect with additional vascular damage (Additional file 3: Table S3).

Outcome analysis

No differences were seen in mortality rates between patients with extremity fracture only and such with associated vascular damage (Table 2). In both groups overall survival was over 90% and death, if any, was due to accompanying head injury, thoracic injury or prolonged course of disease with septic complications. However, a notably high immediate mortality rate (≤24 h) of 13.3% and overall mortality rate of 20% was associated with pelvic fracture with vascular damage. These could, however, not be related to a specific fracture type or vessel involvement (66% arterial/33% venous).

Fracture-associated vascular disruption resulted in longer hospital stay, longer ICU stay and a higher number of revision surgery after the initial procedure for bleeding control and primary fixation (Table 2). Also, the lower extremity amputation rate was significantly higher.

Table 1 Laboratory results and pre-clinical fluid administratio

	Hemoglobin (mg/dl)	Quick (%)	PTT (s)	Fibrinogen (g/l)	Lactate (mmol/l)	Myoglobin (µg/l)	Creatine kinase (U/l)	Crystallines (ml)	Colloids (ml)	Total volume (ml)
Vascular injury group	9.95 ± 2.6	59.2 ± 21.6	41.9 ± 25.2	1.7 ± 0.9	2.1 ± 1.2	1356 ± 1441	393 ± 316	1000 ± 741	500 ± 0	1500 ± 1112
Fracture only group	11.67 ± 2.6	78.0 ± 19.3	35.3 ± 20.7	2.2 ± 0.6	1.8 ± 0.9	855 ± 856	372 ± 337	1000 ± 0	500 ± 0	1000 ± 741
P	0.0004	0.0002	0.002	0.003	0.24	0.24	0.77	0.09	0.64	0.03

The table shows the mean ± standard deviation (SD) or median ± median absolute deviation (MAD) where appropriate (cristalloides; colloides) for each parameter and the P-value for comparison between vascular and control trauma population. Significant P-values are shown in bold. (normal ranges: hemoglobin: 11.5–16 g/dL; prothrombin time according to Quick: 70–120%; activated partial thromboplastin time, PTT: 25–36 s; fibrinogen: 1.6–4.0 g/L; lactate: < 0.5 mmol/L; Myoglobin: < 55 µg/L; creatin kinase: < 170 U/L)

Table 2 Outcome parameters and trauma scores of vascular and control trauma populations

	Overall survival	Hospital stay (d)	ICU stay (d)	Operations (number)	Amputation (leg)	GCS	ISS	RISC I
Vascular injury group	92.5%	36.0 ± 22.1	15.0 ± 14.8	6.0 ± 4.7	25.8%	13.2 ± 3.3	23.4 ± 13.8	81.5 ± 25.1
Fracture only group	91.3%	21.5 ± 13	7.2 ± 7.3	2.9 ± 2.4	–	13.3 ± 3.5	22.7 ± 14.2	86.2 ± 23.1
Effect size Effect type	0.486 hazard	12.5 median diff	5.5 median	2	8.32	0	0	–1.9
Test type	ratio Cox regression	Wilcox-Test	diff Wilcox-Test	median diff Wilcox-Test	odds ratio Fisher's exact-t	median diff Wilcox-Test	median diff Wilcox-Test	median diff Wilcox-Test
P	0.28	0.00002	0.009	0.000003	0.03	0.8	0.74	0.3

The table shows the comparison of the vascular trauma group to the fracture only group, indicating mean ± SD, effect size, effect type and the type of test used, along with their significance. Significant P-values are shown in bold. (GCS, Glasgow Coma Scale, ISS Injury Severity Index, RISC I, Revised Injury Severity Classification Score)

Two amputations were due to primary subtotal above-the-knee amputation during trauma, five were due to severe soft tissue damage and one was due to prolonged ischemia after complicated pelvic fracture with iliac artery occlusion. No upper extremity amputation occurred. The grade of soft tissue damage was, however, comparable for lower and upper extremities (grade IIIC according to Gustilo/Anderson in > 70% of cases). Compartment release had to be done in eight lower and one upper extremity, these cases did not correlate with subsequent need for amputation. These implications were not reflected by either of the trauma scores GCS, ISS or RISC I (Table 2).

Vascular surgical and interventional endovascular means were applied for bleeding control. Open surgical procedures included autologous vein interposition, patch plasty, ligature as well as direct suture and were the method of choice in both extremities (Figs. 1 and 3). Pelvic fracture associated bleedings were mostly treated by endovascular coiling or covered stent implantation in one case (Figs. 1 and 2).

Discussion

Fracture-associated vascular injury of the limbs and especially the pelvis may have severe consequence for the patient. Accurate detection, early treatment and supportive therapy determine the outcome [15].

Mechanisms of vascular trauma include blunt trauma (external force or through fracture fragments), sharp trauma or strain which might lead to disruption or intima damage leading to ischemia (Fig. 3) [16, 17]. Presentation is thus hemorrhage or ischemia, a phenomenon best described for supracondylar humeral fracture or knee trauma [18–20]. The initial clinical symptoms, especially hemodynamic instability, were not available retrospectively in our cohort. Nevertheless, the established algorithm of local CT-angiography in case of suspected severe fracture of the pelvis and the extremities provided good results, since all patients with vascular injury were identified immediately and no late amputations due to ischemia occurred [5, 12, 21].

In 3–9% of fractures a concomitant vascular damage is reported varying due to regional and socioeconomic factors [10, 22–24]. In this single-center cohort we identified an accompanying vascular damage in 7% of the fractures. Required treatments were very heterogeneous, for the fracture-associated vascular injury as well as vascular incidents in general (Fig. 1). Unfortunately, most publications are case reports or case series focusing on a specific entity or treatment, thus not catering for the need for more general data analysis [25]. No conclusive pattern of injury for consecutive vascular damage could be identified in our cohort, in fact, vascular damage has

to be expected regardless of the fracture localization, the impact of trauma or any trauma scores (Table 2).

This data displays a similar incidence of vascular injury in upper/lower extremity and pelvic fractures. Nevertheless, outcomes such as higher immediate mortality in pelvic fractures and significant amputation rates for the lower extremity are area-specific (Fig. 1 and Table 2). The management is considerably influenced by the degree of tissue damage and occasional primary subtotal amputation. Of 15 pelvic fractures, 4 were classified stable while the rest were type B/C fractures (Pennal and Tile classification) possibly yielding additional rupture of the venous plexus. Patients with fractures and vascular injuries also show a longer hospital stay and higher number of operative procedures (Table 2). Elevated immediate mortality in the fracture only group was due to the higher rate of multiple fractures, suggestive of more severely trauma (Table 2 and Additional file 2: Table S2). The additional severity of vascular damage to multi-injured patients is currently not reflected by any trauma score (Table 2).

This study demonstrates the effect of additional vascular damage on the admission laboratory data (Table 1 and Additional file 2:Table S2 and Additional file 3: Table S3). The presented results show similar trends in overall, as well as entitiy-specific analysis (Additional file 2: Table S2). Low hemoglobin, and altered coagulation were, however, associated with an increased need of fluid in the preclinical course. Thus some dilution effect has to be taken into consideration However, the available data in retrospective analysis was not available in all patients, and results have to be interpreted carefully. Nevertheless, substantial fluid administration and low initial hemoglobin, i.e. by rapid blood gas analysis, may raise the attention to direct diagnostics to identifying vascular damage. Trauma-induced coagulation defect is a severe co-morbidity, strongly associated with an increased mortality [26]. Early therapy might also include platelet-directed treatments [27, 28].

Ever since the late stages of World War II, where ligation of arteries and veins was the treatment of choice, surgical and technical abilities have evolved towards a diversified armamentarium, significantly increasing limb salvage and survival rates, nowadays enabling individualized care [29, 30]. Especially rapid endovascular repair for bleeding control has evolved as primary option for certain clinical entities of vascular injury, like embolization in pelvic bleeding, stentgraft implantation in aortic transection or thoracic outlet vessel breach [22, 25, 31, 32]. However, mangled extremities remain a domain of open vascular repair (Fig. 1). Open fracture, eventual contamination and massive tissue loss require autologous reconstruction [9, 33, 34].

Conclusion

This retrospective single-center cohort study we could demonstrate that fracture-associated vascular damage occurs in one of fourteen trauma patients, with a specific clinical impact regarding pre-hospital fluid management, eventual early transfusion and coagulation support. A multidisciplinary approach requires trauma and vascular surgery in combination with interventional radiology to guarantee the best possible outcome for overall survival and limb salvage.

Additional files

Additional file 1: Table S1. Baseline characteristics of vascular and control trauma populations. Both populations have a similar size and show no differences in age, sex and trauma type distribution. The number of patients with multiple fractures is slightly higher in the control trauma population. (DOC 31 kb)

Additional file 2: Table S2. Laboratory results and total preclinical volume comparison between vascular and control trauma population overall and based on area of fracture. The table shows the mean ± SD or median ± MAD where appropriate for each parameter and the P-value for comparison between vascular and control trauma population. Significant P-values are shown in bold. (normal ranges: hemoglobin: 11.5-16 g/dL; prothrombin time according to Quick: 70–120%; activated partial thromboplastin time, PTT: 25–36 s; fibrinogen: 1.6–4.0 g/L; lactate: < 0.5 mmol/L). (DOC 45 kb)

Additional file 3: Table S3. Preclinical fluid administration in dependence of hemoglobin and fibrinogen. Regression results of indicated parameters against total administered volume are shown for the overall study population as well as both patient groups separately. The effect size corresponds to the average volume of required preclinical fluid administration when the examined parameter value is increased by 1. Significant P-values are shown in bold. (DOC 35 kb)

Abbreviations

CT: Computed tomography; CTA: computed tomography angiography; GCS: Glasgow coma scale; ISS: Injury severity index; PTT: Partial thromboplastin time; RISC I: Revised Injury Severity Classification Score

Acknowledgments

We thank S. Duell for administrative help and C. Wagner for help with patient identification in SAP. We especially thank all the nursing and medical staff that makes working in the emergency room possible every day and night.

Funding

This publication was funded by the German Research Foundation (DFG) and the University of Wuerzburg in the funding program Open Access Publishing. Funding includes only the publication fee. No funding for the design of the study, the collection, analysis, and interpretation of data and for writing the manuscript was obtained.

Authors' contributions

FG: made substantial contribution in design an conception of the study, performed acquisition of data and interpretation of data, revisited the manuscript critically CS: performed acquisition of data and interpretation of data CJS: performed acquisition of data and interpretation of data RK: made substantial contribution in design and conception of the study, revisited the manuscript RM: made substantial contribution in design and conception of the study, revisited the manuscript RW: made substantial contribution in design and conception of the study, revisited the manuscript UL: made substantial contribution in design and conception of the study, revisited the manuscript RK: made substantial contribution in design and conception of the study, wrote the manuscript AB: made substantial contribution in design and conception of the study, wrote the manuscript. All authors approved the final version of the manuscript.

Competing interests

The authors declare that they have no competing interests.

Author details

[1]Department of Orthopaedic Trauma, Hand, Plastic and Reconstructive Surgery, University Hospital Würzburg, Würzburg, Germany. [2]Department for General Visceral, Vascular & Paediatric Surgery, University Hospital Würzburg, Würzburg, Germany. [3]Core Unit Systems Medicine IZKF, University Hospital Würzburg, Würzburg, Germany. [4]Department of Diagnostic and Interventional Radiology, University Hospital Würzburg, Würzburg, Germany. [5]Department of Vascular Surgery, Klinikum Fulda, Fulda, Germany. [6]Department for Vascular and Endovascular Surgery Klinikum rechts der Isar, Technical University Munich, Munich, Germany. [7]Department of Trauma Hand Plastic and Reconstructive Surgery, University Munich Germany, Julius-Maximilians-University of Würzburg Oberdürrbacherstr, 6 D-, 97080 Würzburg, Germany.

References

1. Bundesamt D-S. https://www.destatis.de/DE/ZahlenFakten/GesellschaftStaat/Gesundheit/Todesursachen/Todesursachen.html.
2. Tiel Groenestege-Kreb D, van Maarseveen O, Leenen L. Trauma team. Br J Anaesth. 2014;113(2):258–65. https://doi.org/10.1093/bja/aeu236 PubMed PMID: 24980423.
3. Wurmb TE, Fruhwald P, Knuepffer J, et al. Application of standard operating procedures accelerates the process of trauma care in patients with multiple injuries. Eur J Emerg Med. 2008;15(6):311–7. https://doi.org/10.1097/MEJ.0b013e3283036ce6 PubMed PMID: 19078832.
4. Wurmb TE, Fruhwald P, Hopfner W, et al. Whole-body multislice computed tomography as the first line diagnostic tool in patients with multiple injuries: the focus on time. J Trauma. 2009;66(3):658–65. https://doi.org/10.1097/TA.0b013e31817de3f4 PubMed PMID: 19276734.
5. Fung Kon Jin PH, Goslings JC, Ponsen KJ, et al. Assessment of a new trauma workflow concept implementing a sliding CT scanner in the trauma room: the effect on workup times. J Trauma. 2008;64(5):1320–6. https://doi.org/10.1097/TA.0b013e318059b9ae PubMed PMID: 18469657.
6. Sektion Notfall- & Intensivmedizin SNdDGfrUDAT. Jahresbericht 2015. 2015.
7. Hupp T, Eisele R. Traumatic injuries to the extremities including bone and blood vessel damage: priorities, triage and interdisciplinary management. Gefässchirurgie. 2002;7(4):202–7. https://doi.org/10.1007/s00772-002-0242-7.
8. Scalea TM, DuBose J, Moore EE, et al. Western trauma association critical decisions in trauma: management of the mangled extremity. J Trauma Acute Care Surg. 2012;72(1):86–93. https://doi.org/10.1097/TA.0b013e318241ed70 PubMed PMID: 22310120.
9. Rozycki GS, Tremblay LN, Feliciano DV, et al. Blunt vascular trauma in the extremity: diagnosis, management, and outcome. J Trauma. 2003;55(5):814–24. https://doi.org/10.1097/01.TA.0000087807.44105.AE PubMed PMID: 14608150.
10. Marzi I, Lustenberger T. Management of Bleeding Pelvic Fractures. Scandinavian journal of surgery. 2014;103(2):104–11. https://doi.org/10.1177/1457496914525604 PubMed PMID: 24737854.
11. Seamon MJ, Smoger D, Torres DM, et al. A prospective validation of a current practice: the detection of extremity vascular injury with CT angiography. J Trauma 2009;67(2):238–243; discussion 243-4. doi: https://doi.org/10.1097/TA.0b013e3181a51bf9. PubMed PMID: 19667874.
12. Luo W, Hosseini H, Zderic V, et al. Detection and localization of peripheral vascular bleeding using Doppler ultrasound. J Emerg Med. 2011;41(1):64–73. https://doi.org/10.1016/j.jemermed.2010.01.001 PubMed PMID: 20189743.
13. Halvorson JJ, Anz A, Langfitt M, et al. Vascular injury associated with extremity trauma: initial diagnosis and management. J Am Acad Orthop Surg. 2011;19(8):495–504 PubMed PMID: 21807917.
14. Shah SR, Wearden PD, Gaines BA. Pediatric peripheral vascular injuries: a review of our experience. J Surg Res. 2009;153(1):162–6. https://doi.org/10.1016/j.jss.2008.03.006 PubMed PMID: 18541266.

15. Albert B, Gilbert F, Schneemann C, Kickuth R, Meffert R, Kellersmann R, Wildenauer R, Lorenz U. Klinische Implikationen bei Fraktur-assoziierten Gefäßschäden im Schockraum. 134. München: Kongress Deutsche Gesellschaft für Chirurgie ICM; 2017. p. 284. https://goo.gl/Qs3hdH.

16. Linder F, Vollmar J. [The current status of treatment of arterial injuries and their sequelae]. Chirurg 1965;36:55–63. PubMed PMID: 14265784.

17. Larcan A, Fieve G. Louis Sencert, vascular surgeon (1878–1924). J Mal Vasc. 1986;11(Suppl B):68–74 PubMed PMID: 3519817.

18. Wegmann H, Eberl R, Kraus T, et al. The impact of arterial vessel injuries associated with pediatric supracondylar humeral fractures. J Trauma Acute Care Surg. 2014;77(2):381–5. https://doi.org/10.1097/TA.0000000000000306 PubMed PMID: 25058268.

19. Parker S, Handa A, Deakin M, et al. Knee dislocation and vascular injury: 4 year experience at a UK major trauma Centre and vascular hub. Injury. 2015. https://doi.org/10.1016/j.injury.2015.11.014 PubMed PMID: 26652226.

20. Xu YQ, Li Q, Shen TG, et al. Early diagnosis and treatment of trauma in knee joints accompanied with popliteal vascular injury. Int J Clin Exp Med. 2015; 8(6):9421–9 PubMed PMID: 26309604; PubMed Central PMCID: PMCPMC4538002.

21. Linder F, Mani K, Juhlin C, et al. Routine whole body CT of high energy trauma patients leads to excessive radiation exposure. Scand J Trauma Resusc Emerg Med. 2016;24(1):7. https://doi.org/10.1186/s13049-016-0199-2 PubMed PMID: 26817669; PubMed Central PMCID: PMCPMC4729033.

22. Hauschild O, Aghayev E, von Heyden J, et al. Angioembolization for pelvic hemorrhage control: results from the German pelvic injury register. J Trauma Acute Care Surg. 2012;73(3):679–84. https://doi.org/10.1097/TA.0b013e318253b5ba PubMed PMID: 22710767.

23. Poyhonen R, Suominen V, Uurto I, et al. Non-iatrogenic civilian vascular trauma in a well-defined geographical region in Finland. Eur J Trauma Emerg Surg. 2015;41(5):545–9. https://doi.org/10.1007/s00068-014-0460-1 PubMed PMID: 26037992.

24. Galyfos G, Kerasidis S, Stefanidis G, et al. Iatrogenic and non-iatrogenic arterial injuries in an urban level I trauma Centre in Greece. Int Angiol. 2015; 25 PubMed PMID: 26406965.

25. Lustenberger T, Wutzler S, Stormann P, et al. The role of angio-embolization in the acute treatment concept of severe pelvic ring injuries. Injury. 2015; 46(Suppl 4):S33–8. https://doi.org/10.1016/S0020-1383(15)30016-4 PubMed PMID: 26542864.

26. Gando S, Hayakawa M. Pathophysiology of trauma-induced coagulopathy and Management of Critical Bleeding Requiring Massive Transfusion. Semin Thromb Hemost. 2016;42(2):155–65. https://doi.org/10.1055/s-0035-1564831. PubMed PMID: 26716498.

27. Ramsey MT, Fabian TC, Shahan CP, Sharpe JP, Mabry SE, Weinberg JA, Croce MA, Jennings LK. A prospective study of platelet function in trauma patients. J Trauma Acute Care Surg. 2016. https://doi.org/10.1097/TA.0000000000001017. PubMed PMID: 26895088.

28. Fachgesellschaften. AdWM. S3 – Leitlinie Polytrauma/ Schwerverletzten-Behandlung. online publication. 2011 valid till 2016-06-30;AWMF RegNr 012/019.

29. Barr J, Cherry KJ, Rich NM. Vascular surgery in world war II: the shift to repairing arteries. Ann Surg. 2016;263(3):615–20. https://doi.org/10.1097/SLA.0000000000001181 PubMed PMID: 25719811.

30. De BM, Simeone FA. Battle injuries of the arteries in world war II; an analysis of 2,471 cases. Ann Surg. 1946;123:534–79 PubMed PMID: 21024586.

31. Serra R, de Franciscis S, Grande R, et al. Endovascular repair for acute traumatic transection of the descending thoracic aorta: experience of a single centre with a 12-years follow up. J Cardiothorac Surg. 2015;10(1):171. https://doi.org/10.1186/s13019-015-0388-5 PubMed PMID: 26590963; PubMed Central PMCID: PMCPMC4655082.

32. Sinha S, Patterson BO, Ma J, et al. Systematic review and meta-analysis of open surgical and endovascular management of thoracic outlet vascular injuries. Journal of vascular surgery : official publication, the Society for Vascular Surgery [and] International Society for Cardiovascular Surgery. North American Chapter. 2013;57(2):547–567 e8. https://doi.org/10.1016/j.jvs.2012.10.077 PubMed PMID: 23337863.

33. The Lower Extremity Vascular Repairs Outcome Group; Fortuna G, DuBose J, Mendelsberg R, Inaba, K, Haider A, Joseph B, Skarupa D, Selleck MJ, O'Callaghan T, Charlton-Ouw K. Contemporary outcomes of lower extremity vascular repairs extending below the knee: a multicenter retrospective study. J Trauma Acute Care Surg. 2016. https://doi.org/10.1097/TA.0000000000000996. PubMed PMID: 26885995.

34. Scott AR, Gilani R, Tapia NM, et al. Endovascular management of traumatic peripheral arterial injuries. J Surg Res. 2015;199(2):557–63. https://doi.org/10.1016/j.jss.2015.04.086 PubMed PMID: 26115809.

26

The hsa-miR-181a-5p reduces oxidation resistance by controlling SECISBP2 in osteoarthritis

Jianli Xue[1], Zixin Min[2], Zhuqing Xia[3], Bin Cheng[1], Binshang Lan[1], Fujun Zhang[2], Yan Han[2], Kunzheng Wang[1*] and Jian Sun[2]

Abstract

Background: The phenotypes of osteoarthritis (OA) consist of cartilage extracellular matrix (ECM) metabolism disorder and the breakdown of cartilage homeostasis, which are induced by pro-inflammatory factors and oxidative stress. Selenoproteins regulated by selenocysteine insertion sequence binding protein 2 (SBP2) are highly effective antioxidants, but their regulatory mechanisms, particularly the involvement of miRNAs, are not fully understood.

Methods: To explore whether *miR-181a-5p* and *SBP2* are involved in OA pathogenesis, we established an IL-1β model using the chondrocyte SW1353 cell line. Next, we up- or down-regulated *SBP2* and *miRNA-181a-5p* expression in the cells. Finally, we measured the expression of *miRNA-181a-5p*, *SBP2* and three selenoproteins in OA cartilage and peripheral blood.

Results: The results showed that IL-1β increased *hsa-miR-181a-5p* and decreased *SBP2* in a time- and dose-dependent manner. *GPX1* and *GPX4*, which encode crucial glutathione peroxidase antioxidant enzymes, were up-regulated along with *SBP2* and *miR-181a-5p*. Furthermore, *SBP2* showed a significant negative correlation with *miR-181a-5p* during induced ATDC5 cell differentiation. There was lower *GPX1* and *GPX4* mRNA expression and SBP2 protein expression in damaged cartilage than in smooth cartilage from the same OA sample, and *hsa-miR-181a-5p* expression on the contrary. Similar results were observed in peripheral blood. In conclusion, we have reported a novel pathway in which pro-inflammatory factors, miRNA, SBP2 and selenoproteins are associated with oxidation resistance in cartilage.

Conclusion: Overall, this study provides the first comprehensive evidence that pro-inflammatory factors cause changes in the cartilage antioxidant network and describes the discovery of novel mediators of cartilage oxidative stress and OA pathophysiology. Our data suggest that *miR-181a-5p* may be used to develop novel early-stage diagnostic and therapeutic strategies for OA.

Keywords: *miRNA-181a-5p*, SECISBP2, Selenoprotein, Cartilage, Osteoarthritis

Background

Osteoarthritis (OA) may be a response to superfluous mechanical stress or inflammation, and pro-inflammatory factors, including interleukin-1 (IL-1β), interleukin-6 (IL-6), and tumour necrosis factor-α (TNF-α), are involved in OA pathogenesis [1, 2]. The phenotypes of cartilage injury processes induced by pro-inflammatory factors are cartilage extracellular matrix (ECM) metabolic disorder, the disruption of cartilage homeostasis, and enhanced expression of matrix degradation enzymes such as MMP13 [3]. MMP13, a major enzyme hydrolysing type-II collagen (COL2), is a dominant protein component of the cartilage ECM [4, 5] and a biomarker for arthritis progression and therapeutic effects [6–8].

Reactive oxygen species (ROS) are products of aerobic metabolism that injure DNA, proteins, and cellular membranes [9–11]. Oxidative stress plays important roles in the pathogenesis of OA and cartilage degradation, which is induced by ROS, and traumatic loading

* Correspondence: wkzh1955@163.com
[1]Department of Orthopaedics, The Second Affiliated Hospital, Xi'an Jiaotong University Health Science Center, 157 West 5th Road, Xi'an, Shaanxi 710004, People's Republic of China
Full list of author information is available at the end of the article

increases cartilage oxidation and causes cell death [12]. In addition, oxidative stress-mediated regulation of the expression of redox-sensitive proteins is regarded as a key mechanism underlying age-related cellular dysfunction and disease progression [13].

Selenoproteins (Sel) are important members of a network of antioxidant enzymatic systems and minimize damage induced by ROS. They contain selenocysteine (Sec), the 21st proteinogenic amino acid, which is named after the essential biological trace element selenium (Se) and acts as an active-site residue essential for the catalytic activity of selenoproteins [9–11]. The genetic code 'UGA', commonly a termination codon in cells, encodes Sec into selenoproteins [14]. Several special cis-trans elements and trans-acting factors, typically the Sec insertion sequence (SECIS) and Sec insertion sequence binding protein 2 (SECISBP2 or SBP2), regulate selenoprotein biosynthesis [15, 16]. SECIS, which is located in the selenoprotein mRNA 3′-untranslated region (3′-UTR), binds with SBP2. The function of SBP2 is to carry Sec-tRNA^{Sec} into the ribosome 'A site' to recognize 'UGA' as the Sec codon during selenoprotein synthesis [15, 16].

Intriguingly, osteo-chondroprogenitor-specific deletion of the selenocysteinyl tRNA^{Sec} gene results in dyschondroplasia phenotypes, particularly those showing abnormal skeletal development in mice [17]. 'UGA' is recognized as a termination codon, and inactive truncated selenoproteins are produced in the presence of insufficient Sec-tRNA^{Sec} [18]. Similarly, the TrxR1 short inactive fragment, a two-amino-acid truncated C-terminal motif, leads to the death of human lung carcinoma A549 cells [19]. However, little is known about how selenoprotein biosynthesis regulates OA cartilage. In particular, the pathway from pro-inflammatory factors to selenoprotein biosynthesis mediated by SBP2 in cartilage is poorly understood.

Moreover, more than 20 miRNAs, such as the cartilage-specific miR-140-5p, participate in chondrogenesis, cartilage homeostasis and degradation, and chondrocyte metabolism, which are closely associated with OA development [20–22]. Further, miR-9, miR-34a and miR-146a are related with oxidative stress in OA chondrocytes [23, 24]. In a previous study, we identified a repertoire of miRNAs during the development of rat femoral articular cartilage [25] and demonstrated that miR-337 regulates chondrogenesis through a direct target, TGFBR2 [26]. Specifically, miR-181a-5p, a member of the miR-181 family, which is organized into three clusters (miR-181a/b-1, miR-181a/b-2, and miR-181c/d), is positively correlated with chondrogenesis [25]. Meanwhile, non-hypertrophic articular and hypertrophic MSC-derived chondrocytes showed differential expression of miR-181a-5p, suggesting that its expression is altered during successive differentiation stages [27]. Moreover, miR-181a-5p is predicted to be a target of hSBP2 by

TargetScanHuman7.1, and it may inhibit the expression of the important ECM protein aggrecan (ACAN) in chondrocytes, simultaneously acquiring a negative feedback function for cartilage homeostasis [28]. However, further investigation is required to understand the oxidation resistance-associated roles of miR-181a-5p in OA.

In the present study, the glutathione peroxidase-encoding genes GPX1 and GPX4 and the selenoprotein S-encoding gene SELS were examined due to their regulation by SBP2. Hence, we investigated the detailed regulatory relationships among pro-inflammatory factors, miRNA, SBP2 and selenoproteins in the context of oxidation resistance in cartilage. Overall, this study provides the first comprehensive evidence for changes in pro-inflammatory factors in the cartilage antioxidant network during OA and describes the discovery of novel mediators of cartilage oxidative stress and OA pathophysiology. Therefore, our data suggest that miR-181a-5p may be useful for the development of novel early-stage diagnostic and therapeutic strategies for OA.

Methods
Cell culture
The human chondrosarcoma chondrocyte SW1353 cell line was obtained from the Chinese Academy of Sciences (Shanghai, China) and cultured in RPMI-1640 medium (HyClone, USA) with 10% foetal bovine serum (ExCell, China). The murine chondroblast ATDC5 cell line was obtained from the European Collection of Cell Cultures (ECACC) and maintained in Dulbecco's Modified Eagle's medium/Ham's F12 medium (DMEM/F12, HyClone, USA) supplemented with 5% FBS (Gibco, USA). Both cell lines were maintained in a humidified incubator with 5% CO_2 at 37 °C, cultured in monolayers and grown to confluence. The medium contained 1% penicillin/streptomycin (Sigma, USA). The cells were seeded in 12-multiwell plates at 7×10^4 cells/well.

For the cartilage matrix degradation model, SW1353 cells were placed in FBS-free medium for more than 10 h, and then the cells were incubated with 0 (as control), 1, 5, 10 and 20 ng/ml IL-1β (Sino Biological Inc., China) for 12 h, or 10 ng/ml IL-1β for 0 (as control), 6, 12, 24 and 48 h. For the chondrocyte differentiation model, ATDC5 cells were induced with 1× ITS supplement (1 mg/ml insulin, 0.55 mg/ml transferrin and 0.5 μg/ml selenium) added to the medium. The chondrogenic culture medium was changed every day.

Transient transfection of hsa-miR-181a-5p mimics or inhibitor sequences
SW1353 cells were seeded for 24 h, and 50 nM hsa-miR-181a-5p mimics (mimic-181a-5p) or negative control (mimic-NC) (Genepharma, China) and 200 nM hsa-miR-181a-5p inhibitor (inhibitor-181a-5p) or negative control (inhibitor-NC) (Genepharma, China) were transiently

transfected into SW1353 cells by 1.5 μl/well Lipofecta-mine™ 2000 (Invitrogen, USA) according to the manufacturer's instructions. Information about *miR-181a-5p* is provided in Tables 1 and 2.

Transient transfection of siRNAs and plasmids

The full-length human *SBP2* CDS was cloned from SW1353 chondrocyte cDNA and inserted into a *pEFGP-N1* vector (Invitrogen, USA). The primer sequences for the *hSBP2-CDS* clone are listed in Table 3. SW1353 cells were seeded for 24 h, and 1, 1.5, 2 and 4 μg of the *pEFGP-mSBP2-N1* vector or empty vector were transiently transfected into cells by 1.5 μl/well Lipofectamine™ 2000 (Invitrogen, USA). The expression of exogenous and endogenous SBP2 was determined by western blotting with an anti-SBP2 antibody after transfection for 24 h.

Additionally, *hSBP2* siRNA (*si-SBP2*) and control siRNA (*si-NC*) sequences were purchased from Genepharma Biotechnology Inc. (Genepharma, China). Cell transfection was performed according to the manufacturer's instructions. For gene knockdown, SW1353 cells were seeded for 24 h, and 50 nM *si-SBP2* (5′-GAGC CACACUACAUUGAAATT-3′) or *si-NC* was transiently transfected into the cells by 1.5 μl/well Lipofectamine™ 2000 (Invitrogen, USA) according to the manufacturer's instructions. Knockdown efficiency was determined by western blotting after transfection for 48 h.

Patients and articular cartilage collection

OA patients were diagnosed according to the modified Outerbridge classification by The Second Affiliated Hospital, Xi'an Jiaotong University Health Science Center. Articular cartilage samples were obtained at the time of total knee replacement (TKR) from 10 human patients with knee OA (6 women and 4 men; mean ± SEM age: 60 ± 8.3 y) from Shaanxi province, China. All patients were diagnosed with Kellgren and Lawrence grade IV OA. After washing with sterile phosphate buffered saline (PBS), portions of cartilage with a damaged articular surface and portions with a smooth articular surface were used for RNA extraction and immunohistochemistry. Smooth cartilage samples were carefully assessed for any gross signs of degeneration or injury, and only normal-appearing smooth cartilage was used as an internal control (a self control). All cartilage samples were collected without fibrillation. Peripheral blood samples were obtained from 20 OA patients (14 women and 6 men; mean ± SD age:

66.6 ± 5.7 y) and 20 normal control patients (14 women and 6 men; mean ± SD age: 65.9 ± 3.1 y).

Total RNA extraction and quantitative PCR analysis

For RNA extraction, cartilage tissues were harvested from smooth articular surfaces and damaged articular surfaces of the same patient and chopped into pieces that were smaller than 2×2 mm. Then, the pieces were immediately frozen in liquid nitrogen. Total RNA was isolated from cells, tissue pieces or plasma samples using TRIzol® (Invitrogen, USA). cDNA was synthesized from 2 μg of total RNA according to the manufacturer's instructions (RevertAid™; Fermentas, Canada) in a final volume of 20 ml and stored at -20 °C until use. Furthermore, miRNA-cDNA was obtained using the One Step PrimeScript® miRNA cDNA Synthesis Kit (Takara, Japan).

Both mRNA and miRNA expression was tested by 10 μl real-time quantitative PCR (RT-qPCR), which was performed on an iQ5 real-time PCR detection system (Bio-Rad, Hercules, CA, USA) with SYBR® Premix Ex Taq™ II (TaKaRa, Japan). Relative gene expression was normalized against *GAPDH* expression in SW1353 cells or *β-Actin* expression in ATDC5 cells. Additionally, let-7a was used as the internal reference for *miR-181a-5p*. The procedure for miRNA-cDNA qPCR consisted of two-step amplification: pre-denaturation at 95 °C for 10 s, followed by PCR amplification with 40 cycles of 95 °C for 5 s and 60 °C for 20 s. Information about the primers and PCR amplification is provided in Tables 4, 5 and 6.

Protein sample preparation and western blotting

Total protein samples from SW1353 cells or ATDC5 cells (10–20 μg) were separated by 10% SDS-PAGE and transferred to PVDF membranes (EMD Millipore, Darmstadt,

Table 2 Information of Stem-loop *hsa-miR-181a*

ID	Accession	Location	Stem-loop sequence (5'-3')
hsa-mir-181a-1 (*hsa-mir-213*)	MI0000289	1q32.1	UGAGUUUUGAGGUUGCUUC AGUGAACAUUCAACGCUG UCGGUGAGUUUGGAAUUA AAAUCAAAACCAUCGACCGU UGAUUGUACCCUAUGGCUAA CCAUCAUCUACUCCA
hsa-mir-181a-2	MI0000269	9q33.3	AGAAGGGCUAUCAGGCCAG CCUUCAGAGGACUCC AAGGAACAUUCAACGCUG UCGGUGAGUUUGGGAUUUGAAA AAACCACUGACCGUUGACUGU ACCUUGGGGUCCUUA

Table 1 Information of Mature *miR-181a-5p*

ID	Accession	Mature sequence (5'-3')
hsa-miR-181a-5p	MIMAT0000256	AACAUUCAACGCUGUCGGUGAGU
mmu-miR-181a-5p	MIMAT0000210	

Table 3 Information of human primers for *hSBP2-CDS*

Gene	Sequence (5'-3')
hSBP2-CDS-Forward	CAGGTCGGATCCAGA**CCCGGG**gccaccATGGCGTCG GAGGGG
hSBP2-CDS-Reverse	TCTGTAGAATTCGGT**CCCGGG**TAAATTCAAATTCATCAT

Table 4 Information of miRNA-181a-5p for Real-time PCR

MicroRNAs	Accession NO.	Forward primer (5'-3')
hsa-miRNA-181a-5p	MIMAT0000858	CGCAACATTCAACGCTGTC
hsa-let-7a	MIMAT0000774	CGCTGAGGTAGTAGGTTGT
Reverse primer: GTGCAGGGTCCGAGGT		

Germany). After blocking with 3% non-fat milk in TBST buffer, the membranes were incubated with primary antibodies followed by secondary antibodies conjugated to horseradish peroxidase (HRP) and visualized using an ECL detection system (EMD Millipore, Darmstadt, Germany) on a chemiluminescence imaging system. The primary antibodies included anti-SBP2 (1:500, CA, USA), anti-GPX1 (1:2000, CA, USA), anti-MMP13 (1:1000, Abcam, USA) and anti-β-ACTIN (1:2000, Proteintech, China). The following secondary antibodies were purchased from Beyotime Biotech (Jiangsu, China): horseradish peroxidase-coupled anti-rabbit (1:5000) and anti-mouse (1:5000).

Immunohistochemistry staining

After measuring intrinsic peroxidase activity, articular cartilage sections were blocked with 3% hydrogen peroxide (H_2O_2) and then incubated with 1.5% BSA for 1 h. The sections were covered with anti-SBP2 antibodies (1:250, CA, USA) and incubated at 4 °C in a wet box. After 14 h, all sections were rinsed with PBS and then sequentially incubated with biotinylated secondary antibody for 1 h and DAB reagent (Boster, Wuhan, China) for 5 min at room temperature. Chromogenic reactions were terminated once claybank regions were observed under a microscope. Rabbit IgG was used as a negative control.

Statistical analysis

Data are presented as the mean ± SEM. The statistical significance of pathological data was calculated by using the Mann-Whitney U test. Means of two groups were compared using Student's t test, and statistical significance was achieved at $P < 0.05$ in all tests (*: $P < 0.05$, **: $P < 0.01$ and ***: $P < 0.001$). All analyses were performed

Table 5 Information of mouse primers for Real-time PCR

Gene	Sequence (5'-3')	Product size (bp)	Annealing temperature (°X)
Sbp2	Forward:CTGCTCCAAAGGCC AAAG	195	60
	Reverse:GTGATTGCCCTCTG TGTCTTC		
β-Actin	Forward:AACAGTCCGCCTAG AAGCAC	281	60
	Reverse:CGTTGACATCCGTA AAGACC		

Table 6 Information of human primers for Real-time PCR

Gene	Sequence (5'-3')	Product size (bp)	Annealing temperature (°C)
SBP2	Forward: CCGCAGATTCAGGGATTACT	92	60
	Reverse: CTTGGAAACGGACCAGTTCT		
ACAN	Forward: GGCATTTCAGCGGTTCCTTCTC	135	60
	Reverse: AGCAGTTGTCTCCTCTTCTACGG		
MMP13	Forward: AATATCTGAACTGGGTCTTCCAAAA	102	60
	Reverse: CAGACCTGGTTTCCTGAGAACAG		
COL2A1	Forward: TGGACGATCAGGCGAAACC	244	62
	Reverse: GCTGCGGATGCTCTCAATCT		
GPx1	Forward: AAGCTCATCACCTGGTCTCC	124	60
	Reverse: CGATGTCAATGGTCTGGAAG		
GPx4	Forward: GCTGTGGAAGTGGATGAAGA	105	60
	Reverse: TGAGGAACTGTGGAGAGACG		
SELS	Forward: CACCTATGGCTGGTACATCG	130	60
	Reverse: AACATCAGGTTCCACAGCAG		
GAPDH	Forward: CACCCACTCCTCCACCTTTG	110	64
	Reverse: CCACCACCCTGTTGCTGTAG		

using GraphPad Prism 6.0 (GraphPad Software, San Diego, CA, USA).

Results

Both hsa-miR-181a-5p and SBP2 are regulated by IL-1β in chondrocytes

IL-1β was selected to stimulate SW1353 cells, and *hsa-miR-181a-5p* expression levels were determined by stem loop RT-qPCR. The expression of *hsa-miR-181a-5p* and *MMP13* continuously and robustly increased after treatment with 10 ng/ml IL-1β for 0 (as a control), 6, 12, 24 and 48 h in SW1353 cells, while *SBP2* and *GPX1* expression was continuously and sharply reduced at the mRNA level (Fig. 1a). Meanwhile, SBP2, GPX1 and MMP13 expression at the protein level showed the same patterns observed at the mRNA level (Fig. 1b). The expression of *hsa-miR-181a-5p* increased, and the expression of *SBP2* at the mRNA level reduced over time after treatment

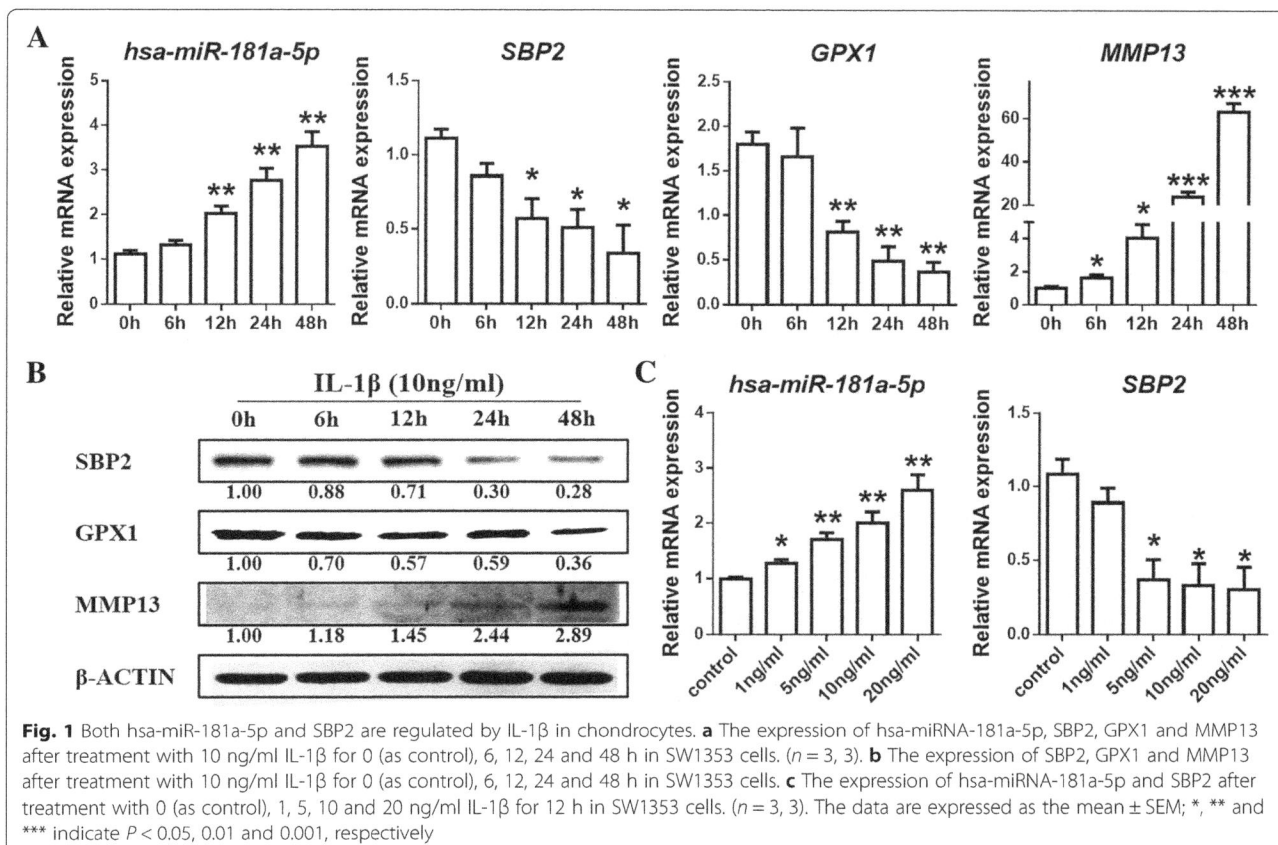

Fig. 1 Both hsa-miR-181a-5p and SBP2 are regulated by IL-1β in chondrocytes. **a** The expression of hsa-miRNA-181a-5p, SBP2, GPX1 and MMP13 after treatment with 10 ng/ml IL-1β for 0 (as control), 6, 12, 24 and 48 h in SW1353 cells. (n = 3, 3). **b** The expression of SBP2, GPX1 and MMP13 after treatment with 10 ng/ml IL-1β for 0 (as control), 6, 12, 24 and 48 h in SW1353 cells. **c** The expression of hsa-miRNA-181a-5p and SBP2 after treatment with 0 (as control), 1, 5, 10 and 20 ng/ml IL-1β for 12 h in SW1353 cells. (n = 3, 3). The data are expressed as the mean ± SEM; *, ** and *** indicate P < 0.05, 0.01 and 0.001, respectively

with 0 (as a control), 1, 5, 10 and 20 ng/ml IL-1β for 12 h (Fig. 1c).

SBP2 regulated the biosynthesis of three selenoproteins and oxidation resistance in chondrocytes

To assess the role of SBP2 in chondrocytes, we constructed recombinant *hSBP2-CDS* clones and *si-SBP2* (Fig. 2a) and transfected these constructs into SW1353 cells. Exogenous *SBP2* (122 kDa, Fig. 2b) showed remarkable concentration-dependent up-regulation with *pEGFP-N1-mSBP2*. Overall, taking into consideration both endogenous *SBP2* (95 kDa, Fig. 2b) and exogenous *SBP2*, 2 μg of *pEGFP-N1-mSBP2* was the most suitable treatment to achieve *SBP2* over-expression. *SBP2* over-expression (P = 0.0003) in SW1353 cells elevated both *GPX1* (P = 0.0064) and *GPX4* (P = 0.0215) mRNA levels, whereas *SELS* (P = 0.4532) induced no evident changes (Fig. 2c). On the other hand, when *SBP2* levels were specifically reduced by *si-SBP2* (P = 0.0087), both *GPX1* (P = 0.0097) and *GPX4* (P = 0.0431) mRNA levels, but not *SELS* levels (P = 0.2093), were also down-regulated significantly (Fig. 2d). Meanwhile, total GPXs activity was increased (P = 0.0097) by *SBP2* over-expression, and total GPXs activity was reduced (P = 0.0023) under *SBP2* knockdown conditions (Fig. 2e).

Transfection of miR-181a-5p affects chondrocyte phenotype and oxidation resistance through SBP2

To confirm the roles of *miR-181a-5p* in chondrocytes, a *miR-181a-5p* mimic (P = 0.0022) or a *miR-181a-5p* inhibitor (P = 0.0108) was applied to alter *miR-181a-5p* levels (Additional file 1: Figure S1). The expression of cartilage-specific genes such as *COL2A1*, *ACAN* and *MMP13* and total GPXs activity were detected in SW1353 cells after transfection for 24 h. First, *mimic-miR-181a-5p* down-regulated *ACAN* (P = 0.0052) and up-regulated *MMP13* (P = 0.0095) (Fig. 3a), while *inhibitor-miR-181a-5p* also significantly up-regulated *MMP13* (P = 0.0319) (Fig. 3b). Furthermore, both *SBP2* (P = 0.0209) and SBP2 were significantly down-regulated in SW1353 cells when *miR-181a-5p* was up-regulated by *mimic-181a-5p* (Fig. 3c and d). In contrast, neither *SBP2* nor SBP2 expression changed when *miR-181a-5p* was down-regulated by *inhibitor-181a-5p* (Fig. 3c and d). Meanwhile, total GPXs activity was reduced (P = 0.0145) by *miR-181a-5p* over-expression, and total GPXs activity was increased (P = 0.0143) under *miR-181a-5p* knockdown conditions (Fig. 3e). In addition, ITS treatment was applied to cultured cells for 14 days as described previously to induce ATDC5 cells to differentiate in vitro [29], and then the expression of *mmu-miR-181a-5p*, *Sbp2* and

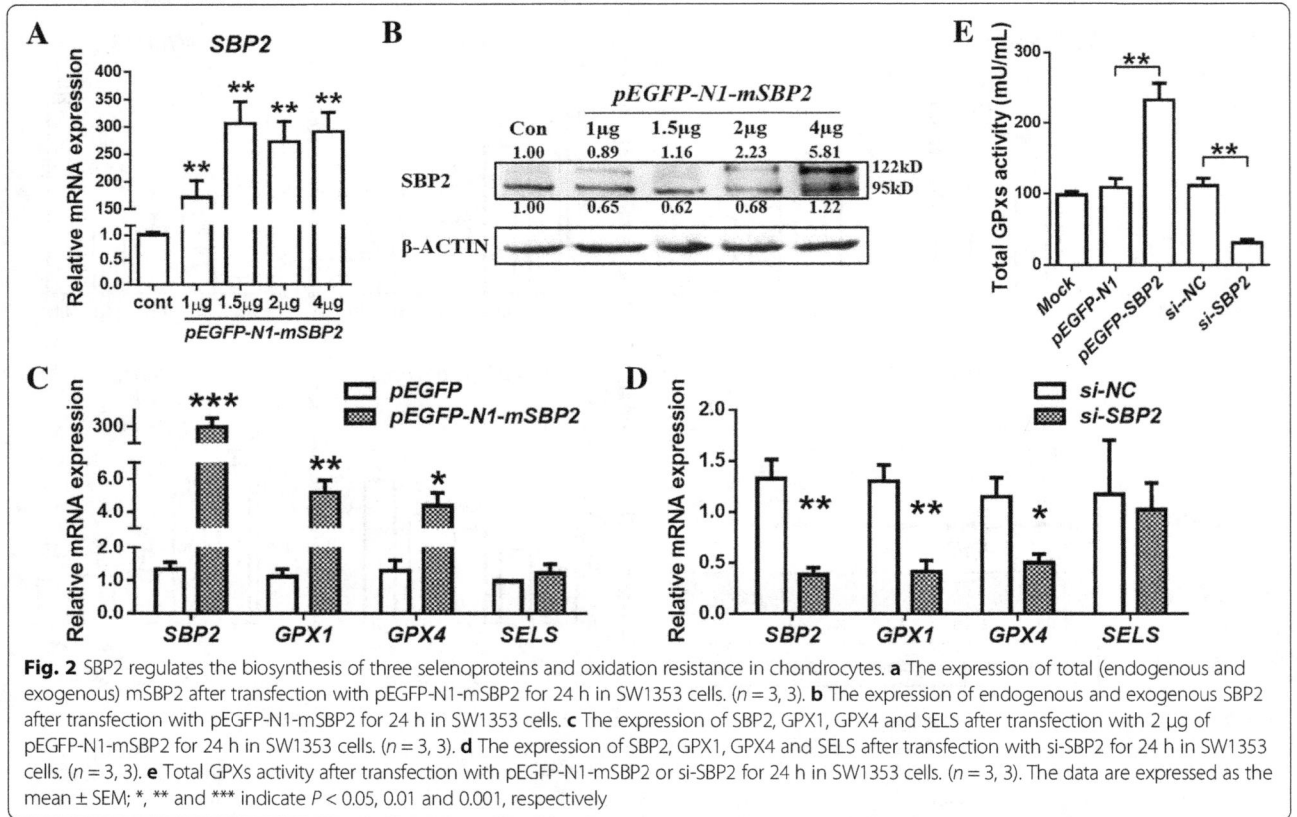

Fig. 2 SBP2 regulates the biosynthesis of three selenoproteins and oxidation resistance in chondrocytes. **a** The expression of total (endogenous and exogenous) mSBP2 after transfection with pEGFP-N1-mSBP2 for 24 h in SW1353 cells. ($n = 3$, 3). **b** The expression of endogenous and exogenous SBP2 after transfection with pEGFP-N1-mSBP2 for 24 h in SW1353 cells. **c** The expression of SBP2, GPX1, GPX4 and SELS after transfection with 2 μg of pEGFP-N1-mSBP2 for 24 h in SW1353 cells. ($n = 3$, 3). **d** The expression of SBP2, GPX1, GPX4 and SELS after transfection with si-SBP2 for 24 h in SW1353 cells. ($n = 3$, 3). **e** Total GPxs activity after transfection with pEGFP-N1-mSBP2 or si-SBP2 for 24 h in SW1353 cells. ($n = 3$, 3). The data are expressed as the mean ± SEM; *, ** and *** indicate $P < 0.05$, 0.01 and 0.001, respectively

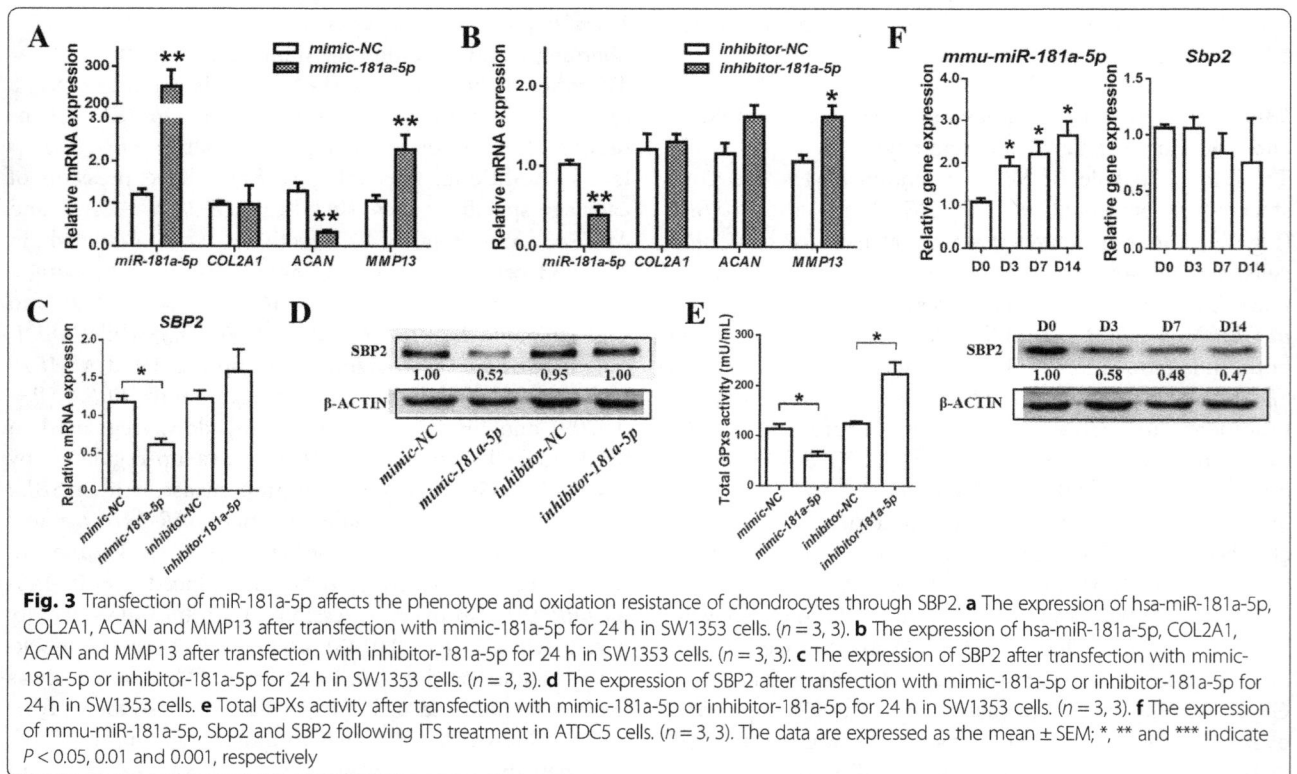

Fig. 3 Transfection of miR-181a-5p affects the phenotype and oxidation resistance of chondrocytes through SBP2. **a** The expression of hsa-miR-181a-5p, COL2A1, ACAN and MMP13 after transfection with mimic-181a-5p for 24 h in SW1353 cells. ($n = 3$, 3). **b** The expression of hsa-miR-181a-5p, COL2A1, ACAN and MMP13 after transfection with inhibitor-181a-5p for 24 h in SW1353 cells. ($n = 3$, 3). **c** The expression of SBP2 after transfection with mimic-181a-5p or inhibitor-181a-5p for 24 h in SW1353 cells. ($n = 3$, 3). **d** The expression of SBP2 after transfection with mimic-181a-5p or inhibitor-181a-5p for 24 h in SW1353 cells. **e** Total GPxs activity after transfection with mimic-181a-5p or inhibitor-181a-5p for 24 h in SW1353 cells. ($n = 3$, 3). **f** The expression of mmu-miR-181a-5p, Sbp2 and SBP2 following ITS treatment in ATDC5 cells. ($n = 3$, 3). The data are expressed as the mean ± SEM; *, ** and *** indicate $P < 0.05$, 0.01 and 0.001, respectively

SBP2 was detected. With chondrocyte differentiation, the expression of *mmu-miR-181a-5p* showed remarkable up-regulation at D3 ($P = 0.0258$), D7 ($P = 0.0178$) and D14 ($P = 0.0103$), while SBP2 protein expression was significantly reduced, although the expression of *Sbp2* was almost constant (Fig. 3f).

The expression of hsa-miRNA-181a-5p, SBP2 and selenoproteins in OA cartilage

Cartilage tissues were obtained from 8 OA patients to detect the expression of *miRNA-181a-5p*, SBP2 and three pivotal selenoproteins. OA smooth cartilage and damaged cartilage from the same patients undergoing TKR were separated (Fig. 4a). Total RNA was extracted, and RT-qPCR was performed. According to a paired Student's t test, *miRNA-181a-5p* expression levels were significantly higher ($P = 0.0114$) in damaged cartilage than in smooth cartilage of OA patients (Fig. 4b). Meanwhile, although *SBP2* mRNA expression was unattenuated in damaged cartilage (Fig. 4c), SBP2 protein expression was reduced in damaged cartilage (Fig. 4d). Furthermore, *GPX1* ($P = 0.0183$) and *GPX4* ($P = 0.0149$) were down-regulated in damaged OA cartilage (Fig. 4e), while *SELS* showed no significant changes (Fig. 4e).

The expression of hsa-miRNA-181a-5p, SBP2 and selenoproteins in peripheral blood

Peripheral blood was collected from 20 healthy controls and 20 OA patients. To detect the expression of *miR-NA-181a-5p*, *SBP2*, *GPX1*, *GPX4* and *SELS*, total RNA from peripheral blood was extracted, and RT-qPCR was performed. The expression of *hsa-miRNA-181a-5p* ($P = 0.0329$) in OA peripheral blood was significantly higher than that in normal controls (Fig. 5a), while *SBP2* ($P = 0.0061$) and *GPX1* ($P = 0.0111$) were both lower in OA peripheral blood than in normal controls (Fig. 5b and c). In addition, *SELS* ($P = 0.8160$) showed no statistically significant differences (Fig. 5d), and *GPX4* was not detected (data not shown). These results suggested that *hsa-miR-NA-181a-5p* is a potential diagnostic biomarker for OA.

Discussion

To explore whether *miR-181a-5p* and *SBP2* are involved in OA pathogenesis, we established an IL-1β model

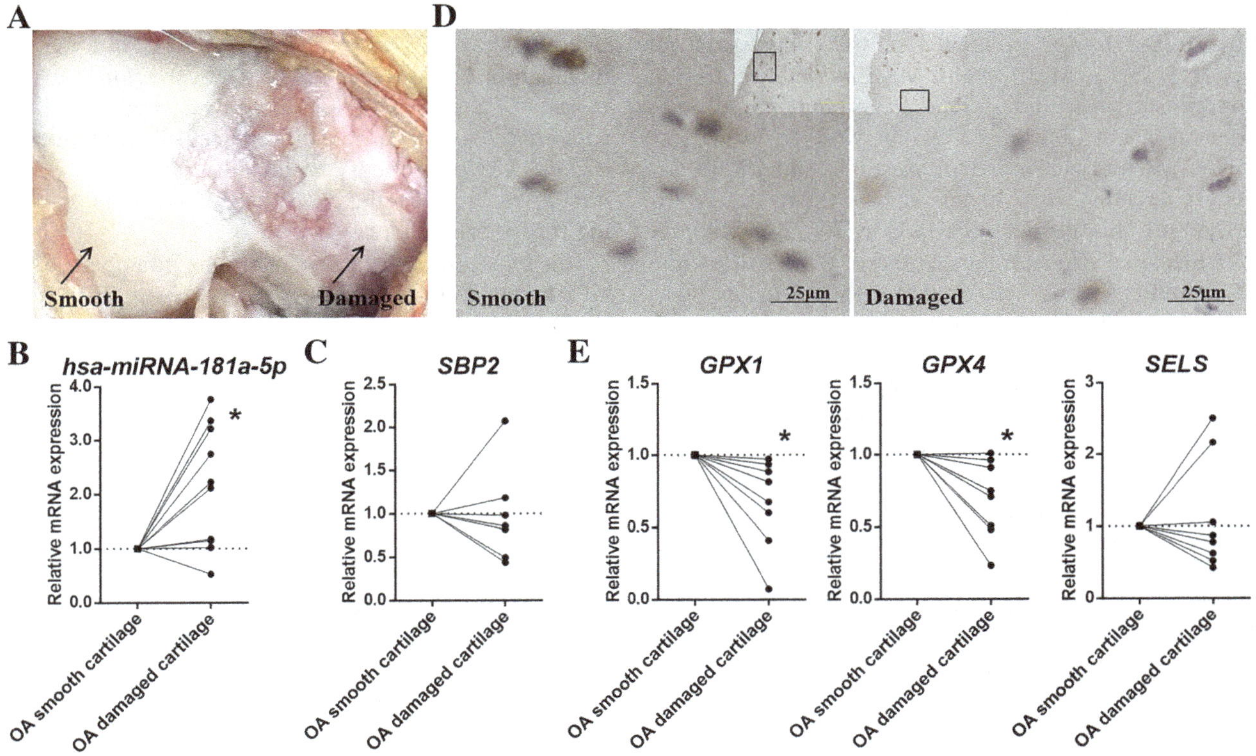

Fig. 4 The expression of hsa-miRNA-181a-5p, SBP2 and selenoproteins in OA cartilage. **a** OA smooth cartilage and damaged cartilage from the same patients undergoing total knee replacement. **b** The expression of *hsa-miRNA-181a-5p* in smooth cartilage and damaged cartilage from the same OA cartilage sample. ($n = 10$). **c** The expression of *SBP2* in smooth cartilage and damaged cartilage from the same OA cartilage sample. ($n = 7$). **d** The expression of SBP2 in smooth cartilage and damaged cartilage from the same OA cartilage sample. **e** The expression of *GPX1*, *GPX4* and *SELS* in smooth cartilage and damaged cartilage from the same OA cartilage sample. ($n = 8$). The data were expressed as the mean ± SEM; *, ** and *** indicate $P < 0.05$, 0.01 and 0.001, respectively

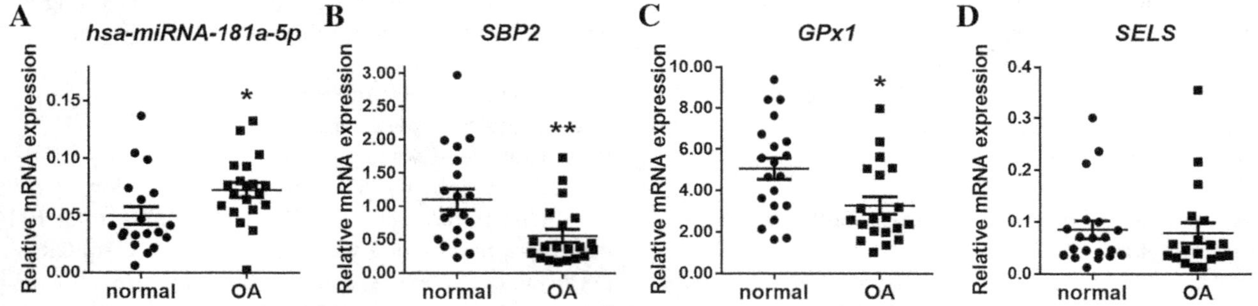

Fig. 5 The expression of hsa-miRNA-181a-5p, SBP2 and selenoproteins in peripheral blood. **a** The expression of hsa-miRNA-181a-5p in the peripheral blood of healthy controls and OA patients. (n = 19, 20). **b** The expression of SBP2 in the peripheral blood of healthy controls and OA patients. (n = 20, 20). **c** The expression of GPX1 in the peripheral blood of healthy controls and OA patients. (n = 20, 20). **d** The expression of SELS in the peripheral blood of healthy controls and OA patients. (n = 20, 19). The data are expressed as the mean ± SEM; *, ** and *** indicate P < 0.05, 0.01 and 0.001, respectively

using the chondrocyte SW1353 cell line. The results showed that IL-1β increased *hsa-miR-181a-5p* and decreased *SBP2* in a time- and dose-dependent manner, while both *hsa-miR-181a-5p* and *SBP2* seemed to participate in the catabolism pathway and oxidative stress in chondrocytes induced by IL-1β. This finding is in line with our expectation that pro-inflammatory cytokines induce *miR-181a-5p* up-regulation in chondrocytes along with SBP2 down-regulation. Coincidentally, *miR-181a-5p* up-regulates the expression of caspase-3, PARP, MMP-2, and MMP-9 while repressing chondrocyte proliferation and promoting chondrocyte apoptosis in OA [22, 30].

Next, we used recombinant plasmids and siRNA sequences targeting *SBP2* to up- or down-regulate the expression of this gene in SW1353 cells. To investigate SBP2-mediated selenoprotein synthesis, *GPX1*, *GPX4* and *SELS* were selected as representative selenoproteins expressed by chondrocytes in this study not only because these proteins exhibit differential cellular localization and fulfil different functions in physiological and pathological processes in various cells but also because the affinity of their SECIS binding with 'UGA' recoding has been categorized as strong, moderate and weak, respectively [31, 32]

As crucial antioxidant enzymes, *GPX1* and *GPX4* were regulated by *SBP2* up- or down-regulation, while *SELS* expression levels were always stabilized; these expression patterns are attributable to the differential SECIS affinities and SBP2 binding efficiencies of these proteins. Our findings suggest that *SBP2* expression did not align with selenoprotein expression regulation, which affected total GPXs activity and oxidation resistance in chondrocytes. Oxidative damage due to the concomitant overproduction of ROS is present in ageing and OA cartilage [33]. Predictably, oxidative stress destroys normal physiological signalling and contributes to OA [13]. The synergy between blocked selenoprotein expression and disordered metabolism of the articular cartilage ECM

induces chondrocyte apoptosis and contributes to cartilage destruction [9, 34] In summary, selenoprotein biosynthesis leads to decreased antioxidant stress.

Additionally, we modulated *miR-181a-5p* expression by using mimic and inhibitor sequences in SW1353 cells. The expression of *miR-181a-5p* showed remarkable up-regulation, while SBP2 protein expression was significantly reduced. Unexpectedly, SBP2 expression did not change after *miR-181a-5p* knockdown, which implies that a very complex regulatory network and multiple modulators are involved in SBP2 expression. Furthermore, *SBP2* showed a significant negative correlation with *miR-181a-5p* during the induced differentiation of ATDC5 cells. These results suggest that *hsa-miR-181a-5p* affects the chondrocyte phenotype by altering oxidation resistance.

The most effective antioxidants are members of the GPx family, but the mechanisms underlying their effects on OA chondrocytes under oxidative stress are not yet fully understood [9]. Our results established that *miR-181a-5p* regulated total GPXs activity by decreasing the expression of *SBP2* in cartilage, leading to chondrocyte apoptosis and cellular damage induced by ROS. SBP2 is required for protection against ROS-induced cellular damage and increased cell survival [35]. For instance, gene mutations in *SBP2* decreased the expression of several selenoproteins, resulting in a complex multisystem selenoprotein deficiency disorder in humans [36], and lipid peroxidation products mediated by free radicals increased in the blood [37]. Further, miR-34a, miR-146a, SOD2, CAT, GPXs and NRF2 are subjected to H_2O_2 stimulus in OA chondrocytes [24]. Meanwhile, miR-9 is a OA-related effects of oxidative stress in chondrocytes through targets SIRT1 [23].

Finally, we discovered that *miRNA-181a-5p* expression was increased, and SBP2 protein and *GPX1* and *GPX4* mRNA expression were reduced in damaged cartilage. These results suggest that *hsa-miRNA-181a-5p*, *GPX1*,

GPX4 and SBP2 all participate in the OA cartilage damage process to a certain extent. Despite the inadequate number of samples, our peripheral blood data partly support the hypothesis that *miR-181a-5p* is released in plasma and may facilitate early-stage diagnosis of OA because it induces ROS to damage cartilage proteins. Currently, few blood-based tests are used for the detection of early-stage OA.

Conclusions

We have reported a novel pathway in cartilage. Pro-inflammatory factors mediate *miR-181a-5p* expression, and then *miR-181a-5p* regulates the pivotal selenoproteins GPX1 and GPX4 through its target SBP2, resulting in alterations to the overall activity of GPXs, which are the most important oxidation resistance proteins in cartilage. Oxidation resistance involves a series of antioxidants that overcome ROS-related stress to maintain ECM metabolism balance and protect the essential physiological functions of cartilage.

Abbreviations
ACAN: Aggrecan; COL2: type-II collagen; ECM metabolic: Extracellular matrix; HRP: Horseradish peroxidase; IL-1β: Including interleukin-1; IL-6: Interleukin-6; inhibitor-181a-5p: miR-181a-5p inhibitor; mimic-181a-5p: miR-181a-5p mimics; OA: Osteoarthritis; PBS: Phosphate buffered saline; ROS: Reactive oxygen species; Se: Selenium; Sec: Selenocysteine; SECIS: Sec insertion sequence; SECISBP2 or SBP2: Sec insertion sequence binding protein 2; Sel: Selenoprotein; TKR: Total knee replacement; TNF-α: Tumour necrosis factor-α

Funding
This work was supported by grants from the National Natural Science Foundation of China (Project No. 81371986, 81772410), the Shaanxi province science and technology project (2016SF-187).

Authors' contributions
All authors have made substantial contributions to: (1) the conception and design of the study, or acquisition of data, or analysis and interpretation of data, (2) drafting the article or revising it critically for important intellectual content, (3) final approval of the version to be submitted. JX finished the most of experiments, analysis and interpretation of the data and wrote the original manuscript. ZM was involved in conception and design of the study, analysis and interpretation of the data, drafting of the article, critical revision of the article for important intellectual content, and final approval of the article. ZX was involved in the acquisition, analysis (the miRNA expression) and interpretation of the data, assembly of the data, critical revision of the article for important intellectual content, and final approval of the article. BC was involved in the analysis and interpretation of the data, collection and assembly of the data, critical revision of the article for important intellectual content, and final approval of the article. BL was involved in the collection the samples and interpretation of the data, collection and assembly of the data, critical revision of the article for important intellectual content, and final approval of the article. FZ was involved in the analysis (histological examination by staining with IHC) and interpretation of the data, assembly of the data, critical revision of the article for important intellectual content, and final approval of the article. YH was involved in the analysis (cell culture) and interpretation of the data, assembly of the data, logistical support, critical revision of the article for important intellectual content, and final approval of the article. KW critically revised the article for important intellectual content, take responsibility for the integrity of the work as a whole. JS was involved in conception and design of the study, got the funds, analysis and interpretation of the data, critical revision of the article for important intellectual content, and final approval of the article.

Authors' information
Kunzheng Wang, the corresponding author, is the Chairman of Chinese Orthopedic Association.

Competing interests
The authors declare that they have no competing interests.

Author details
Department of Orthopaedics, The Second Affiliated Hospital, Xi'an Jiaotong University Health Science Center, 157 West 5th Road, Xi'an, Shaanxi 710004, People's Republic of China. ²Department of Biochemistry and Molecular Biology, School of Basic Medical Sciences, Xi'an Jiaotong University Health Science Center, Xi'an, Shaanxi 710061, People's Republic of China. ³Beaurau of healthcare, Shaanxi Health and Family Planning Commission, Xi'an, Shaanxi 710000, People's Republic of China.

References
1. Loeser RF, Collins JA, Diekman BO. Ageing and the pathogenesis of osteoarthritis. Nat Rev Rheumatol. 2016;12(7):412–20.
2. Mobasheri A, Rayman MP, Gualillo O, Sellam J, van der Kraan P, Fearon U. The role of metabolism in the pathogenesis of osteoarthritis. Nat Rev Rheumatol. 2017;13(5):302–11.
3. Kapoor M, Martel-Pelletier J, Lajeunesse D, Pelletier JP, Fahmi H. Role of proinflammatory cytokines in the pathophysiology of osteoarthritis. Nat Rev Rheumatol. 2011;7(1):33–42.
4. Mitchell PG, Magna HA, Reeves LM, Lopresti-Morrow LL, Yocum SA, Rosner PJ, Geoghegan KF, Hambor JE. Cloning, expression, and type II collagenolytic activity of matrix metalloproteinase-13 from human osteoarthritic cartilage. J Clin Invest. 1996;97(3):761–8.
5. Wang M, Sampson ER, Jin H, Li J, Ke QH, Im HJ, Chen D. MMP13 is a critical target gene during the progression of osteoarthritis. Arthritis Res Ther. 2013; 15(1):R5.
6. Kim JH, Jeon J, Shin M, Won Y, Lee M, Kwak JS, Lee G, Rhee J, Ryu JH, Chun CH, et al. Regulation of the catabolic cascade in osteoarthritis by the zinc-ZIP8-MTF1 axis. Cell. 2014;156(4):730–43.
7. Corciulo C, Lendhey M, Wilder T, Schoen H, Cornelissen AS, Chang G, Kennedy OD, Cronstein BN. Endogenous adenosine maintains cartilage homeostasis and exogenous adenosine inhibits osteoarthritis progression. Nat Commun. 2017;8:15019.
8. Jeon OH, Kim C, Laberge RM, Demaria M, Rathod S, Vasserot AP, Chung JW, Kim DH, Poon Y, David N, et al. Local clearance of senescent cells attenuates the development of post-traumatic osteoarthritis and creates a pro-regenerative environment. Nat Med. 2017;23(6):775–81.
9. Labunskyy VM, Hatfield DL, Gladyshev VN. Selenoproteins: molecular pathways and physiological roles. Physiol Rev. 2014;94(3):739–77.
10. Kryukov GV, Castellano S, Novoselov SV, Lobanov AV, Zehtab O, Guigo R, Gladyshev VN. Characterization of mammalian selenoproteomes. Science. 2003;300(5624):1439–43.
11. Lu J, Holmgren A. Selenoproteins. J Biol Chem. 2009;284(2):723–7.
12. Issa R, Boeving M, Kinter M, Griffin TM. Effect of biomechanical stress on endogenous antioxidant networks in bovine articular cartilage. J Orthop Res. 2018;36(2):760–9.
13. Collins JA, Wood ST, Nelson KJ, Rowe MA, Carlson CS, Chubinskaya S, Poole LB, Furdui CM, Loeser RF. Oxidative stress promotes Peroxiredoxin Hyperoxidation and attenuates pro-survival signaling in aging chondrocytes. J Biol Chem. 2016;291(13):6641–54.
14. Driscoll DM, Copeland PR. Mechanism and regulation of selenoprotein synthesis. Annu Rev Nutr. 2003;23:17–40.
15. Takeuchi A, Schmitt D, Chapple C, Babaylova E, Karpova G, Guigo R, Krol A, Allmang C. A short motif in Drosophila SECIS binding protein 2 provides differential binding affinity to SECIS RNA hairpins. Nucleic Acids Res. 2009; 37(7):2126–41.
16. Donovan J, Caban K, Ranaweera R, Gonzalez-Flores JN, Copeland PR. A novel protein domain induces high affinity selenocysteine insertion sequence binding and elongation factor recruitment. J Biol Chem. 2008; 283(50):35129–39.
17. Downey CM, Horton CR, Carlson BA, Parsons TE, Hatfield DL, Hallgrimsson B, Jirik FR. Osteo-chondroprogenitor-specific deletion of the selenocysteine

tRNA gene, Trsp, leads to chondronecrosis and abnormal skeletal development: a putative model for Kashin-Beck disease. PLoS Genet. 2009; 5(8):e1000616.

18. Papp LV, Wang J, Kennedy D, Boucher D, Zhang Y, Gladyshev VN, Singh RN, Khanna KK. Functional characterization of alternatively spliced human SECISBP2 transcript variants. Nucleic Acids Res. 2008;36(22):7192–206.

19. Anestal K, Arner ES. Rapid induction of cell death by selenium-compromised thioredoxin reductase 1 but not by the fully active enzyme containing selenocysteine. J Biol Chem. 2003;278(18):15966–72.

20. Vicente R, Noel D, Pers YM, Apparailly F, Jorgensen C. Deregulation and therapeutic potential of microRNAs in arthritic diseases. Nat Rev Rheumatol. 2015.

21. Nugent M. MicroRNAs: exploring new horizons in osteoarthritis: Osteoarthritis and cartilage / OARS, Osteoarthritis Research Society; 2015.

22. Nakamura A, Rampersaud YR, Sharma A, Lewis SJ, Wu B, Datta P, Sundararajan K, Endisha H, Rossomacha E, Rockel JS, et al. Identification of microRNA-181a-5p and microRNA-4454 as mediators of facet cartilage degeneration. JCI insight. 2016;1(12):e86820.

23. D'Adamo S, Cetrullo S, Guidotti S, Borzi RM, Flamigni F. Hydroxytyrosol modulates the levels of microRNA-9 and its target sirtuin-1 thereby counteracting oxidative stress-induced chondrocyte death. Osteoarthr Cartil. 2017;25(4):600–10.

24. Cheleschi S, De Palma A, Pascarelli NA, Giordano N, Galeazzi M, Tenti S, Fioravanti A. Could Oxidative Stress Regulate the Expression of MicroRNA-146a and MicroRNA-34a in Human Osteoarthritic Chondrocyte Cultures? Int J Mol Sci. 2017;18(12).

25. Sun J, Zhong N, Li Q, Min Z, Zhao W, Sun Q, Tian L, Yu H, Shi Q, Zhang F, et al. MicroRNAs of rat articular cartilage at different developmental stages identified by Solexa sequencing. Osteoarthr Cartil. 2011;19(10):1237–45.

26. Zhong N, Sun J, Min Z, Zhao W, Zhang R, Wang W, Tian J, Tian L, Ma J, Li D, et al. MicroRNA-337 is associated with chondrogenesis through regulating TGFBR2 expression. Osteoarthr Cartil. 2012;20(6):593–602.

27. Gabler J, Ruetze M, Kynast KL, Grossner T, Diederichs S, Richter W. Stage-specific miRs in chondrocyte maturation: differentiation-dependent and hypertrophy-related miR clusters and the miR-181 family. Tissue Eng A. 2015;21(23–24):2840–51.

28. Sumiyoshi K, Kubota S, Ohgawara T, Kawata K, Abd El Kader T, Nishida T, Ikeda N, Shimo T, Yamashiro T, Takigawa M. Novel role of miR-181a in cartilage metabolism. J Cell Biochem. 2013;114(9):2094–100.

29. Xu J, Jiang C, Zhu W, Wang B, Yan J, Min Z, Geng M, Han Y, Ning Q, Zhang F, et al. NOD2 pathway via RIPK2 and TBK1 is involved in the aberrant catabolism induced by T-2 toxin in chondrocytes. Osteoarthr Cartil. 2015; 23(9):1575–85.

30. Wu XF, Zhou ZH, Zou J. MicroRNA-181 inhibits proliferation and promotes apoptosis of chondrocytes in osteoarthritis by targeting PTEN. Biochem Cell Biol. 2017;95(3):437–44.

31. Latreche L, Jean-Jean O, Driscoll DM, Chavatte L. Novel structural determinants in human SECIS elements modulate the translational recoding of UGA as selenocysteine. Nucleic Acids Res. 2009;37(17):5868–80.

32. Touat-Hamici Z, Legrain Y, Bulteau AL, Chavatte L. Selective up-regulation of human selenoproteins in response to oxidative stress. J Biol Chem. 2014; 289(21):14750–61.

33. Loeser RF, Carlson CS, Del Carlo M, Cole A. Detection of nitrotyrosine in aging and osteoarthritic cartilage: correlation of oxidative damage with the presence of interleukin-1beta and with chondrocyte resistance to insulin-like growth factor 1. Arthritis Rheum. 2002;46(9):2349–57.

34. Min Z, Zhao W, Zhong N, Guo Y, Sun M, Wang Q, Zhang R, Yan J, Tian L, Zhang F, et al. Abnormality of epiphyseal plate induced by selenium deficiency diet in two generation DA rats. APMIS. 2015;123(8):697–705.

35. Papp LV, Lu J, Bolderson E, Boucher D, Singh R, Holmgren A, Khanna KK. SECIS-binding protein 2 promotes cell survival by protecting against oxidative stress. Antioxid Redox Signal. 2010;12(7):797–808.

36. Schoenmakers E, Agostini M, Mitchell C, Schoenmakers N, Papp L, Rajanayagam O, Padidela R, Ceron-Gutierrez L, Doffinger R, Prevosto C, et al. Mutations in the selenocysteine insertion sequence-binding protein 2 gene lead to a multisystem selenoprotein deficiency disorder in humans. J Clin Invest. 2010;120(12):4220–35.

37. Saito Y, Shichiri M, Hamajima T, Ishida N, Mita Y, Nakao S, Hagihara Y, Yoshida Y, Takahashi K, Niki E, et al. Enhancement of lipid peroxidation and its amelioration by vitamin E in a subject with mutations in the SBP2 gene. J Lipid Res. 2015;56(11):2172–82.

Permissions

The contributors of this book come from diverse backgrounds, making this book a truly international effort. This book will bring forth new frontiers with its revolutionizing research information and detailed analysis of the nascent developments around the world.

We would like to thank all the contributing authors for lending their expertise to make the book truly unique. They have played a crucial role in the development of this book. Without their invaluable contributions this book wouldn't have been possible. They have made vital efforts to compile up to date information on the varied aspects of this subject to make this book a valuable addition to the collection of many professionals and students.

This book was conceptualized with the vision of imparting up-to-date information and advanced data in this field. To ensure the same, a matchless editorial board was set up. Every individual on the board went through rigorous rounds of assessment to prove their worth. After which they invested a large part of their time researching and compiling the most relevant data for our readers.

The editorial board has been involved in producing this book since its inception. They have spent rigorous hours researching and exploring the diverse topics which have resulted in the successful publishing of this book. They have passed on their knowledge of decades through this book. To expedite this challenging task, the publisher supported the team at every step. A small team of assistant editors was also appointed to further simplify the editing procedure and attain best results for the readers.

Apart from the editorial board, the designing team has also invested a significant amount of their time in understanding the subject and creating the most relevant covers. They scrutinized every image to scout for the most suitable representation of the subject and create an appropriate cover for the book.

The publishing team has been an ardent support to the editorial, designing and production team. Their endless efforts to recruit the best for this project, has resulted in the accomplishment of this book. They are a veteran in the field of academics and their pool of knowledge is as vast as their experience in printing. Their expertise and guidance has proved useful at every step. Their uncompromising quality standards have made this book an exceptional effort. Their encouragement from time to time has been an inspiration for everyone.

The publisher and the editorial board hope that this book will prove to be a valuable piece of knowledge for researchers, students, practitioners and scholars across the globe.

List of Contributors

Kaja Smedbråten, Britt Elin Øiestad and Yngve Røe
Department of Physiotherapy, Faculty of Health Sciences, OsloMet – Oslo Metropolitan University, Pb 4, St. Olavs plass, 0130 Oslo, Norway

Umile Giuseppe Longo
Department of Orthopaedic and Trauma Surgery, Campus Bio-Medico University, Via Alvaro del Portillo, 200, 00128 Rome, Italy
Shoulder Unit, Hospital of St John and St Elizabeth, 60 Grove End Road, London, UK

Steven Corbett and Philip Michael Ahrens
Shoulder Unit, Hospital of St John and St Elizabeth, 60 Grove End Road, London, UK

Fengping Gan, Jianzhong Jiang, Zhaolin Xie, Shengbin Huang, Ying Li, Guoping Chen and Haitao Tan
Department of Orthopaedics, Guigang City People's Hospital, No. 99-1 Zhongshan Rd, Guigang 537100, People's Republic of China

Wen Jie Choy
Faculty of Medicine, University of New South Wales (UNSW), Sydney, Australia
NeuroSpine Surgery Research Group (NSURG), Prince of Wales Private Hospital, Sydney, Australia

Kevin Phan and Ralph J. Mobbs
Faculty of Medicine, University of New South Wales (UNSW), Sydney, Australia
NeuroSpine Surgery Research Group (NSURG), Prince of Wales Private Hospital, Sydney, Australia
Department of Neurosurgery, Prince of Wales Private Hospital, Sydney, Australia

Ashish D. Diwan
Spine Service, Department of Orthopaedic Surgery, St. George and Sutherland Clinical School, University of New South Wales, Kogarah 2217, New South Wales, Australia

Chon Sum Ong
Newcastle University Medicine Malaysia (NUMed), Johor, Malaysia

Masahito Oshina, Yasushi Oshima, Yoshitaka Matsubayashi, Yuki Taniguchi, Hirotaka Chikuda and Sakae Tanaka
Department of Orthopaedic Surgery, The University of Tokyo Hospital, 7-3-1, Hongo, Bunkyo-Ku, Tokyo 113-8655, Japan

Kiehyun Daniel Riew
Department of Orthopedic Surgery, Columbia University, New York, NY, USA

Christoph Biehl, Thomas Braun, Ulrich Thormann and Gabor Szalay
Klinik und Poliklinik für Unfall-, Hand- und Wiederherstellungschirurgie -Operative Notaufnahme, UKGM Gießen, Rudolf-Buchheim-Str. 7, 35392 Giessen, Germany

Amir Oda
Klinik für orthopädische Chirurgie der unteren Extremitäten und Endoprothetik, Krankenhaus Rummelsberg GmbH, Rummelsberg 71, 90592, Schwarzenbruck, Germany

Stefan Rehart
Klinik für Orthopädie und Unfallchirurgie, AGAPLESION MARKUS KRANKENHAUS, Chefarzt Prof. Dr. med. Stefan Rehart, Wilhelm–Epstein–Straße 4, D-60431 Frankfurt am Main, Germany

Ziyang Sun
Department of Orthopaedics, Shanghai Jiao Tong University Affiliated Sixth People's Hospital, 600 Yishan Road, Shanghai 200233, People's Republic of China

Cunyi Fan
Department of Orthopaedics, Shanghai Jiao Tong University Affiliated Sixth People's Hospital, 600 Yishan Road, Shanghai 200233, People's Republic of China
Department of Orthopaedics, Shanghai Sixth People's Hospital East Affiliated to Shanghai University of Medicine and Health Sciences, Shanghai, People's Republic of China

Xin Lu and Jin Lin
Department of Orthopaedics, Peking Union Medical College Hospital, Chinese Academy of Medical Sciences and Peking Union Medical College, Beijing, China

Elżbieta Domka-Jopek
Institute of Physiotherapy, Faculty of Medicine, University of Rzeszow, ul. Hoffmanowej 25, 35-016 Rzeszow, Poland

Agnieszka Bejer and Mirosław Probachta
Institute of Physiotherapy, Faculty of Medicine, University of Rzeszow, ul. Hoffmanowej 25, 35-016 Rzeszow, Poland

The Holy Family Specialist Hospital, Rudna Mała, Poland

Marek Kulczyk
The Holy Family Specialist Hospital, Rudna Mała, Poland

Jędrzej Płocki
The Holy Family Specialist Hospital, Rudna Mała, Poland
Faculty of Medicine, University of Information Technology and Management, Rzeszow, Poland

Sharon Griffin
Fowler Kennedy Sport Medicine Clinic, University of Western Ontario, London, Canada

Nam Hoon Moon
Department of Orthopedic Surgery, Pusan National University Hospital, Pusan National University School of Medicine, Busan, Republic of Korea

Won Chul Shin, Min Uk Do, Seung Hun Woo, Seung Min Son and Kuen Tak Suh
Department of Orthopedic Surgery, Research Institute for Convergence of Biomedical Science and Technology, Pusan National University Yangsan Hospital, Pusan National University School of Medicine, 20 Geumo-ro, Mulgeum-eup, Yangsan, Gyeongsangnam-do 626-770, Republic of Korea

Moon Jong Chang, Min Kyu Song, Min Gyu Kyung, Jae Hoon Shin, Chong Bum Chang and Seung-Baik Kang
Department of Orthopedic Surgery, Seoul National University College of Medicine, SMG-SNU Boramae Medical Center, 5 Gil 20, Boramae-road, Dongjak-gu, Seoul 07061, South Korea

Melissa D. Garganta
Medical University of South Carolina, Greenville, SC, USA

Sarah S. Jaser, Jonathan G. Schoenecker, Erin Cobry and Stephen R. Hays
Vanderbilt University Medical Center, Nashville, TN, USA

Jill H. Simmons
Vanderbilt University Medical Center, Nashville, TN, USA
Division of Pediatric Endocrinology and Diabetes, Village at Vanderbilt, 1500 21st Avenue South, Suite 1514, Nashville, TN 37212-3157, USA

Margot A. Lazow
Cincinnati Children's Hospital Medical Center, Cincinnati, OH, USA

Anisha B. Dua
Section of Rheumatology, University of Chicago, 5841 S Maryland Ave, MC0930, Chicago, IL 60637, USA

Tuhina Neogi
Section of Clinical Epidemiology Research and Training Unit, Boston University School of Medicine, Boston, MA, USA
Section of Rheumatology, University of Chicago, 5841 S Maryland Ave, MC0930, Chicago, IL 60637, USA

Rachel A. Mikolaitis
InventIv Health, Clinical, Abbvie, Chicago, IL, USA

Joel A. Block and Najia Shakoor
Division of Rheumatology, Rush Medical College, Chicago, IL, USA

Kristine Godziuk
Faculty of Rehabilitation Medicine, University of Alberta, 8205 – 114 Street, 2-64 Corbett Hall, Edmonton, AB T6G 2G4, Canada

Carla M. Prado
Division of Human Nutrition, Faculty of Agricultural, Life and Environmental Sciences, University of Alberta, Edmonton, AB, Canada

Linda J. Woodhouse
Department of Physical Therapy, Faculty of Rehabilitation Medicine, University of Alberta, Edmonton, AB, Canada

Mary Forhan
Department of Occupational Therapy, Faculty of Rehabilitation Medicine, University of Alberta, Edmonton, AB, Canada

Akira M. Murakami, Andrew J. Kompel and Ali Guermazi
Section of Musculoskeletal Imaging, Department of Radiology, Boston University School of Medicine, FGH Building, 3rd Floor, 820 Harrison Ave., Boston, MA 02118, USA

Michel D. Crema
Section of Musculoskeletal Imaging, Department of Radiology, Boston University School of Medicine, FGH Building, 3rd Floor, 820 Harrison Ave., Boston, MA 02118, USA

Department of Sports Medicine, National Institute of Sports (INSEP), Paris, France
Department of Radiology, Saint-Antoine Hospital, University Paris VI, Paris, France

Daichi Hayashi
Section of Musculoskeletal Imaging, Department of Radiology, Boston University School of Medicine, FGH Building, 3rd Floor, 820 Harrison Ave., Boston, MA 02118, USA
Department of Radiology, Stony Brook Medicine, Stony Brook, NY, USA

Mohamed Jarraya
Section of Musculoskeletal Imaging, Department of Radiology, Boston University School of Medicine, FGH Building, 3rd Floor, 820 Harrison Ave., Boston, MA 02118, USA
Department of Radiology, Mercy Catholic Medical Center, Darby, PA, USA

Frank W. Roemer
Section of Musculoskeletal Imaging, Department of Radiology, Boston University School of Medicine, FGH Building, 3rd Floor, 820 Harrison Ave., Boston, MA 02118, USA
Department of Radiology, University of Erlangen-Nuremberg, Erlangen, Germany

Lars Engebretsen
Medical and Scientific Department, International Olympic Committee, Lausanne, Switzerland
Oslo Sports Trauma Research Center, Department of Sports Medicine, Norwegian School of Sport Sciences, Oslo, Norway
Department of Orthopedic Surgery, Oslo University Hospital, University of Oslo, Oslo, Norway

Xinning Li
Department of Orthopaedic Surgery, Boston University School of Medicine, Boston, MA, USA

Bruce B. Forster
Department of Radiology, University of British Columbia, Vancouver, BC, Canada

Yeliz Prior and Alison Hammond
Centre for Health Sciences Research, University of Salford, Salford, UK

Alan Tennant
Swiss Paraplegic Research, Nottwil, Switzerland

Sarah Tyson
Division of Nursing, Midwifery and Social Work, University of Manchester, Manchester, UK

Ingvild Kjeken
Department of Occupational Therapy, Prosthetics and Orthotics, Oslo and Akershus University College of Applied Sciences, Oslo, Norway

Kristin Alves
Harvard Combined Orthopaedic Surgery Residency Program, Boston, MA, USA
Department of Orthopaedic Surgery, Brigham and Women's Hospital, Boston, MA, USA

Norgrove Penny
Department of Orthopaedic Surgery, University of British Colombia, Victoria, Canada

John Ekure
Kumi Orthopaedic Center, Kumi, Uganda

Robert Olupot
Kumi Hospital, Kumi, Uganda

Olive Kobusingye
Makerere University School of Public Health, Kampala, Uganda

Jeffrey N. Katz
Department of Orthopaedic Surgery, Brigham and Women's Hospital, Boston, MA, USA

Coleen S. Sabatini
University of California San Francisco Department of Orthopaedic Surgery, UCSF Benioff Children's Hospital Oakland, 747 52nd Street, OPC 1st Floor, Oakland, CA 94609, USA

JuHong Lee, SungIl Wang and KiBum Kim
Department Of Orthopaedic Surgery, Chonbuk National University Hospital, 20, Geonji-ro, Deokjin-gu, Jeonju 54907, South Korea

Alfred C. Gellhorn, Carly A. Creelman and Rachel Welbel
Department of Rehabilitation Medicine, Weill Cornell Medicine, 525 E 68th Street, B16, New York, NY 10065, USA

Jordan M. Stumph
Albert Einstein College of Medicine, New York, NY, USA

Hashem E. Zikry
Icahn School of Medicine at Mount Sinai, New York, NY, USA

Mattia Morri, Cristiana Forni, Riccardo Ruisi, Tiziana Giamboi and Fabrizio Giacomella
Servizio di Assistenza Infermieristica, Tecnica e della Riabilitazione, IRCCS Istituto Ortopedico Rizzoli, Via Pupilli 1, 40136 Bologna, Italy

Davide Maria Donati
Clinica Ortopedica e Traumatologica III a prevalente indirizzo Oncologico, IRCCS Istituto Ortopedico Rizzoli, Bologna, Italy

Maria Grazia Benedetti
Servizio di Medicina Fisica e Riabilitativa, IRCCS Istituto Ortopedico Rizzoli, Bologna, Italy

Ki Hyuk Sung, Chin Youb Chung, Kyoung Min Lee and Moon Seok Park
Department of Orthopaedic Surgery, Seoul National University Bundang Hospital, 82 Gumi-ro 173 Beon-gil, Bundang-Gu, Sungnam, Gyeonggi 13620, South Korea

Soon-Sun Kwon
Department of Mathematics, College of Natural Sciences, Ajou University, Suwon, Gyeonggi, South Korea

Jaeyoung Kim
Department of Orthopaedic Surgery, H Plus Yangji Hospital, Seoul, South Korea

Jan Klouda
Department of Orthopaedics, Hospital Nemocnice České Budějovice, a.s., České Budějovice, Czech Republic
Department of Orthopaedics, First Faculty of Medicine, Charles University and Motol University Hospital, Prague, Czech Republic

Stanislav Popelka Jr, Stanislav Popelka and Ivan Landor
Department of Orthopaedics, First Faculty of Medicine, Charles University and Motol University Hospital, Prague, Czech Republic

Rastislav Hromádka
Department of Orthopaedics, First Faculty of Medicine, Charles University and Motol University Hospital, Prague, Czech Republic
Institute of Anatomy, First Faculty of Medicine, Charles University, Prague, Czech Republic

Simona Šoffová
Institute of Anatomy, First Faculty of Medicine, Charles University, Prague, Czech Republic

Keshav Poonit, Xijie Zhou, Bin Zhao, Chao Sun, Chenglun Yao and Hede Yan
Department of Orthopedics (Division of Plastic and Hand Surgery), The Second Affiliated Hospital and Yuying Children's Hospital of Wenzhou Medical University, Key Laboratory of Orthopedics of Zhejiang Province Wenzhou, China, 109 West Xueyuan Road, Lucheng District, Wenzhou 325027, Zhejiang Province, China

Feng Zhang
Joseph M. Still Burn and Reconstructive Center, 346 Crossgates Blvd, Suite, Brandon, MS 202, USA

Jingwei Zheng
Department of Clinical Research Center, The Affiliated Eye Hospital of Wenzhou Medical University, Wenzhou, China

Giovanni Balato, Maria Rizzo, Francesco Smeraglia and Massimo Mariconda
Department of Public Health, Section of Orthopaedic Surgery, "Federico II" University, Via S. Pansini 5, Building 12, 80131 Naples, Italy

Tiziana Ascione
Department of Infectious Diseases, D. Cotugno Hospital - AORN dei Colli, Naples, Italy

R. H. Meffert
Department of Orthopaedic Trauma, Hand, Plastic and Reconstructive Surgery, University Hospital Würzburg, Würzburg, Germany

F. Gilbert
Department of Orthopaedic Trauma, Hand, Plastic and Reconstructive Surgery, University Hospital Würzburg, Würzburg, Germany
Department of Trauma Hand Plastic and Reconstructive Surgery, University Munich Germany, Julius-Maximilians-University of Würzburg Oberdürrbacherstr, 6 D-, 97080 Würzburg, Germany

C. Schneemann, R. Wildenauer and U. Lorenz
Department for General Visceral, Vascular and Paediatric Surgery, University Hospital Würzburg, Würzburg, Germany

A. Busch
Department for General Visceral, Vascular and Paediatric Surgery, University Hospital Würzburg, Würzburg, Germany
Department for Vascular and Endovascular Surgery Klinikum rechts der Isar, Technical University Munich, Munich, Germany

C. J. Scholz
Core Unit Systems Medicine IZKF, University Hospital Würzburg, Würzburg, Germany

R. Kickuth
Department of Diagnostic and Interventional Radiology, University Hospital Würzburg, Würzburg, Germany

R. Kellersmann
Department of Vascular Surgery, Klinikum Fulda, Fulda, Germany

Jianli Xue, Bin Cheng, Binshang Lan and Kunzheng Wang
Department of Orthopaedics, The Second Affiliated Hospital, Xi'an Jiaotong University Health Science Center, 157 West 5th Road, Xi'an, Shaanxi 710004, People's Republic of China

Zixin Min, Fujun Zhang, Yan Han and Jian Sun
Department of Biochemistry and Molecular Biology, School of Basic Medical Sciences, Xi'an Jiaotong University Health Science Center, Xi'an, Shaanxi 710061, People's Republic of China

Zhuqing Xia
Beaurau of healthcare, Shaanxi Health and Family Planning Commission, Xi'an, Shaanxi 710000, People's Republic of China

Index

www.ingramcontent.com/pod-product-compliance
Lightning Source LLC
Chambersburg PA
CBHW080531200326
41458CB00012B/4400